DYNAMICS OF
ARTERIAL FLOW

ADVANCES IN EXPERIMENTAL MEDICINE AND BIOLOGY

DYNAMICS OF ARTERIAL FLOW

Edited by

Stewart Wolf
St. Luke's Hospital
Bethlehem, Pennsylvania

and

Nicholas T. Werthessen
The Office of Naval Research
Boston, Massachusetts

SPRINGER SCIENCE+BUSINESS MEDIA, LLC

Library of Congress Cataloging in Publication Data

Totts Gap Colloquium on Dynamics of Arterial Flow, 1976.
   Dynamics of arterial flow.

   (Advances in experimental medicine and biology; v. 115)
   Proceedings of the Totts Gap Colloquium on Dynamics of Arterial Flow, held
in Delaware Water Gap, Pa., June 1976.
   Includes index.
   1. Hemodynamics – Congresses. 2. Arteries – Congresses. 3. Blood flow –
Congresses. I. Wolf, Stewart George, 1914-   II. Werthessen, Nicholas The-
odore, 1911-   III. Totts Gap Institute. IV. Title. V. Series.
QP105.T67 1976   616.1'36'071   79-9770
ISBN 978-1-4684-7510-4   ISBN 978-1-4684-7508-1 (eBook)
DOI 10.1007/978-1-4684-7508-1

Proceedings of the Totts Gap Colloquium on Dynamics of Arterial Flow,
held in Delaware Water Gap, Pennsylvania, June 7–9, 1976

© 1979 Springer Science+Business Media New York
Originally published by Plenum Press, New York in 1979
Softcover reprint of the hardcover 1st edition   1979
A Division of Plenum Publishing Corporation
227 West 17th Street, New York, N.Y. 10011

Preface

This volume contains the edited transcript of the Second
Topical Colloquium based on leads developed at the original
conference on the artery and the process of arteriosclerosis
(the Lindau Conference of 1970). The first follow-up colloquium
on "The Smooth Muscle of the Artery" was held in Heidelberg in
1973. Planning for the present one was undertaken by the editors
with Dr. C. Forbes Dewey, Department of Mechanical Engineering,
Massachusetts Institute of Technology, Cambridge, Massachusetts.

The meeting itself was held June, 1976 at the Delaware
Water Gap, Pennsylvania, under the joint sponsorship of Totts
Gap Institute and the Massachusetts Institute of Technology
with financial support from the American Heart Association,
the Office of Naval Research, and the Smith, Kline and French
Company.

The objective of the series of meetings, beginning at
Lindau has been to examine from an interdisciplinary and
international point of view the fundamental physiologic and
pathophysiologic processes pertinent to the development of
arteriosclerosis. This colloquium sought to examine critically
the evidence relating hemodynamic forces to atherogenesis, to
reconcile disparate findings and interpretations in so far as
possible; and to make a synthesis of the present state of
knowledge of the dynamics of arterial flow.

Grateful acknowledgement is made for the valuable assistance
of Joan Martin and Helen Goodell in the entire editorial process.
The editors acknowledge with thanks the secretarial assistance
of Moira Martin, Colleen Nagle, Cindy Carter and Pat Ide. Special
thanks are due Joy Lowe who executed the entire final manuscript.

Participants

S. BJORKERUD, Sweden
T. CAREW, U.S.A.
C. CARO, England
S. CHIEN, U.S.A.
C. COLTON, U.S.A
R. COX, U.S.A.
F. DEWEY, U.S.A.
D. FRY, U.S.A.
H. GREENE, U.S.A.
D. KENYON, U.S.A.
K. LEE, U.S.A.

A. MALLIANI, Italy
P. MANSFIELD, U.S.A.
W. MEYER, Germany
R. NEREM, U.S.A.
C. SCHWARTZ, U.S.A.
E. SMITH, Scotland
L. STONE, U.S.A.
B. TAYLOR, U.S.A.
S. WEINBAUM, U.S.A.
N. WERTHESSEN, U.S.A.
S. WOLF, U.S.A.

Contents

Chapter 1 ANATOMICAL AND PHYSIOLOGICAL CHARACTERISTICS OF ARTERIES

DR. SCHWARTZ: First let us review the light microscopic structure of a variety of arteries derived from differing anatomical sites. The common iliac artery, for example, contains numerous smooth muscle cells, and only a few

Muscular and Elastic Arteries

fine ramifying elastic processes. This artery is typical of those classfied as "muscular" arteries. An anatomical neighbor, the external iliac artery, is also predominantly muscular with but few elastic processes. It is interesting to note the tendency for a double type of internal elastic lamina in this artery, the pathological or physiological significance of which remains uncertain. The internal iliac artery is an intermediate musculo-elastic artery with quite a significant amount of elastin present relative to the external or common iliac arteries.

DR. WERTHESSEN: You have used the name iliac continuously. Are these from different people or from different sections of the same artery?

DR. SCHWARTZ: Different branches of a single major arterial trunk. The common carotid artery is classically described as being an elastic type artery with considerable elastin in its media. More peripherally, its major branch, the internal carotid artery, undergoes morphological transformation and where it enters the skull is predominantly muscular in configuration. Also intriguing is the marked concentration of elastin in the innermost media. The reason for this structural appearance has yet to be explained. Another important vessel to the brain, the vertebral artery, is predominantly muscular in type. It is thus apparent that some arteries are predominantly elastic, some are predominantly muscular, and others have an intermediate structure, to which we ascribe the category, musculo-elastic. These structural types have been described in detail previously (1). There is no clear cut correlation between the muscularity or elastic composition of the artery and the propensity to

*Studies reported here done in collaboration with Ross G. Gerrity, Ph.D. Department of Pathology, McMaster University, Hamilton, Ontario, Canada.

develop atherosclerosis. Some muscular arteries develop
severe disease, as do some elastic arteries. Why then are
there these dramatic differences in structure? What are
their functional correlates, if any?

Now let us turn to the development and ultrastructure
of the arterial media. Histologically, if one compares the
structure of an elastic
Arterial Development   artery (such as the aorta)
from a newborn animal with the
same artery from a mature animal, several distinct differences
emerge. There is a 2-3 fold increase in wall thickness
which is not due to an increase in the number of elastic and
muscular laminae, which remains constant (2), but rather, to
a marked increase in the volume occupied by elastin, and, to
a lesser extent, collagen. For example, in the rat aorta,
the volume of aortic media occupied by elastic tissue
increases from about 12% in the newborn to 52% at three
months of age; collagen content (volume) increases from 2%
to about 20% in the same time span (2). The volume occupied
by smooth muscle cells in the same period shows an inverse
relationship to the total connective tissue volume, dropping
from about 60-70% in the newborn to about 20% in the adult
rat (2). Subsequent thickening in old age in the absence of
lesion formation occurs to some extent in the media, but to
a greater extent in the intima, which frequently exhibits a
diffuse thickening which, in some areas, can increase wall
thickness by a factor of three to five (3).

Ultrastructurally the newborn to one-week-old rat aorta
reveals very little collagen or elastin relative to a more
adult vessel (Fig. 1-1).
Formation of Collagen   Numerous elongated, spindle-
and Elastin   shaped cells with copious
endoplasmic reticulum (ER) and
prominent Golgi are present. There are a few discernible
myofilaments in the peripheral cytoplasm of these cells, but
at this stage of development medial cells are morphologically
more like fibroblasts than smooth muscle cells. At two weeks
of age the ER and Golgi remain conspicuous, but myofilaments
are now readily discernible (Fig. 1-2). Extracellularly,
there is a distinct increase in the amount of elastin, and
scattered clumps of collagen fibrils begin to make their
appearance. At four weeks of age (Fig. 1-3) the lamellae are
wider, and branches of elastin extend between cells. There
is also an increased amount of collagen present in the media
at this point in time, mainly pericellular.

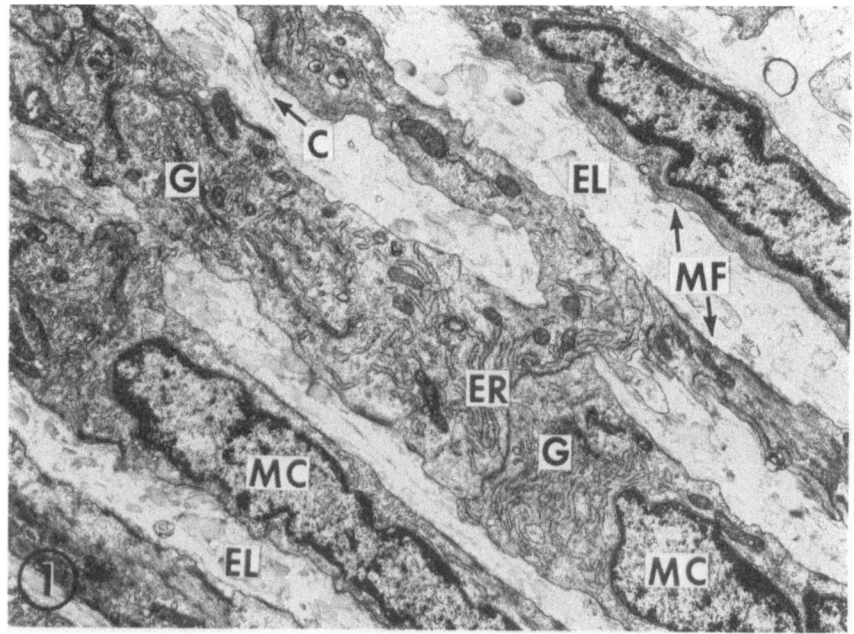

Fig. 1-1: Transmission electron micrograph of the aortic media of newborn rat. Medial cells (MC) resemble fibroblasts, with prominent Golgi (G), rough endoplasmic reticulum (ER), and only a few myofilaments (MF) in the peripheral cytoplasm. Only a few collagen fibrils (C) and elastic tissue bundles (EL) are visible. X 10,000.

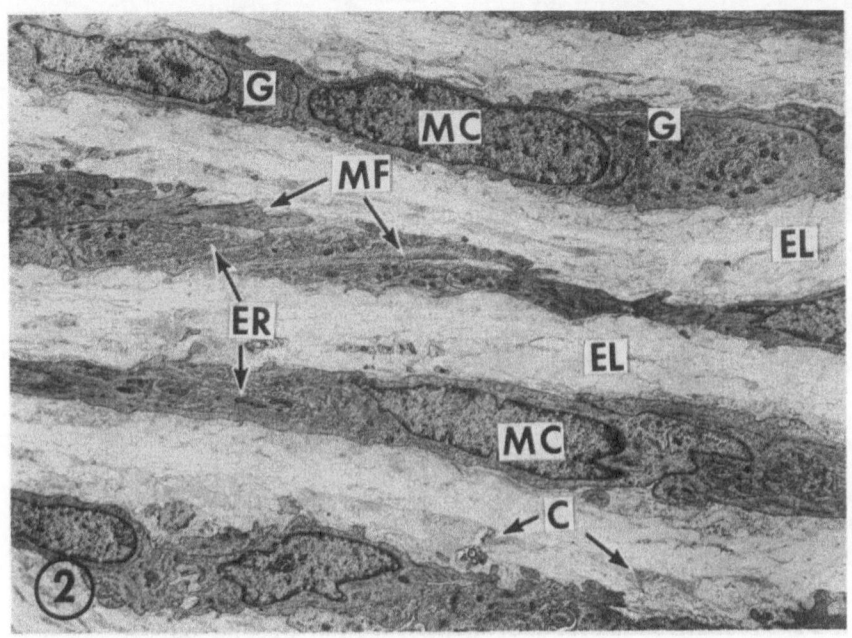

Fig. 1-2: Transmission electron micrograph of aortic media
from a two-week-old rat. Golgi (G) and endoplasmic reticulum
(ER) are very prominent in medial cells (MC), but myofilaments
(MF) are more numerous than in the newborn, and cells are
more spindle-shaped. Elastic tissue (EL) now fills the
laminae between cells, and collagen (C) is visible interspersed
in it. X 6,000.

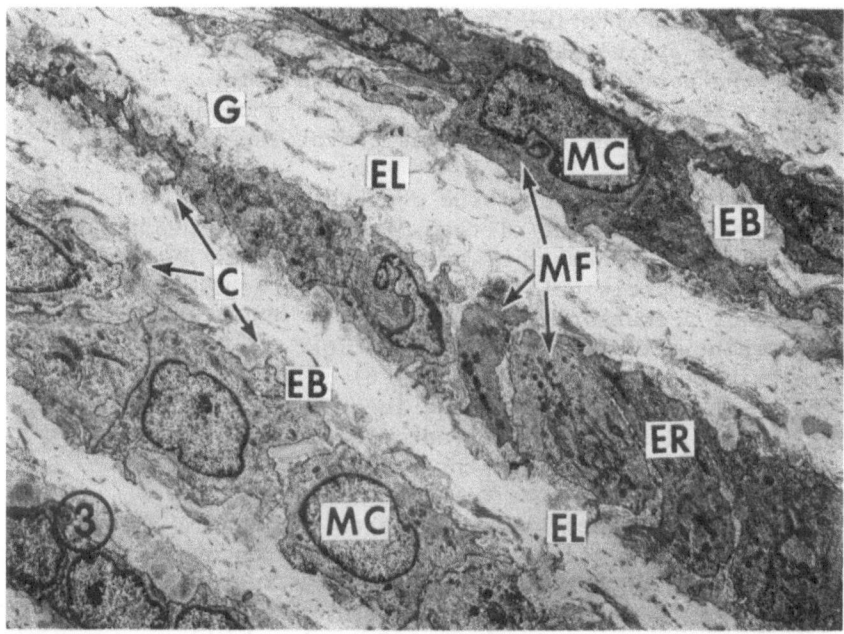

Fig. 1-3: Transmission electron micrograph of the aortic media of a four-week-old rat. Medial cells (MC) are more irregular in outline than previously seen. Golgi (G) and endoplasmic reticulum (ER) are less prominent, and myofilaments (MF) fill much of the cytoplasm. Elastic laminae (EL) are widened, and branches (EB) from them extend between cells. Collagen (C) is seen in moderate quantities at the cell periphery. X, 6000.

Medial cells are decidely more irregular in shape than they
were in the earlier stages of development. The ER and Golgi
are less prominent. Myofilaments are present in large
amounts in the medial cells, which are now identifiable as
smooth muscle cells, although at 4 weeks they are still not
fully differentiated. As further differentiation occurs,
the cytoplasm fills with myofilaments, and the ER and Golgi
are less evident (Fig. 1-4). In the eight-week-old aorta
(Fig. 1-5) the trends are similar to those already described.
At eight weeks the rat is essentially a mature animal, both
sexually and from an arterial structural point of view.
Connective tissue synthesis and in particular, elastin
synthesis in the aorta, has plateaued at this point. Medial
cells are very readily identifiable as mature smooth muscle
cells, with prominent and characteristic myofilaments.

     Returning to connective tissue synthesis briefly, after
a single pulse of H-proline fifteen minutes before death,
in a 4-week-old rat, a number of grains are visible within
the medial smooth muscle cells, indicating intracellular
incorporation of precursor (Fig. 1-6). Three hours after the
pulse some grains are intracellular, and most are present
within the extracellular space (Fig. 1-6).   In other words,
the H-proline has been taken up and incorporated by smooth
muscle cells (SMC), into collagen and elastin, which are
exteriorized or secreted within three hours.

     By six months of age, there are other changes in the
aorta. Large irregular medial SMC are packed with myofilaments
(Fig. 1-7) and considerable thinning of the elastic laminae
                              has occurred. Some cellular
Changes During Aging   degeneration is visible.
                              There is distinctly more
collagen relative to elastin than at earlier ages. It
appears that in aging, as distinct from development, the
relative proportions of arterial collagen and elastin are
reversed, with more collagen and less elastin in the older
artery. At one year of age (Fig. 1-8) the appearances are
essentially similar to those described for the six-month-old
aorta. Now, however, cellular debris and dying cells are
seen scattered throughout the media together with granulo-
vesicular material. At both six months and one year the
Golgi and the ER are clearly more prominent than in the
younger mature aorta (8-12 weeks), probably reflecting
increased synthetic activity.

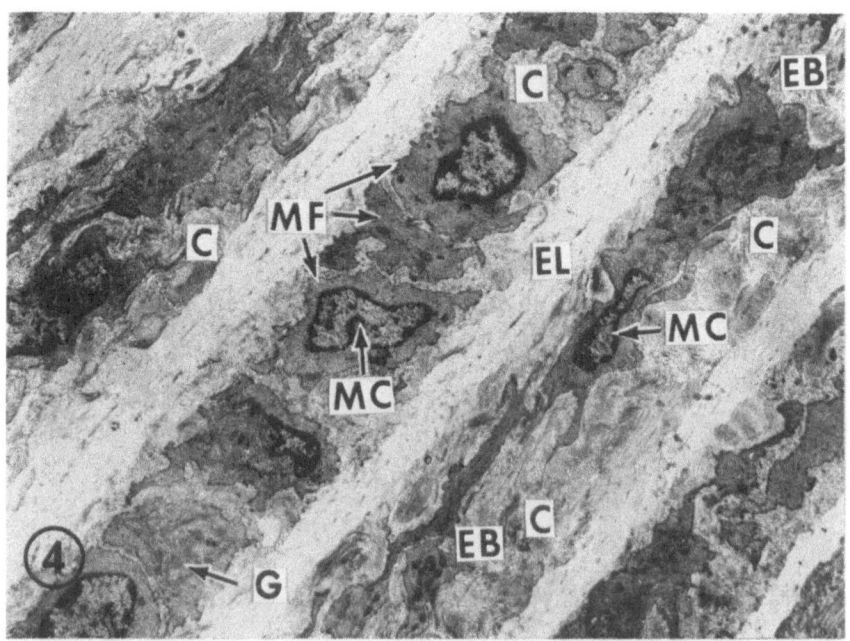

Fig. 1-4: Transmission electron micrograph of the aortic
media of an eight-week-old rat. Medial cells (MC) are now
readily identifiable as arterial smooth muscle cells and
their cytoplasm is filled with myofilaments (MF). The Golgi
(G) is infrequently seen, and the endoplasmic reticulum (ER)
is poorly developed. Collagen (C) fibrils now surround medial
cells, interspersed with elastic tissue branches (EB) separated
from the elastic laminae (E.). X 6,000.

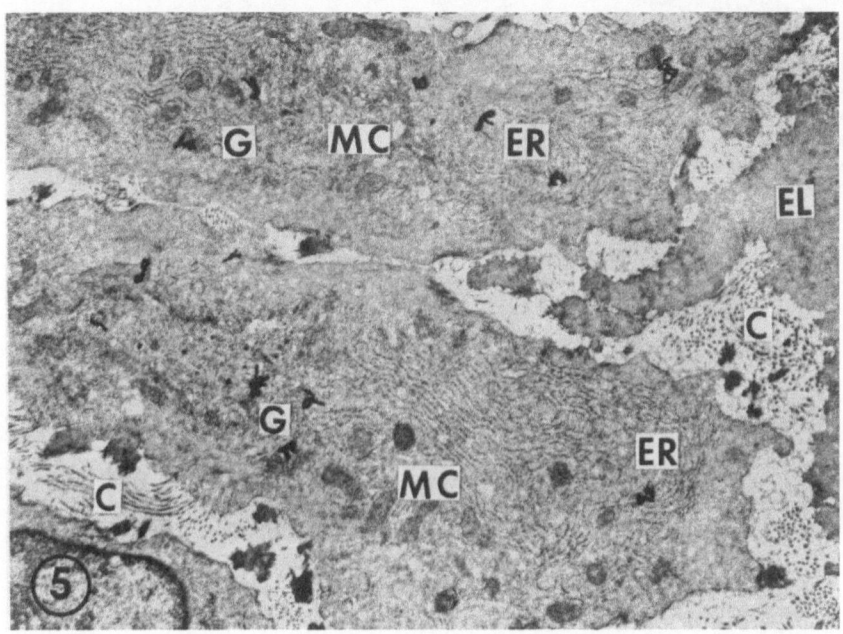

Fig. 1-5: Electron autoradiograph of aortic medial cells (MC),
15 minutes after intravenous injection of ^{3}H-proline. Grains
are visible overlying Golgi (G) and endoplasmic reticulum (ER)
of the cells, but collagen (C) and elastic tissue (EL) are
not labelled. X 8,000.

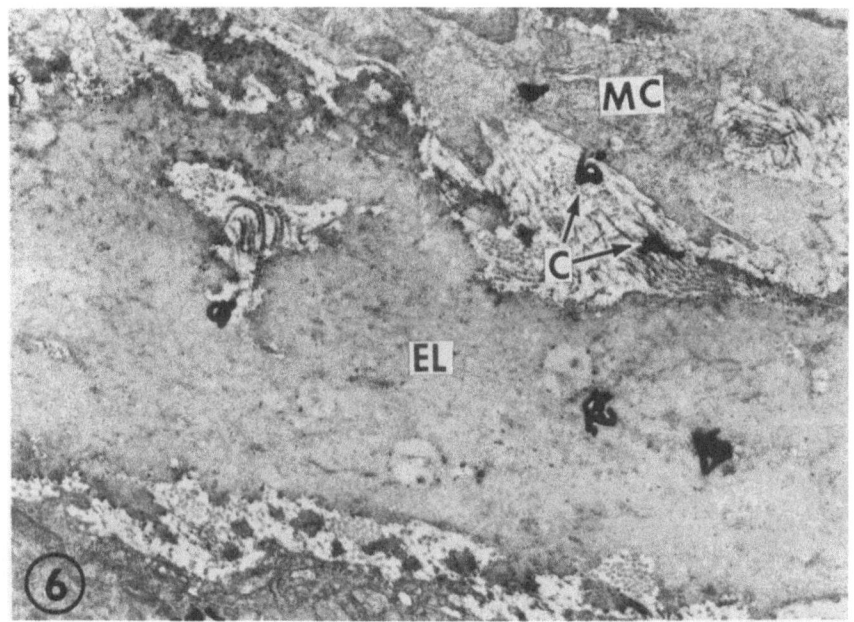

Fig. 1-6: Electron autoradiograph of the aortic media 3 hours after the injection of ^{3}H-proline. Grains are still visible overlying medial smooth muscle (MC), but most grains overlie collagen (C) and elastic tissue (EL). X 15,000.

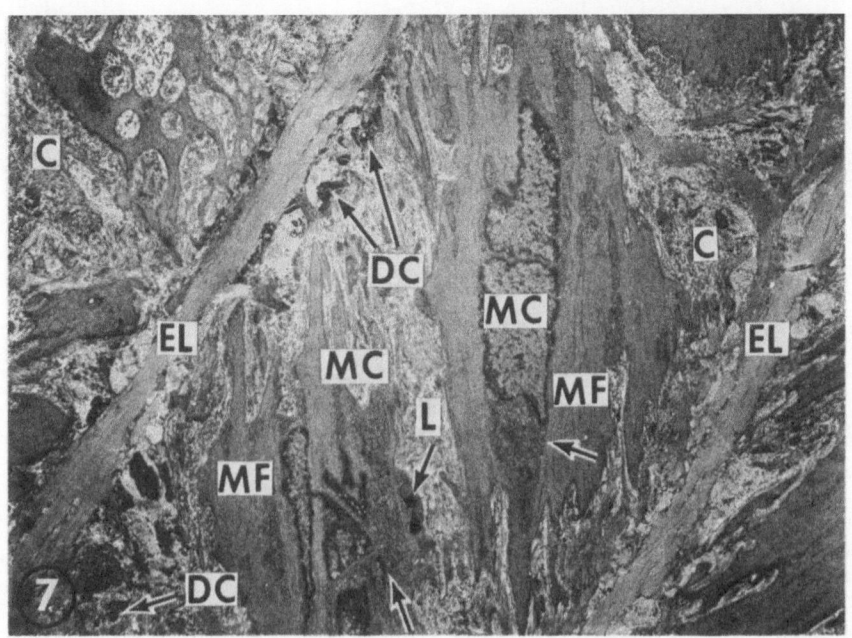

Fig. 1-7: Transmission electron micrograph of the aortic
media of a six-month-old rat. Medial smooth muscle cells (MC)
are large, and irregular in outline. Their cytoplasm is
largely filled with myofilaments (MF), while endoplasmic
reticulum, Golgi and mitochondria are perinuclear (arrows).
Intracytoplasmic lipid inclusions (L) are often seen. There
is thinning of the elastic laminae (EL), collagen (C) is
prevalent, and cellular debris (DC) is visible in the extracellular spaces. X 6,000.

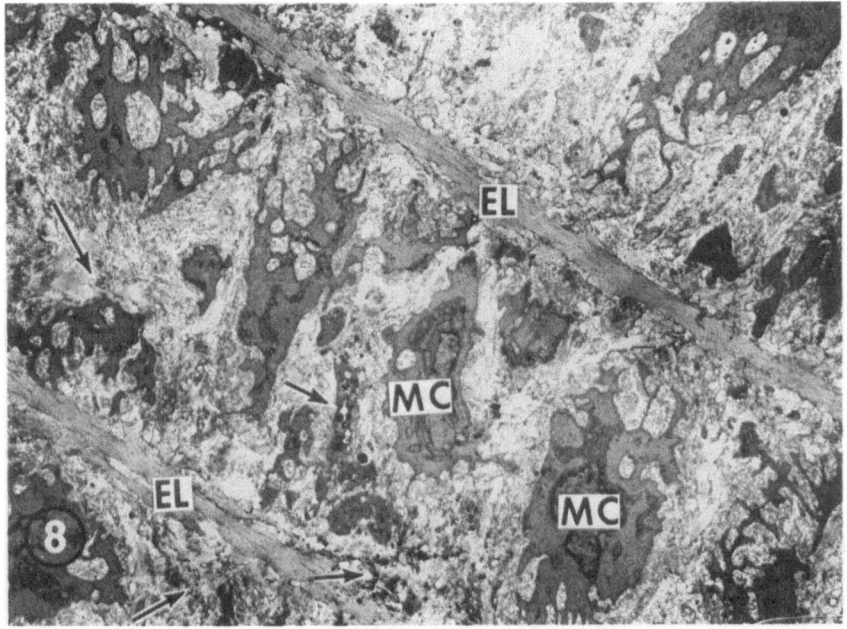

Fig. 1-8: As in Fig. 1-7, but from a one-year-old rat.
Much cellular and granulo-vesicular debris (arrows) is present,
and remaining medial cells (MC) are highly vacuolated. Elastic
laminae (EL) are tenuous and irregular. X 6,000.

As the aorta gets older, the medial cells become larger and
more irregular in shape with many more processes. This
gradual increase in cellular degeneration with normal aging
is interesting, particularly as it corresponds temporarily
with hypertrophy of remaining cells, and hyperplasia of
synthetic organelles in these cells. This pattern continues
and becomes more pronounced in two and three-year-old rats
(4).

DR. STONE: Dr. Schwartz, when you begin to see cell
death, is there any actual indication of a decrease in
protein synthetic capability at that point?

DR. SCHWARTZ: No, the evidence would point to the
contrary. However, there is no simple answer because even
at that time when one is starting to observe cell death, the
Golgi and the ER are becoming more prominent, and remaining
cells are becoming larger. There is also an increasing
amount of collagen being formed, but we have no evidence
that medial cells are dividing. It would appear that the
cells undergo hypertrophy rather than hyperplasia in order
to compensate for the death of adjoining cells. This
phenomenon appears to be a factor in biological aging of the
artery in the absence of disease.

DR. STONE: That is the question. Because the anatomical
evidence of synthesis is there, is there actual synthesis
taking place?

DR. SCHWARTZ: Yes, I believe so. But I think we
should be more specific –what is being synthesized? Obviously,
if cells are undergoing hypertrophy, we can expect that
cellular components and membranes are being produced. Also,
our data show an increase in collagen content of the media
from 24% at 12 weeks to 31% at 26 weeks on a dry weight
basis.

DR. STONE: If there is actual synthesis taking place
with thymidine labeling do you see any increased incorporation
into nuclear DNA?

DR. SCHWARTZ: Yes, but I believe we should be able to
get a comprehensive answer to that from K.T. Lee.

DR. LEE: Are you asking about thymidine incorporation
at that time?

DR. STONE: Yes, in other words, for nuclear activity.

DR. LEE: Usually when cells are dying the vessel
tries to compensate by putting
Cell Renewal   new cells out to maintain the
strength of the vessel wall.
So it is likely that we have regenerating cells there and at
that particular time you will see thymidine incorporation.

DR. WERTHESSEN: But have you actually measured it?

DR. LEE; What do you mean, measured it?

DR. WERTHESSEN: By thymidine. Has anybody measured
it? You can expect it but it doesn't necessarily have to
happen.

DR. LEE: There are two ways of doing this. One way
is to get the labelling indices by counting labelled cells
and baseline cells and the other way is to measure chemically
the content of the thymidine. Probably the chemical method
may be simpler. If a large number of cells die in a vessel
and they are not replaced, the wall is weakened and results
in aneurysmal dilation or rupture. Those dying cells must be
replaced by new cells. However, we have not actually measured
thymidine incorporation in aging vessels.

DR. WOLF: I will summarize this to be sure that we
are all on the same page of the hymn book. What you are
saying is that in association with aging there is increased
cell death accompanied by increased evidence of synthesis.
Fair?

DR. SCHWARTZ: Yes, but the ultrastructural evidence of
increased synthesis is circumstantial, not affirmative. It
indicates that the mechanism for synthesis is present.

DR. WOLF: And that is why we brought these other
people into the conversation. Now are we clear on that, Dr.
Lee?

DR. LEE: I think that is what I have said.

DR. WOLF: Do you have the evidence?

DR. LEE: My statement is based on our observations in vessels stimulated by dietary means for the production of atherosclerosis. In physiological aging, however, I am sure the situation is different from vessels stimulated by dietary means. But, common sense wise, if many cells in the vessel wall die without replacement, sooner or later the vessel will be weakened and rupture.

DR. WOLF: Fair enough, you brought it into focus. Dr. Cox.

DR. COX: We have performed some studies in dogs and rats on the effects of aging on secondary branches of the aorta such as the carotid and the iliac. In general, we have found that the total connective tissue content increases in the aging animal. The cellular content, the smooth muscle cell content, decreases. There are associated with these changes decreases in contractile function as measured by the ability of smooth muscles to generate force on a per unit area basis. So from our results in dogs and rats, and again these may be findings which are species dependent, there seems to be a reduction in cellularity with aging and in the aged. There certainly doesn't seem to be a one-for-one replacement.

DR. BJORKERUD: The rat is a difficult example because the rat is growing very late in life and during the growing phase the cell has an increasing territory. Then the cell increases its synthetic capacity to cope with the increasing territory. If you study differences in synthetic capacities, we have studied, for instance, the synthesis of phospholipids, there is a relationship between the increase of extracellular tissue per cell and a corresponding increase in the rate of phospholipid synthesis per cell. I am not certain when the rat stops growing and when the senile phase starts. One should clearly distinguish between these two phases. I think your discussion is pertinent for the senile phase. That the two phases might overlap each other makes the problem even worse.

Phases of Growth versus Senility

DR. SCHWARTZ: That is a good point. I have tried to indicate developmental changes on the one hand and aging changes on the other, and I made the point that at eight weeks the rat is considered to be a mature animal. There are clearly many changes which are developmental up to the age of eight weeks.

Just precisely what changes are part of growth and development and what changes are degenerative or senescent, or where the cut-off lies, is an extremely difficult question.

At the end of the spectrum, we are obviously dealing with changes in the one to three-year-old rats that are associated with aging, possibly including an increased turnover of medial SMC, as well as documented increases in collagen relative to elastin. It should also be pointed out that only about 5% of these rats live beyond two years of age. Beyond this age we are therefore looking at a select population, and the changes we are observing may well be associated with their ability to live to this advanced age.

DR. WOLF: I think Dr. Elspeth Smith has a comment.

DR. SMITH: I want to make a comment to Dr. Cox. When you say total connective tissue increases and smooth muscle cells decrease, is this relative to each other on a concentration basis, or per unit segment of total artery?

DR. COX: It is on a basis of per unit weight.

DR. SMITH: On a per unit weight basis if one increases the other must by definition, decrease. But do you know what happens supposing you take a unit segment of an artery. In that given segment, are there fewer smooth muscle cells? Or the same number of smooth muscle cells or more smooth muscle cells? Because I think this is one of the problems we are up against. The concentration gives a distorted picture to some extent and you don't really know whether one thing is decreasing and another thing increasing relative to each other or whether in the whole structure there is an absolute increase or decrease.

DR. COX: This is a very difficult question to answer, because of the problem of delineating a unit structure. I think it is particularly
Species Differences   difficult by virtue of the
                                     fact that so many people are
studying different animals, the rat being, with Nathan Shock's group, the principle animal that is used to study the effects of aging on the cardiovascular system. The differences that we have found in the rat and the dog are considerable. I would say it is very difficult to answer that question because of the species variability. In the case of the dog, the changes in body size going from a young adult, say a two year old dog, to a ten or fifteen year old animal are relatively small.

Compare that to the rat, which as we heard continues to
increase in size from the adult stage to the senescent
stage, there is a very large difference in what one would
see in the thoracic aorta. Certainly the size of the thoracic
aorta would increase in the rat. It would not change
significantly in the dog. The wall thickness of arteries
certainly increases with age. That is one of the considerations. In terms of total concept of muscle cells, I really
don't know how to answer that because I don't have the
quantitative information. We have not looked at it on any
other basis besides concentration.

DR. SCHWARTZ: Now I wish to consider changes occurring
in the arterial endothelium during growth, development and
aging. As a prelude, let me
Changes in Endothelium   briefly emphasize that arterial
endothelium has a wide variety
of functions, which are summarized in Table 1. The endothelium
provides a fascinating blood-tissue interface with a regulatory
role in permeability, both in terms of influx into the
vessel and efflux from the vessel. The endothelial cell is
capable of regeneration both in vivo and in tissue culture
(5,6). It may exert some kind of metabolic control over the
underlying media as suggested by recent studies (7). There
may be specific receptor sites on the surface, perhaps
relating to immunologic or pharmacological reactions or to a
variety of other mechanisms, including the internalization
of macromolecules. The endothelium may be contractile. It
certainly contains contractile filaments (3,8) as probably
do most other cells, but the biological significance of
endothelial contraction has yet to be determined. The
spectrum of functions of vascular endothelium is considerable
(Table 1). One needs, however, to enter a note of caution.
Many studies have, for obvious reasons, been undertaken
using capillary endothelium. This exhibits a range of structural
differences consistent with the functional specialization of
the different organs (9). As illustrated by Rhodin (10) the
capillary endothelium may be continuous, fenestrated, or
discontinuous with large gaps. These differences must be
considered in studying transport phenomena. Furthermore,
extrapolation of data derived from studies on capillaries to
the arterial endothelium may be inappropriate, or indeed
misleading.

RAT   When one examines the aortic endothelium of a newborn
rat sectioned "en face" (Fig. 1-9), an extensive endoplasmic
reticulum and numerous mitochondria and free ribosomes are
readily seen. By 2 months of age (Fig. 1-10) the ER is
fragmented with much shorter profiles.

TABLE I
SOME PROPERTIES OF NORMAL VASCULAR ENDOTHELIUM

1. Regeneration, replication.

    a) In arteries or veins
    b) In tissue culture-venous or arterial endothelium

2. Control of macromolecular transport and permeability.

3. Synthesis of platelet inhibitor substances.

4. Contraction, contractile protein.

5. Plasminogen activator, fibrinolysin.

6. Tissue thromboplastin.

7. Heparin and heparatin sulphate.

8. Factor VIII synthesis.

9. Prostaglandin E synthesis and release.

10. Basement membrane formation.

11. Angiotensin conversion.

12. Serotonin uptake.

13. Histamine synthesis.

14. Phagocytosis.

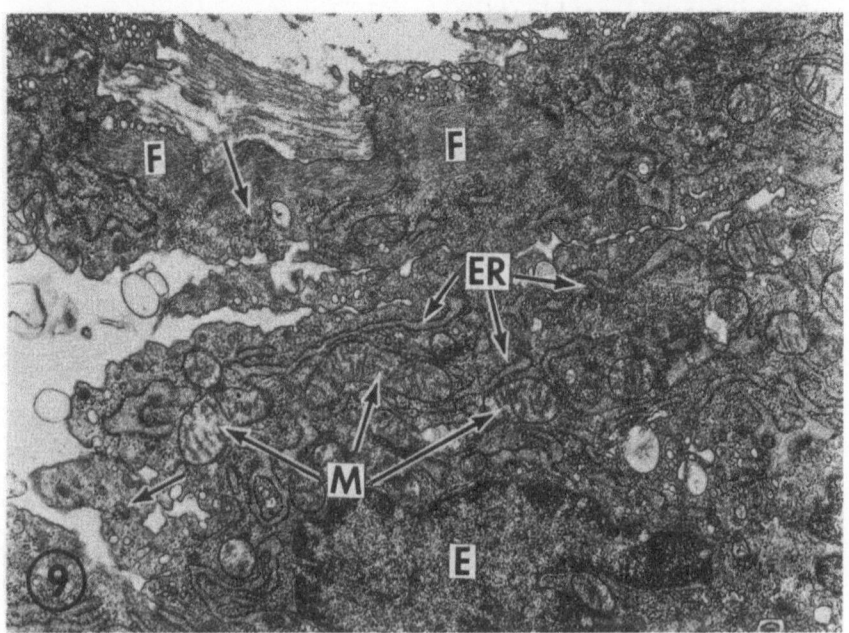

Fig. 1-9: Transmission electron micrograph of an "en face"
section through the aortic endothelium (E) of a newborn rat.
The endoplasmic reticulum (ER) is extensive, and mitochondria
(M) are numerous. Free ribosomes are numerous (arrows) and
cytoplasmic filaments (F) are frequently found in the peripheral
cytoplasm. X 15,000.

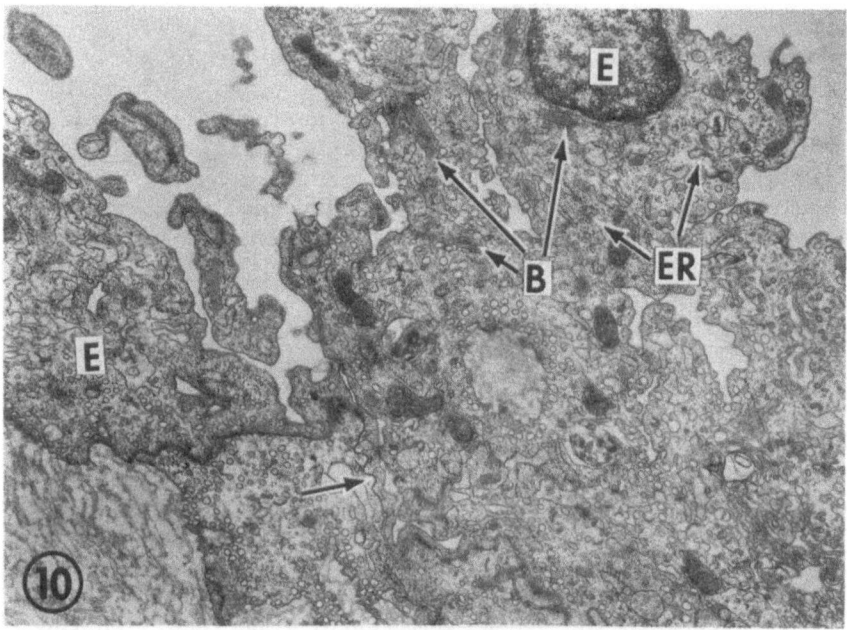

Fig. 1-10: As in Fig. 1-9, but through the aortic endothelium (E) from a two-month-old rat. The endoplasmic reticulum (ER) is fragmented and less prominent than in the newborn rat. Weibel-Palade bodies (B) are frequently seen in the mature rat, and a tight junction (arrow) is visible. X 12,000.

Copious plasmalemmal vesicles are apparent at all ages.
Tight intercellular junctions are present at all ages studied.
Weibel-Palade bodies are present with a variable frequency
in the mature aorta. However, they are not normally seen
with any frequency in immature animals, and also exhibit a
significant species difference with respect to frequency.
PIG Thus, they may be unreliable markers of endothelium in
tissue culture, and in our experience are rare in porcine
arterial endothelium. Some multi-vesicular bodies may be
precursors of Weibel-Palade bodies (11). Their roles,
albeit uncertain, may relate to the fibrinolytic system, or
to the development of tissue thromboplastins (12,13).

Now continuing with the mature rat aorta sectioned
"en face," the very large number of plasmalemmal vesicles is
readily apparent (Fig. 1-9,1-10), and needs emphasis,
particularly as one sees only a relatively small number of
vesicles in transverse sections. The frequency of plasmalemmal
vesicles is not age dependent (2).

Endothelial mitosis was for many years regarded as a
                          rare phenomenon, but is regularly
Mitosis   seen up to approximately three weeks
                          of age in the arterial endothelium.
Endothelial cell division is definitely an age-dependent
phenomenon, the mitotic frequency declining in mature
animals,

Contractile filaments tend to have either a distinctive
perinuclear orientation in the endothelium, or alternatively,
are associated with the plasma membranes. "En face," in the
rat aorta, cytoplasmic myofilaments, sometimes with dense
bodies across them, may be seen (Fig. 1-9,1-10,1-11). They
are frequently parallel to the subendothelial anchoring
filaments which attach to the connective tissue in the subendothelium (Fig. 11). These anchoring filaments are also
present in veins, arteries, capillaries and lymphatics
(14,15).

    DR. DEWEY: Dr. Schwartz, with regard to these anchoring
                    filaments, to what extent do they penetrate
Filaments   the sub-endothelial tissue?

    DR. SCHWARTZ: To the best of my knowledge, and I
can't be dogmatic on this, they are quite superficial. They
emerge and attach to the connective tissue in the innermost
part of the subendothelial space.

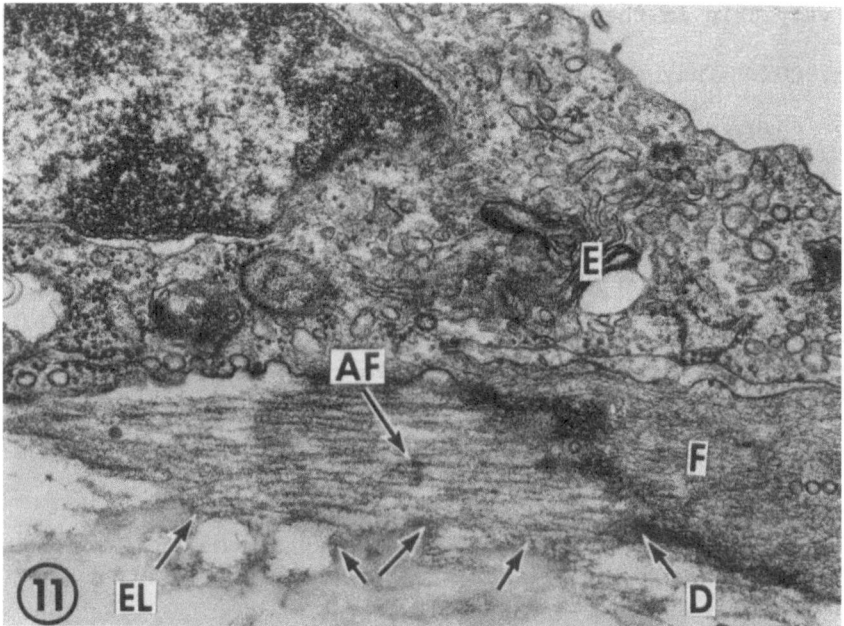

Fig. 1-11: Transmission electron micrograph of an oblique
section through the endothelium (E) of a three-month-old rat
aorta. Cytoplasmic filaments (F) appear to merge with dense
areas (D) along the plasma membrane, and are aligned with
anchoring filaments (AF) in the subendothelial space. The
latter filaments are closely associated with (arrows), and are
similar in diameter to, the protofibrils surrounding elastic
tissue (EL). X 25,000.

In young and mature animals in which the endothelium is not
widely separated from the internal elastic lamina, these
filaments merge with the protofibrils seen at the edges of
elastic tissue bundles. Don, can you comment on this?

DR. FRY: If one looks at transverse sections, one
does not see these structures. It is apparently only by
this tangential sectioning technique that they are made
visible. They must lie in the plane of the subendothelium
and be very thin in the radial direction.

DR. COX: They are extracellular?

DR. SCHWARTZ: Yes: the filaments are extracellular;
they are parallel with the intracellular filaments and fuse
into a dense body at the plasma membrane. It is impossible
to tell whether they are continuous with the cytoplasmic
filaments, or whether both types of filament attach to their
respective side of the plasma membrane.

DR. KENYON: Is there any evidence that the number of
attachment sites, if you could call them that, is a function
of the age of the endothelial layer?

DR. SCHWARTZ: I can't answer that.

DR. CHIEN: Just a comment about Dr. Cox's question.
Since the vesicles are about seven hundred angstroms in
diameter, these anchoring filaments or fibers probably are
on the order of one hundred angstroms.

DR. SCHWARTZ: That is not an unreasonable estimate.
Let us turn now to a final aspect of this part of the presentation. Within the subendothelial
Subendothelial Changes   space there is generally more
than one morphologic cell type
visible, even in the immature animal. Some of these cells
are readily identified as smooth muscle cells, while others
are undifferentiated and less readily identifiable. This
becomes important later when one begins to think about
atherogenesis and examines the spectrum of changes in the
endothelium and subendothelial space associated with aging.
In the 3-year-old rat aorta (Fig. 1-12), the endothelial
nuclei are dense and crenated, and irregular blebbing is
frequently seen on the surface of the endothelium. Droplets
of variable electron density, which are thought to be lipid,

are often present within the endothelial cytoplasm, sometimes
associated with lysosomes or the Golgi apparatus.
The 3-year-old rat endothelium, when viewed obliquely,
exhibits a tremendous number of cytoplasmic processes
projecting into the lumen, which may increase the surface
area considerably (Fig. 1-12). As the processes also contain
copious numbers of plasmalemmal vesicles, this change may
increase the effective number of vesicles exposed to the
lumen. At three years of age it is also of interest that
lymphocytes are often attached to the endothelial surface.
This phenomenon becomes more frequent in aging animals. The
reasons for this lymphocytic attachment have yet to be
explained.

The aortic subendothelial space of aged animals usually
demonstrates a diffuse intimal thickening in the absence of
any discernible lesions (2,16). When viewed "en face"
sections through the intima, the subendothelial space is
seen to be filled with amorphous granulo-vesicular material
of varying electron density (Fig. 1-13). Cellular debris
and ghost-bodies, presumably caused by the complete dissolution of cells, are prevalent. Other cells containing
large inclusions appear to be phagocytising this material
(Fig. 1-13).

Crystalline bodies may be seen in the subendothelial
space from approximately 18 months of age onward (Fig. 1-14).
Some are intracellular, but most are extracellular and have
a two-dimensional periodicity of 5.67 nm (2).

They do not appear to be viruses, and their role and significance
is uncertain. Finally, one should mention the considerable
fraying of the internal elastic lamina which occurs "pari
passu" with thinning of the medial elastic laminae with
aging.

So far, we have briefly described a sequence of changes
in the media, endothelium, and subendothelial space which
occur during growth and development on the one hand, and
aging on the other.

I will review some aspects of endothelial structure and
function, with particular references to permeability later
on in chapter 6.

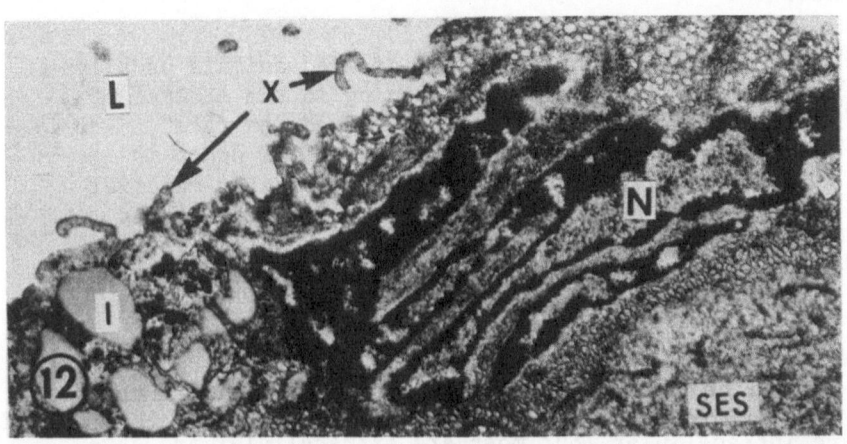

Fig. 1-12: Transmission electron micrograph of an oblique
section through the aortic endothelium of a three-year-old
rat. The nucleus (N) is electron dense and tortuous in outline, and there are many cellular extensions (X) into the
lumen (L). Many lipid inclusions (I) are visible in the
cytoplasm, which appear to be associated with dense lysosomes
(arrow). The subendothelial space (SES) contains flocculent
material. X 18,500.

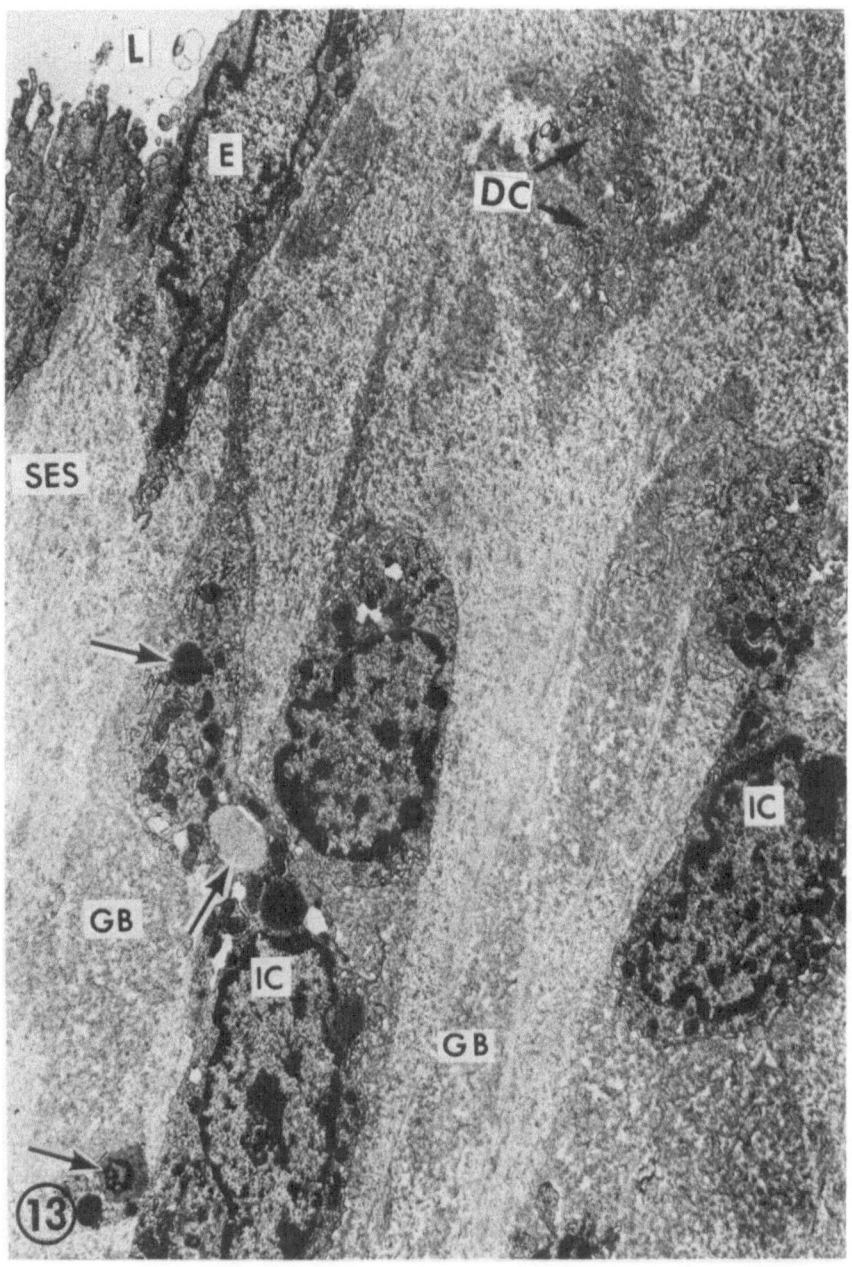

Fig. 1-13: Transmission electron micrograph of an en face section
through the aortic subendothelial space (SES) of a two-year-old
rat. Endothelium (E) and lumn (L) are at top left. Ghost bodies
(GB), cellular debris (DE), and intimal cells (IC) containing
large inclusions (arrows) are embedded in a matrix of granulo-
vesicular material of varying electron density. X 6,400.

Fig. 1-14: Transmission electron micrograph of a crystalline
body in the aortic subendothelial space of a two-year-old rat.
Two dimensional periodicity has a spacing of 5.67 nm. X 134,400

DR. KENYON: My work concentrates on certain gross features of blood vessel force and deformation relationships. This point of view may be used to interpret some aspects of arterial disease, but without accounting for altered vessel wall constituents. In other words, I take the continuun viewpoint for the most part. That is to view the arterial wall as an equivalent homogeneous deformable material. I look for some interesting behavior of this structure near bifurcations, for example, and other illustrations that I will get into later. I use this continuum concept not because of its completeness but because I think it represents an area where not enough attention has been focused up to now. Being from the Fluid Mechanics Laboratory at M.I.T. we have emphasized fluid stresses on the endothelial surfaces and on the vessels themselves. I would also like to make a plea for studying the effects of what we might call the "solid stress" in the vessel itself.

Effects of Shear Stress and Other Hydrodynamic Forces on Arterial Structure

Let me try to introduce some of the very simple notions that are fairly standard in the engineering literature but which deserve to be distributed to a wider audience so that in your own studies you might better appreciate the effects of force and deformation.

Figure 1-15 is a longitudinal section of a human descending thoracic aorta from a standard histology textbook. I only want to use it to illustrate the terminology of vessel wall stresses. The force in the axial direction i.e. perpendicular to the figure per unit area is the longitudinal stress. The hoop stress represents the force per unit area acting perpendicular to the wall thickness and is absorbed by the layers of medial tissue. We have already seen in Colin Schartz's earlier talk the detailed structure of the vessels themselves so that this does not need reiteration at this time. What I would point out here is that the models I will be talking about probably are useful, if anywhere, for blood vessels which are more or less homogeneous and I think an elastic artery, before it becomes highly thickened, is more homogeneous than say a typical distributing artery. So if we are talking about macroscopic stress versus deformation relationships they are probably going to be most meaningful before significant arterial disease has occurred.   Figure 1-16 simply represents a similar section from the same book for a distributing artery, a highly inhomogeneous structure. This has been stained on the left for the muscular constituents (a) and for elastin stain on the right (b).

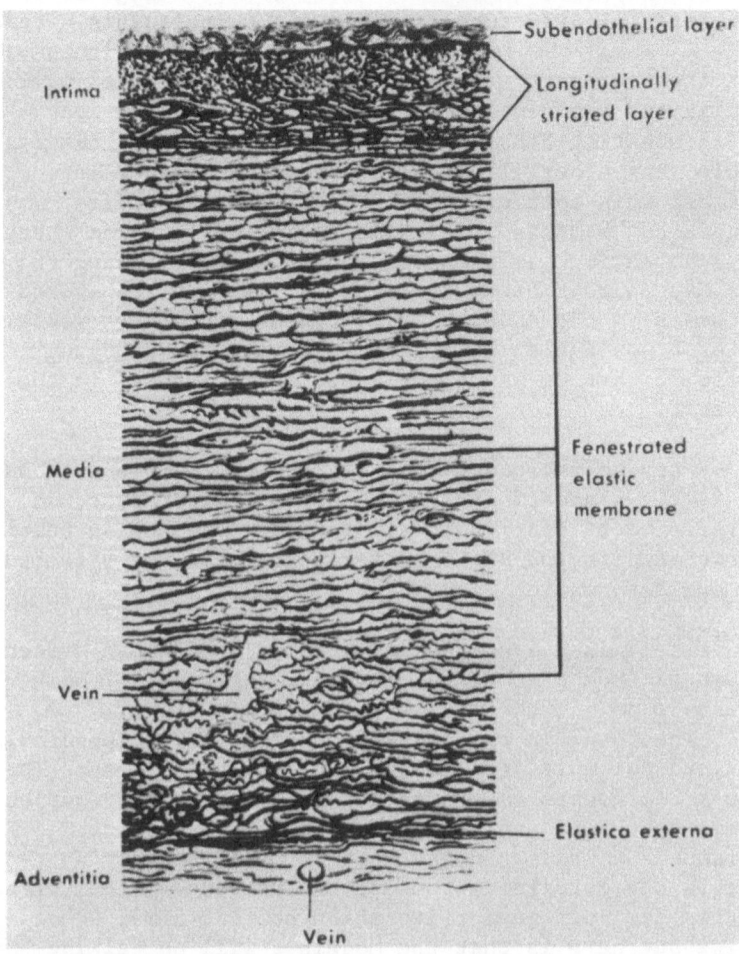

Fig. 1-15: Longitudinal section through posterior wall of human descending aorta. Elastic tissuents are not shown clearly. Elastic fiber stain. X 85 (After Koolliker and von Ebner).

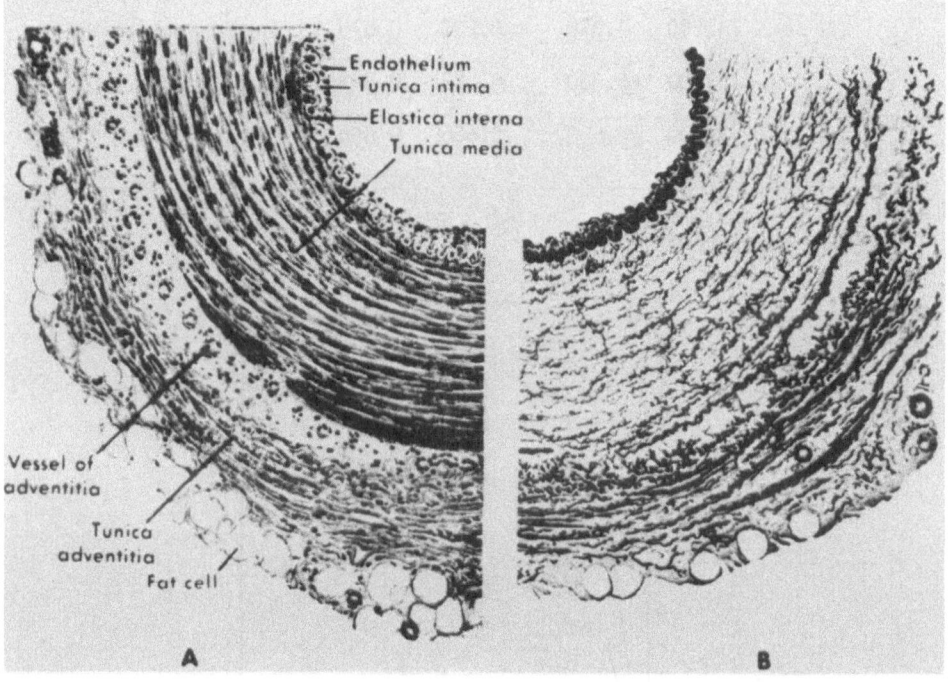

Fig. 1-16: Sectors of two cross sections of the volar digital artery of man. A. Stained with hematoxylin and eosin. B. Stained with orcein to show elastic tissue. X 80. (Slightly modified from Schaffer.)

TABLE 1.   Parameter values for stress-strain law

$$\sigma_{\theta\theta} \;=\; A\left(1 - \frac{\lambda_0}{\lambda_\theta}\right) e^{\kappa\lambda_\theta}$$

Artery	$A^\dagger$		λ_0		κ	
	NEpi	KCN	NEpi	KCN	NEpi	KCN
1	11,800	4,350	0.233	0.579	4.0	4.5
3	13,100	46,800	0.222	0.549	5.2	3.1
5	7,100	10,500	0.665	0.696	5.7	4.8

†Units in dyne/cm^2

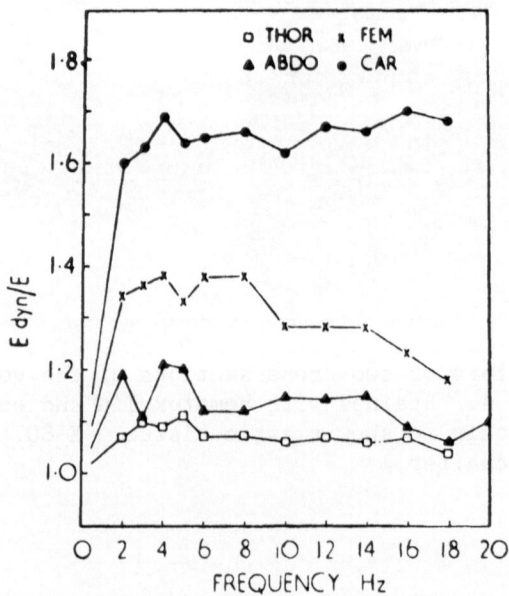

Fig. 1-17:   Viscoelasticity of Canine Aorta (Bergel, 1961).

This particular artery looks as though it has a more difficult characterization in terms of the ability of the elastin to withstand stress because it almost looks as if it is fragmented. It is very difficult, I think, to assign a mechanical role to the elastin in this particular vessel. In general, I have come to the conclusion that the small distributing arteries are going to be very difficult to model with any meaningful precision from the concepts that I will be talking about right now.

When there are roughly five significant engineering behavior modes that appear, the first one of importance is nonlinearity in the observed versus strain law. If an artery is excised and allowed to contract and is then pressurized the observed diameter versus pressure relationship is highly nonlinear, and the engineering concept of finite strain has to be applied. This circumferential strain is based on an at-rest dimension, radius, for example. The data shown in Table 1 are taken from a paper by Doyle and Dobrin (17) in which they found that they could mechanically characterize their canine carotids DOG using an empirical factor of A (units and stress) and another empirical factor kappa (dimensionless). As you can see, the application of norepinephrine as a muscular stimulant greatly increases the stress A compared to the application of KCN, a muscular poison. Thus in the canine carotid the smooth muscle cell, a fairly significant influence on the stress deformation exerts relationship.

The next important property that physiologists and engineers have examined in blood vessel mechanics is the ability of the blood vessel to exhibit a time Stress versus Strain dependent stress versus strain behavior. I am not sure (for a typical vessel) what this is really caused by in terms of a micro-constituent. I am tempted to suggest that it is due to the smooth muscles, and how fast they can relax. I am sure there are people here who can comment on the relative importance of smooth muscle in stress relaxation. Thus, the artery is a viscoelastic material. If I stress the artery with an internal pressure, the diameter does not immediately respond, or if I stress it in a time dependent fashion there is a phase vessel. In Fig. 1-17 some original data of Bergel (18) reveals that there is an asymptotic behavior in vessels such as that at about two Hertz and above the artery is more or less elastic in character. That is, there is no subsequent interesting or significant further dependence on the applied frequency.

Since this is for a dog where the normal heart rate is at
least on the order of 2 Hertz for those vessels of investigation,
it is probably a good assumption to make that at the fundamental
heart rate and all the higher harmonics the vessel properties
are governed by these asymptotic properties, such that the
dynamic stiffness modulus is about 1.7 times the static
modulus. The carotid apparently has much more frequency
DOG dependent behavior, as presumably it has more smooth muscles,
and I think these smooth muscles are allowing the material
to behave stiffer dynamically compared to its static property
than say the thoracic or even the abdominal aorta, which are
more elastic-type vessels. So it would appear as though the
smooth muscle constituent is, in part, responsible for
allowing the more peripheral arteries to behave in a much
more time dependent fashion. However, at least above two
Hertz in the dog the properties are relatively unchanged
with frequency.

Fig 1-18 provides data from a recent paper by Azuma on
more or less the same topic (19). Azuma took strips of
arteries in both longitudinal
Stress Relaxation   and ring specimens. These
were five millimeter wide
strips. The samples were subjected to an applied constant
stretch and the force required to hold it at that position diminished as a function of time. This is called
stress relaxation and stress relaxation is again another
measure of some constituent in the vessel wall allowing
itself to relax with time. The longitudinal sections,
sections along the axis of the vessel, have been stressed in
the direction that blood flows. The arch of the aorta
exhibits almost no stress relaxation for this particular
sample. In fact the only obvious amount of longitudinal
relaxation occurs in the abdominal aorta. However, the ring
sections, which are circumferential strips, exhibit somewhat
the same pattern for the more elastic arteries but as we
proceed distally, the iliac artery exhibits a very pronounced
circumferential stress relaxation and apparently this is due
again to the predominance of both tension and smooth muscle
in ring-type configurations as you proceed distally. Now the
time constants of interest here can't really be seen from
Fig. 1-18 because it is too coarse but this is a one
minute time bar, so it would appear as though the relaxations
went on within the very small part of a minute, perhaps even
on the order of a heart rate. Thus, a great part of what we
would do to attribute as gross viscoelastic character of
arteries is due to the ability of smooth muscle cells to
relax under stress. So, therefore, the proliferation of
smooth muscles with age and with disease could be very

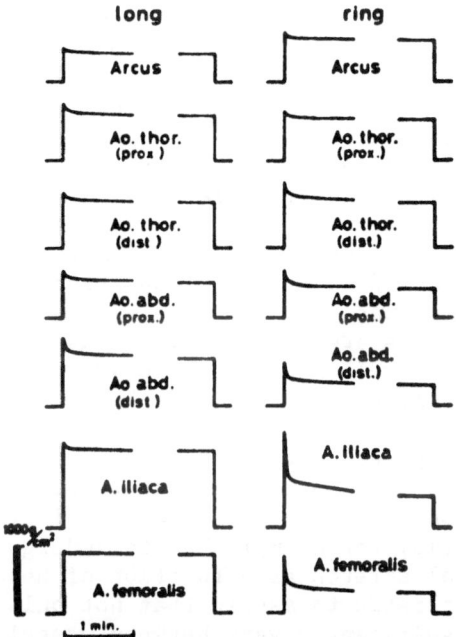

Fig. 1-18: Stress relaxation in canine arterial segments.
(Azuma, 1972).

important in controlling their elastic characteristics,
apart from the obvious changes in collagen to elastin which
also may play a lesser role in viscoelasticity.

The third mechanical property obtained from the existing
literature says that there is a pronounced anisotropy of the
vessels. Now anisotropy, in engineering usage, means that
the stretch versus deformation relation of an element depends
on the orientation of the element before stressing. If I
do not get the same value for force versus deformation, I
call the material anisotropic. There are some data for
canine aortas from Patel (Fig. 1-19) which should look
familiar to most of you (20-27). The hoop modulus E's is
about (7-12) X 10 9M/Cm at heart rate frequencies. The
axial modulus E's for this particular test was about twice
as large. We would conclude from this particular test that
within the incremental conditions of this test, the arteries
should be about twice as stiff axially as circumferentially.
Now this does not agree with some measurements of wave
speeds in the canine carotid obtained by Moritz and Anliker
(21) Their wave speed data was only consistent with a hoop
stress modulus which was roughly twice as big as the axial
modulus. These results are completely at odds for these two
vessels. Now it may well be that there are functional needs
for these two vessels which vary, and therefore, we would
not expect a consistent pattern of relative stiffness in the
axial direction compared to the circumferential. On the
other hand, I would also point out that these values are
highly dependent on the state of pre-stress in the vessel
and that the carotid, for example has to undergo quite
severe longitudinal stretch as a function of head position.
It seems quite realistic to assume that not only is anisotropy
very likely to significantly vary between vessels but within
any one vessel it is very likely to be a function of what
one might call the physiologic state.

The prime notation of Fig. 1-20 is a measure of whether
the deformation occurs in phase with applied force or out of
phase and the values of the out of phase components for
either the hoop stress, the axial stress or the radial
stresses appear to be very small compared to the real part.
So in a very crude sense, these vessels are anisotropic
and they are roughly within 10% of being perfectly incrementally
elastic.

  DR. DEWEY: What artery was the Anliker data on?

  DR. KENYON: Carotid.

  DR. DEWEY: And this is the aorta?

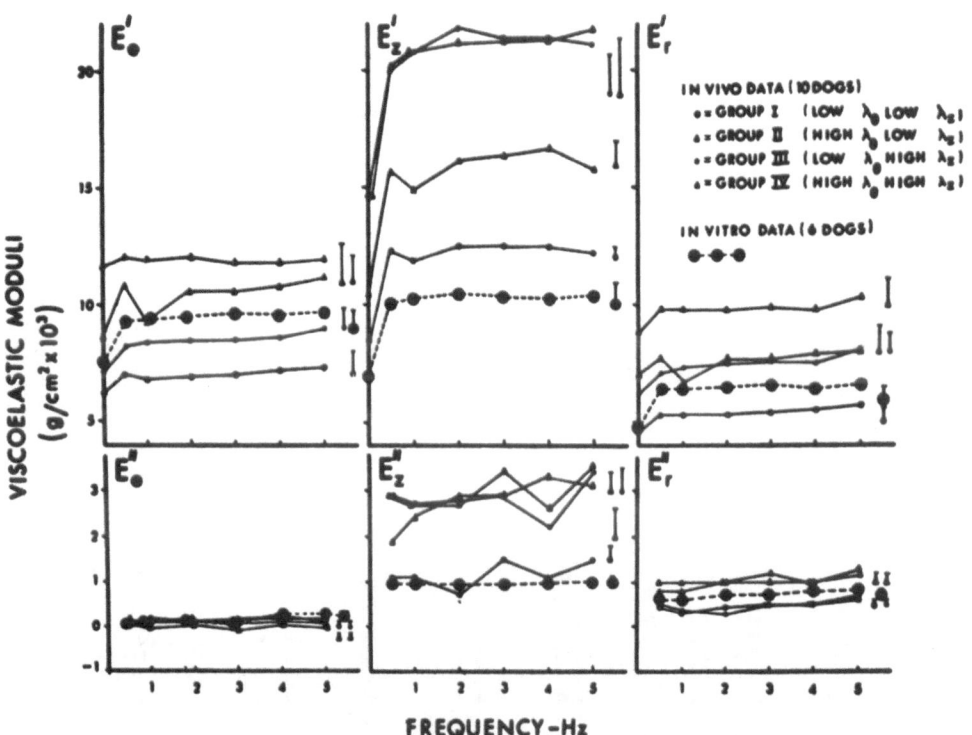

Fig. 1-19: Anisotropy of canine aorta (Patel, 1973).

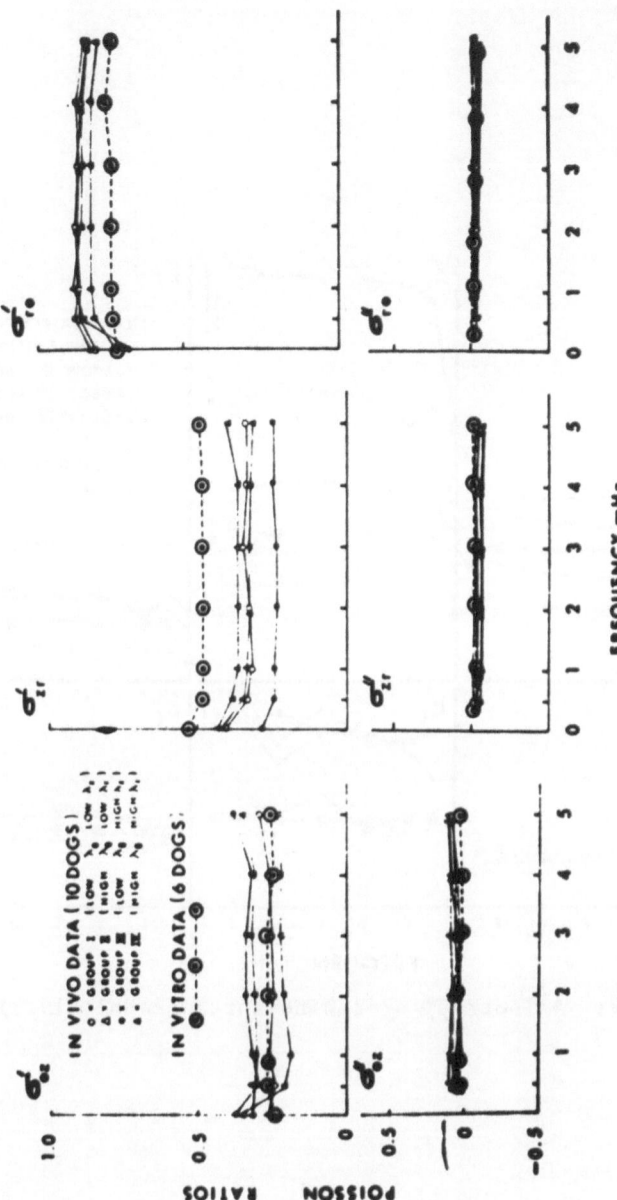

Fig. 1-20: Anistropy of canine aorta (Patel, 1973).

DR. KENYON: Yes, apparently it seems not to be
consistent between those two.   If you want to characterize,
and I think it is a valid thing for one to do, the anisotropic
properties of the vessels, you have to be very careful which
one you are talking about and how you perform your tests.
For example, do you leave the vessel in the animal when you
make your longitudinal displacement measurement, or do you
excise it? I would believe that there is a significant
amount of longitudinal strengthening of at least some vessels
in situ. This may account for some of the discrepancy but
again the comparison between Patel, and Moritz and Anliker
should be quite close because, after all, they were both in
situ measurements.

DR. CAREW: Just a short comment. There are some
older data that tell an interesting story with regard to
wave speed and that is the observation of the amount of
longitudinal displacement during the cardiac cycle. These
are data back in the early 60's. In the thoracic aorta,
Hall et al showed a lengthening with passage of the pressure
faults underneath that particular site which was being
measured. But in the abdominal aorta just the points of
attachment, the initial stretch on the vessels as well as
perhaps the inherent properties can vary enormously from
site to site.

DR. KENYON: I cannot really justify the differences I
see reported in the literature, variations in values may be
due to experimental technique.   None the less, I think
there are some real fundamental differences in each vessel.
Fig. 1-20 is of more recent vintage but is a generalization
of an earlier study of corresponding static properties.

DR. FRY: Yes, there was a series of papers about that
time from our laboratory by Patel and co-workers in which
they studied systematically the geometry; longitudinal
vascular tethering; elastic symmetry; and the anisotropic,
static and dynamic rheologic properties of the aorta, (Fig.
22-26) (Fig. 1-5). Later, Vaishnav, Young, and Patel
studied the nonlinear viscoelastic properties of the aorta
(27). Many of these studies are summarized by Patel and
Vaishnav in review articles (28,29).

DR. KENYON: That takes us through three fairly conventional
engineering descriptions of blood vessel rheology. I think
                              the next important point to
Retraction of Cut Vessel   make about blood vessels is
                              that they do appear to be
under a state of pre-stress and this is a fairly common

observation of the physician, or the physiologist, that when
he snips a vessel it contracts. It seems to withdraw. I
have always wondered why it should be. I have read through
Bergel's article very carefully and he said that it might be
due to a polymerization process within the vessel during its
maturation and that there are certain internal stresses set
up in the vessel leading to longitudinal stress. However,
there is another concept that may be involved. I imagine
the systemic circulation as being some kind of very peculiar
shaped glove in which you have an aorta, as "wrist," say,
and a peripheral circulation of small distributing arteries
and capillary networks as fingers with many small perforations.
One concept which could explain the longitudinal pre-stress
in the vessel is to visualize how one could maintain equilibrium
in the system assuming there is no restraint on this glove
due to the tissue around it. The wall tension that would
exist in the vessel under normal hydrostatic pressures,
systemic circulation, is about the right order of magnitude
to explain the pre-stress in the vessel. Now I am not
saying that this is what happens, in fact, because I don't
know what the time mean value of the tethering in the longitudinal
direction is from systemic circulation, but I do think that
it offers a mechanical reason for "pre-stress" longitudinally.
Whatever vessel we are looking at, it would appear to be
necessary to maintain equilibrium with a longitudinal tensile
force in the wall.

DR. CARO: Could a very simple minded biologist comment?
I can't think of any tissue in the body that isn't pre-
stressed, much less those of the blood vessels.

DR. WOLF: There are other alternative explanations
that take into account the innervation of the arterial wall
The trauma of snipping may stimulate the nerve network to
bring about the retraction you observe.

DR. KENYON: I quite accept your comments as pertinent.
This survey completes the picture for this particular view
of the blood vessel and its dynamic and anisotropic properties.
One comment I would like to make on this view of arteries in
general is that you have to make some assumptions about the
mechanical behavior of the vessel under pulsatile strain,
and the assumptions that were made by Patel and others were
these. First that the vessel is incompressible under rapid
changes of pressure (heart rate frequency). The second
assumption is that the artery is in a state of stress such
that excursions are defined by a free energy function for
the vessel.

While I can accept the concept of incompressibility for
rapid load changes, I find it much more difficult to appreciate
the pertinence or mechanical correctness of the assumption
that these changes are dominated or controlled by energy
function. That does not follow from thermodynamics because
this is a highly memory-sensitive system.

I would also like to mention the fifth and final property
of blood vessels which has been described, the permeability
function. Permeability, we think, is probably control for
the large particles determined by the vesicular transport
mechanisms. On the other hand, we know that the arteries
are capable of supporting a water flux through the wall.
This water flux is extremely small and is therefore very
difficult to measure ...a typical number might be 10 to the
minus 6 centimeters per second or about 1/100th a micron per
second. It is a very, very small fraction of the endothelial
cell thickness per second. An interesting calculation you
can do is to use the Palade data and calculate a flux
of water using their vesicular transport rates and you come
up with about the same number. That is, it would appear
that you could account for all the water flux in a typical
endothelial cell just by assuming that everytime a vesicle
came up to the surface that it gulped in mostly water. It
may be low molecular weight, it may be L.D.L. or whatever,
but some way or other arteries are able to transmit a small
and yet measurable water flux through their surface. Now
the quantity that controls this rate of flux is the hydraulic
permeability and I will denote it as K/μ . For arteries it
is about ten to the minus thirteen. The units are square
centimeters per second. This represents the water flux on a
bulk area basis produced by a unit pressure drop across the
unit thickness of tissue, and the relative smallness of this
number has important implications for the assumption of
incompressibility. If you make a model of the arterial wall
of two phase material capable of exuding water, then it
exudes it at a rate which, in part, is determined by this
number. The other quantity which enters into this exudation
rate is the compliance of the tissue itself. The relative
smallness of the permeability is in part responsible, I
should think, for the success with which the artery may be
viewed as incompressible for short term loading. For long-
time loading, I am much less secure about the assumption of
constant volume. You don't have to squeeze an artery between
two porous plates for example, to exclude water. I believe
it is possible to change its volume if you wait long enough,
by producing a variety of load patterns which is not a
concept which I think many people have previously considered.

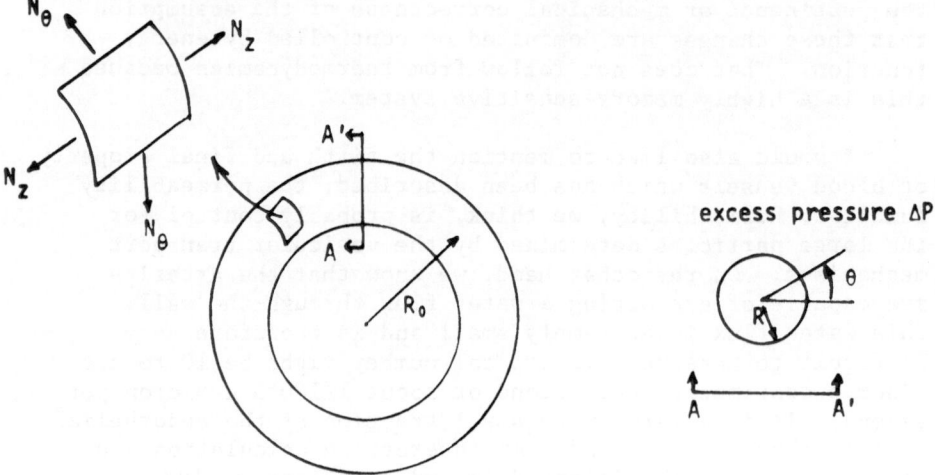

Fig. 1-21: Model for aortic arch.

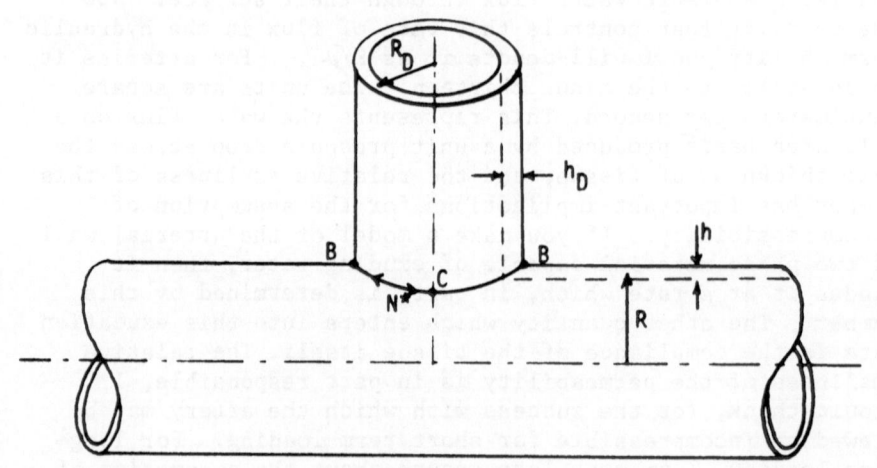

Fig. 1-22: T-junction geometry.

I first of all want to get into some very simple-minded
concepts of stress at places in the arterial system which
are points of interest which are likely to develop plaques.
Fig. 1-21 is a model of the aortic arch and I assume that
the aorta is isotropic and linearly elastic. I can use
known solutions to find the hoop stresses in the arch under
a small excursion of pressure. There is an axial hoop
stress, i.e., a stress along the flow direction. There is
also stress in the circumferential or hoop direction,
N_θ . Now it turns out that the value of this hoop stress
is a function of position around the hoop and it is greater
on the inside of the bend and least on the outside of the
bend.   The difference between the maximum and the minimum
hoop stress divided by their mean value is equal to twice
the ratio of vessel radius to the radius of the bend, R/Ro.
If as typical data for the aortic arch R = 1.5 cm. Ro = 5
cm., then you should get about a 60% increase in hoop
stress on the inside of the turn in the aorta compared to as
opposed to the outside. I am neglecting bifurcations and
all the other obvious complications which would make it very
difficult to solve this precisely. But this indicates, for
a crude approximation, how we could view the difference in
uptake, for example, between inside and outside of a turn.
I do not intend that this be considered complete but it does
indicate an interesting trend.

The next model I want to talk about is a model of a T-
branch (Fig. 1-22) as representative of something we can
actually calculate.
The increase in vessel stress
is at the branch point
itself. The Y-branch is also

Model for Stress
Concentration

of interest but is very difficult to calculate. It should be
done experimentally first, I think. Fig. 1-22 represents a
geometry solved in an approximate way and verified with a
photoelastic model. We may view this, for example, as the
aorta with the intercostal branchings. This has been solved
for a number of ratios of parent vessel radius to daughter
radius, and as a function of parent vessel thickness to
daughter thickness. In this particular solution it was
assumed that there was no strengthening of the material
locally at the bifurcation, so naturally we would expect
some elevated stresses. For example the hoop stress N*,
which represents the membrane stress at the point at which
these two cylinders intersect is quite high. And in fact
one can picture this mechanically by considering the effect
of a "hole" in the parent tube. Slice it along the bottom
surface longitudinally, open it up, and then stretch it.

We have an equivalent to what the engineering literature calls stress concentration due to a hole in a plate. The stresses at the hole are a function of position around the hole. The membrane stresses are most severe at point B. The theoretical solution for a plate predicts an increment of stress at point B of three times the hoop stress far away from the junction. Again, however, I must emphasize that this assumes there is no extra material thickening at the junction. Table 2 gives the stress concentration factor K. (30). K here represents the ratio of predicted stress at point B from that which would occur if there were no junction present. The numbers are, I think, interesting. These are certainly factors which seem to be more important than taking account for example, thick vessel effects or vessel inhomogeneity which have been suggested as important to atherosclerosis. These results suggest to me that it would be worthwhile to do some geometric mappings of bifurcations and make models of these materials to find out what is the stress distribution at these sites because it looks to me as though they are also points where there is augmentation of shear stress and these two mechanical factors may "complement" one another at bifurcations. The theory shown here relates only to unstiffened junctions for various radius ratios and thickness ratios. Results for what might be called structural reinforcement at the junction have been worked out.

DR. CARO: I haven't studied this in detail but I have the impression, indeed strong impression, from casts that the intercostal junction which you mentioned is not really a T junction. It is a Y junction, it seems as if the daughter vessel is coming off at right angles to the parent, but in fact, its initial course is tangential to it, and then it rapidly turns through 90 degrees.

DR. KENYON: The geometry (Fig. 1-22) is highly idealized for use in physiological junctions. But I think the numbers would still be something quite interesting in the more physiological geometrics.

DR. CARO: I am sure you are right, but would that modify your conclusions?

DR. KENYON: Yes, very much. The angle of bifurcation is a very strong factor in the stress concentrations. A Y configuration would reduce the stress on the inside of the bend. Thank you for bringing that out.

TABLE 2

Diameter ratio a^B/a^M	Stress ratio $a^B T/a^M t$	Main-vessel thickness ratio $2a^M/T$	K (theory)	K_1 (exp.) [1, 2]	Deviation $\dfrac{K-K_1}{K_1}\%$	Model
0.50	0.98	13.4	3.74	3.50	7	E-4
0.50	0.99	13.2	3.73	3.50	7	E-4B
0.50	0.98	13.3	3.73	3.74	0	E-4E
0.80	1.00	13.0	4.32	4.10	5	C-7A
1.00	1.00	13.0	4.40	3.90	13	C-8A
0.28	1.23	26.9	3.54	4.00	-12	C
0.63	0.92	19.0	4.52	5.00	-10	R
1.00	1.00	19.0	5.06	5.43	-7	S
0.34	1.02	98.0	6.53	5.70	15	
0.29	0.56	13.1	2.66	3.32	-20	E-1
0.29	0.59	12.9	2.67	2.90	-8	E-2
0.29	0.58	13.0	2.67	3.28	-18	E-3
0.29	0.56	13.3	2.67	3.36	-20	E-7
0.57	0.41	13.1	2.56	2.70	-5	C-5H
0.30	0.48	26.9	3.24	3.00	8	B
0.50	0.512	30.0	9.02	8.33	8	C-1

Arteries do have their permeability, and they also have
their ability to withstand normal force, and when you put
                                    these two together you come
Contribution of Arterial   out with a model that was
Permeability   originally developed in soil
                                    mechanics, incidentally, called
Consolidation Theory. This means that if an elastic material
with a pore structure squeezed it, it doesn't empty spontaneously.
It takes time for the liquid to squeeze through the pores
and the time it takes is a function of how fine the pores
are. If you model the artery as a two-phase material with a
compliance and permeability of correct order of magnitude,
one estimates that it takes a time on the order of several
minutes at least, to release water from an artery when
suddently squashed and this is due to its relatively fine
pore structure. The consequence of this is that the volume
change is really very small during normal rates of application
of pulsatile blood pressure. But that volume change, if it
occurs at all, is going to be confined to those areas of the
vessel that have, what you might call, free access to fluid
the lumen end at the capillary network between the media and
adventitia. This suggests that in pulsatile studies there
may be a time dependent volume change locally of a very
small amount, such that if you are interested in mass transfers,
this could be significant. Now why is it significant?
Because it is a small distance through which these volume
changes are propagated. Incidentally, it is governed by a
diffusion equation. The volume change within an artery
satisfies the diffusion equation. And yet the diffusion
constant itself is on the order of ten to the minus 6 square
centimeters per second. So during one heart beat the diffusion
distance is the square root of this diffusion coefficient
divided by frequency. The volume change during each heart
beat will propagate about ten microns.

This is a theoretical calculation. It reveals that the
region undergoing volume change is such a small fraction of
the vessel thickness that the incompressibility assumption
would be a good one. Yet having the ability to distribute
forces that vary significantly over a ten micron distance,
means that I will have a potential for a large transfer via
the water flux at those points and only at those points. If
you have ever done any heat transfer problems, here is an
analogy. In heat transfer we might think of how much heat
flux occurs if sinusoidal temperature variation of high
frequency exits at the surface.

If the material has a fairly low thermal diffusion constant, it means that all the temperature gradients are established over a very thin surface layer and that means that the heat flux which accomapnies that applied temperature difference is going to be extremely large. The same concept, at least in theory, applies to the artery. By establishing significant pressure differences over small thicknesses we have in principle a mechanism for very high augmentation of water flux during the heart beat.

All of the approximations which have been made here are important because the artery is not homogeneous. If there is any surface resistance to the water flow this would be extremely important to account for. The model would then be an approximation for a vessel denuded of endothelium.

The system of hoop stress and liquid stress which is produced by this model is shown in Fig. 1-23 The thickness to radius ratio is denoted by ($3 = h/R$) With a two-phase view of an artery we have to somehow distribute this stress system to the fluid and solid constituents. If you assume that the solid is both isotropic and elastic, then there is an incremental hoop tension of amount. There is a radial compression of $\Delta P/23$ amount. On the other hand there is a system of fluid stresses and, of course, the stress in fluid is the same in all directions on a bulk basis. It is also of amount $\Delta P/23$ and it is a <u>tension</u>. It is extremely important to realize that if I apply internal pressurization ΔP against the lumen that I actually reduce the fluid inside the vessel, (where there is no significant amount of fluid flow). The pressure drop occurs over thickness, which is on the order of ten microns. I think you can see what is happening. We have the potential for a highly augmented plasma flux within this superficial intimal layer.

These results are summarized in Fig. 1-24. We have at the lumen of the blood vessel an applied pressure increment ΔP, and I have normalized the associated incremental liquid pressures, ΔP, within the artery to the magnitude of applied pressure, ΔP. P rapidly drops to a value which is about $-5\Delta P$. It stays constant throughout the thickness of the vessel because for those deep regions of the vessel no significant volume change occurs in the time between heart beats. There is not enough time for significant fluid flux to occur. During diastole, on the other hand, applied pressure is reversed inside and according to this model, plasma flows back to the lumen. Mechanically, this is due to a kind of "wringing out" of the surface layer during diastole.

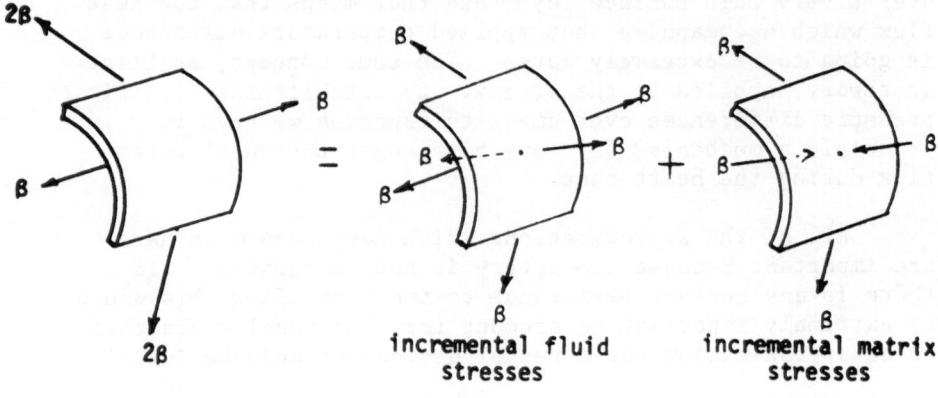

$$\beta \equiv \Delta P/2\zeta$$

Fig. 1-23: Incremental stresses (two phases).

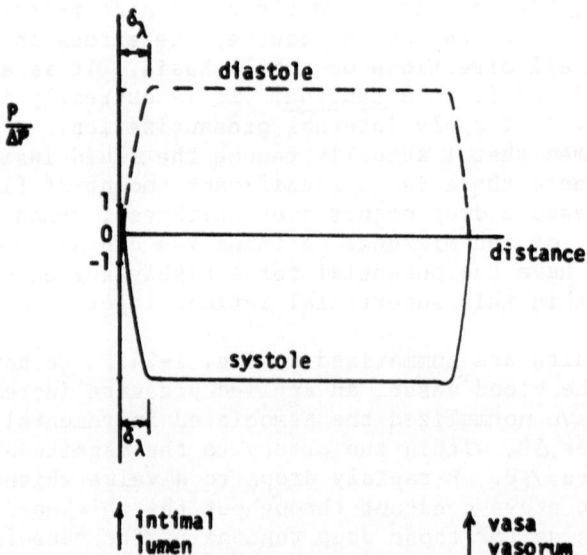

Fig. 1-24: Pulsatile plasma pressure distribution.

So there is with this model a sponge-like property of the intima which could be quite relevant to plasma wall flux. I would like to leave time for questions because I think apart from its highly speculative outlook, I would like to convey to you that even though we think that the permeability is controlled by events on a molecular scale, there are circumstances where this motion could be affected by plasma squeezing. Thus, continuum mechanics at this stage can offer some interesting if not formative descriptions of what we might call vessel rheology. This is only a start. The problems yet to be solved depend very intimately on detailed architecture of the wall at the point under investigation and the magnitude of the forces in the longitudinal direction, which I do not yet know how to estimate.

DR. STONE: Peterson (31) showed quite a few years ago that there was about a one percent change during the cardiac cycle in the radius of the carotid artery in the in situ-artery.   Conversely, Arndt (32) showed to the contrary that there was an average of 15 percent change in that same location, but the artery had not been handled before measurement. So we are now not only talking about in vitro, in vivo, in situ but intact as well.   There seemed to be a large discrepancy in these radius change figures from the intact to in vitro experiments.

DR. KENYON: I am aware of the discrepancy and I failed to point out that in fact the X-ray and ultrasonic determinations of compliance for a cat, at least, seemed to indicate that it is more flexible in the body than out.   But on the other hand, I think Strandness has done some measurements which indicate that there is not that much difference.   I still think that there is a possibility that the Arndt data (32) on cats are not necessarily invalid because there is yet to be an exact determination of in vivo compliance data. My intuition suggests that, if anything, the vessel should be stiffer circumferentially in situ and in vivo than in vitro. I don't know...There is an interaction between the radial and the longitudinal behavior and you have to snip a significant amount of tissue away from the artery to make your in situ determination, and that in itself may affect the stretch during pressure excursions.

DR. STONE: You will get a tremendous vasoconstrictor response when you manipulate most blood vessels. It lasts for extended periods of time so, to me, anyway, it seems like my reaction would be just the reverse of yours.

Vasomotor Effects

That the vessel would be much more compliant normally than
it is once it has been manipulated.

DR. KENYON: I think it is a question of how much more.
I think there are compliance data where it was about twelve
to one, I don't think it was quite that bad...

DR. STONE: Arndt's data showed some 15 percent change
in carotid radius with the cardiac cycle as opposed to 1
percent for Peterson.

DR. KENYON: It is believed, but I am sure more people
here can testify than I can, that to make a diameter determination
in a vessel undergoing pressurization, the vessels don't
remain round and the action of your gauge is sometimes
uncertain...

DR. NEREM: Would you comment on the difference between
the coronary system and the aorta from the viewpoint that
you are bringing us?

DR. KENYON: I am excited about the potential importance
of strain on coronaries because it seems as though the
distributing arteries and coronary vessel remain relatively
disease free when they dive into the myocardium. This
therefore, suggests that if the artery is free to distend
under pressure, it might undergo larger changes in longitudinal
or axial strain, than when it is imbedded in a highly dense
tissue. But I am only speculating. In terms of this permeability
process, it is going to be very difficult to establish the
pressures within the arterial wall by any experimental means
I can think of.

DR. COX: I had a couple of comments, with regard to
your questions about deformation, the magnitude of deformation,
and comparing Arndt's and Peterson's work. (32,31) There
are many factors that can contribute to the determination of
values of circumferential strain during the cardiac cycle.
One of the most important of these is the value of mean
pressure that exists at the time of measurement. Peterson's
measurements were in an anesthetized dog. As soon as you
start tampering with an unanesthetized animal, you get
moderatly severe hypertension, 130 to 150 mm Hg arterial
pressure are not unusual. This would result in an increase
in stiffness due to the nonlinear nature of vascular elasticity
and you would certainly expect a smaller value of wall
strain.

With regard to Arndt's work, he used two types of measurements, one using an ultrasonic transducer on the carotid artery which he subsequently used on the aorta, and for some other measurements he used radiographs. He measured wall diameter from radiographs at different pressures and used these data to define values of strain. To some extent there are methodolo-gical reasons for the differences in wall strain which he reported to an extent in comparing Arndt's data with other data in the literature especially data on the thoracic aorta, the effects of thoracotomy, of surgery in general, of trauma, all contribute to a determination of the value of radial wall strain both directly and indirectly. You also have to consider that the value of the pulse pressure which is dependent on the physiological state of the animal, also is affected by thoracotomy, by fluid loss, the state of hydration, by the nature of blood loss in an animal. These factors also contribute to wall strain. So just saying wall strain is 5% or 10% is really meaningless because of these large numbers of factors. It must be related to both mean and pulsatile pressure under the conditions of measurement.

The other comment I had was concerned with the continuum models you were talking about. One of the things I think you have to remember is that the blood vessel is an amazingly complex structure that has an autoregulatory capacity.

By autoregulation I mean a structural autoregulatory capacity. The smooth muscle cells apparently respond to the state of wall strain, or rate at which connective tissue elements are synthesized and extruded into the extracellular space. One of the determinents of that rate of synthesis is growth. During growth and development when there are large increases, for example, in bone size, I am sure you can expect increases in the axial strain of blood vessels in the axial direction through increased connective tissue synthesis. Also in some of your models with complicated geometry and stress concentrations at certain points, one would expect that smooth muscle cells in those areas that sense the elevated wall stress or elevated deformation would increase locally the synthesis of connective tissue proteins, to minimize differences in wall stress. This would be expected to be true at complicated geometry such as branching and curvature. Also, the movement of the heart and the associated deformation of coronary arteries with cardiac contraction would produce time varying changes in deformation of coronary arteries. These may also be signals to coronary artery smooth muscle which would control connective tissue synthesis.

So, for example, in aging as we get dilatation of the cardiac chamber there may be different signals impinging on coronary artery smooth muscle cells that may regulate their synthesis of connective tissue proteins and this, instead of having a negative feedback effect may produce a positive feedback effect at least in the direction of coronary artery pathology.

DR. KENYON: I think I am a convert to your point of view in the sense that it would appear that we would really like to know something more about the actual stress distribution within the arteries as they exist. I am perfectly sympathetic to your qualifications that must be put on these models. I would reiterate, they were only presented, not in completeness but because I hope they will stimulate further serious investigation of what I consider physiologically important applications of continuum mechanics to rheology of blood vessels. The finite strain models are interesting in a sense but they are not, of themselves, necessarily going to shed light on how the day-by-day physiological state of arteries is affected by stress. That is just a personal point of view. In other words, the natural state of the artery is not something, that to my mind can be achieved by letting it come to rest in a beaker.

DR. CARO: I believe I found a slight discrepancy. I think you said that you account for the observed water transport by vesicular movement. But my unpublished data on sodium acetate transport, indicate that it is transported at a far higher rate than protein and because of its small size and low lipid solubility I expect it to be transported mainly via the endothelial intercell clefts rather than the vesicles. Thus, I suspect that vesicle transport is by comparison quite slow.

DR. KENYON: Perhaps I was misunderstood. A long time ago I made the calculation but I assumed that what was being transported was some volume of material of a water-like nature. When I used the average vesicular density in the apparent front movement (as pointed out in the transmission electron micrographs of Pallade) that it would appear to account for most of the water flux, not necessarily the protein flux. It was a very crude calculation and it was only interesting in comparison to measured water fluxes. That is really what I was estimating, not the protein.

DR. WEINBAUM: We have been interested, as you might guess, in the viscoelastic behavior of the endothelial cells. At least three different relaxation times are involved. There is going to be a viscous motion of intracellular fluid contents and an associated relaxation time. There is also a membrane flow, relaxation time, and finally a longer time volume change effect of the nature that you are talking about. What I find really interesting is that the relaxation time you find in your macroscopic models is of the order of half a second or a second. This time is of the same order that Shu Chien and Dick Skalak observe in their studies of the viscoelastic behavior of a red cell. In the red cell this time is associated with membrane flow. My intuition would be that the behavior you are observing that corresponds to that is viscoelastic membrane behavior integrated now over many cells. I would like to hear your own thoughts on this.

Viscoelastic Behavior of Endothelial Cells

DR. KENYON: Could be. But I just thought it could be due to internal mechanisms in smooth muscle itself. Whatever its source, it appears to be associated with the muscular constituent because it appeared as though it had the most dramatic and long-lasting relaxation pattern compared to, for example, the more pure collagen type tissue or the more pure elastintype tissue, which apparently have a shorter and less dramatic relaxation problem. I don't know what the relative role of the three major constituents is. Let us not forget mucopolysaccharide. I think to some extent it might contribute to viscoelastic phenomena on perhaps a longer time scale.

DR. DEWEY: One of the interesting things to come out of Dr. Kenyon's calculations is that there is, by virtue of the structure of the artery, a tremendous potential to drive the fluid into and out of the vessel. I emphasize the word potential because in the presence of an intact endothelial barrier it appears that the transport mechanisms are reduced by as much as one to two orders of magnitude. In the absence of an intact endothelial barrier, however, the pressure gradients which are produced by the stretch in the artery, and the fact that the fluid has to enter the artery to accommodate this incompressible condition, movement of water would be relatively great, perhaps one to two orders of magnitude greater with every heart beat but over a distance of only a few tenths of a micron at the most.

DR. KENYON: I would suggest that if endothelial cells
were ever susceptible to the ballooning mechanism that I
just illustrated you might well get a little more water flux
there than you would account for if you just used the mean
driving force for fluid flow. Apparently you only need to
move them apart a little bit to obtain fluid flow but when
they are on the order of 40 to 50 angstroms at their junctions,
it is very difficult to get through them at high rates. In
fact, here again you can estimate what the typical mean
pressure drop is across the endothelial cell for the observed
flux and it turns out to be in the neighborhood of 10 millimeters
of mercury, a significant fraction of the total plasma
pressure drop which may well occur across the endothelial
junction.

BIBLIOGRAPHY

1.   Mitchell, J.P.A. and Schwartz, C.J.: In "Arterial Disease"
      Blackwell Scientific Publications, Oxford, England,
      1965.

2.   Gerrity, R.G. and Cliff, W.J.: The aortic tunica media of
      the developing rat. I. Quantitative sterologic and
      biochemical analysis. Lab. Invest. 32: 585-600, 1975.

3.   Gerrity, R.G. and Cliff, W.J.: The aortic tunica intima in
      young and aging rats. Exp. Molec. Pathol. 16: 382-402,
      1973.

4.   Cliff, W.J.: The aortic tunica media in aging rats. Exp.
      Molec. Pathol. 13: 172-189, 1970.

5.   Schwartz, S.M. and Benditt, E.P.: Cell replication in the
      aortic endothelium: A new method for study of the
      problem. Lab. Invest. 28: 699-707, 1973.

6.   Jaffee, E.A., Nachman, R.L., Becker, C.G., and Minick, C.R.:
      Culture of human endothelial cells derived from
      umbilical veins. J. Clin. Invest. 52: 2745-2756, 1973.

7.   Morrison, A.D., Berwick, L., Orci, L., and Winegrad, A.L.:
      Morphology and metabolism of an aortic intima-media
      preparation in which an intact endothelium is
      preserved. J. Clin. Invest. 57: 650-667, 1976.

8. Gabbiani, G., Badonnel, M.C., and Rona, G.: Cytoplasmic contractile apparatus in aortic endothelial cells of hypertensive rats. Lab. Invest. 32: 227-234, 1975.

9. Majno, G.: Ultrastructure of the vascular membrane. In "Circulation." Handbook of Physiology. Amer. Physiol. Soc., Washington D.C., Vol. 3, 1965.

10. Rhodin, J.A.G.: In "Histology. A Text and Atlas." Oxford University Press, New York, pp. 331-370, 1974.

11. Sengel, A. and Stoebner, P.: Golgi origin of tubular inclusions of endothelial cells. J. Cell Biol. 44: 223-226, 1970.

12. Astrup, T. and Buluk, K.: Thromboplastic and fibrinolytic activities in vessels of animals. Circ. Res. 13: 252-260, 1963.

13. Warren, B.A.: Fibrinolytic properties of vascular endothelium. Brit. J. Exp. Pathol. 44: 365-372, 1963.

14. Leak, L.V. and Burke, J.F.: Ultrastructural studies on the lymphatic anchoring filaments. J. Cell Biol. 36: 129-149, 1968.

15. Ts'Ao, C. and Glagov, S.: Basal endothelial attachment. Tenacity at cytoplasmic dense zones in the rabbit aorta. Lab. Invest. 23: 510-516, 1970.

16. Moss, N.S. and Benditt, E.P.: The ultrastructure of spontaneous and experimentally induced arterial lesions. Lab. Invest. 23: 231-245, 1970.

17. Doyle, J.M., and Dobrin, P.B.: "Finite deformation analysis of the relaxed and contracted dog carotid artery." Microvascular Research 3: 400-415, 1971.

18. Bergel, D.H.: "The dynamic elastic properties of the arterial wall." J. Physiol. 156: 445-457, 1961.

19. Azuma, T., et al: Viscoelastic properties of large arteries Proc. 5th. International Congress of Rheology, Vol. 2 University of Tokyo, 1969.

20. Patel, D.J., et al: Static anisotropic elastic properties of the aorta in living dogs. Circ. Res. 25: 765-779, 1969.

21. Moritz, W.E., and Anliker, M.A.: Wave transmission
     characteristics and anisotrophy of canine carotid
     arteries. J. Biomechanics 7: 151-154, 1974.

22. Patel, D.J., Mallos, A.J., and Fry, D.L.: Aortic mechanics
     in the living dog. J. Appl. Physiol. 16: 293-299,
     1961.

23. Patel, D.J., and Fry, D.L.: Longitudinal tethering dogs.
     Circ. Res. 19: 1011-1021, 1966.

24. Patel, D.J., and Fry, D.L.: The elastic symmetry of arterial
     segments in dogs. Circ. Res. 24: 1-8, 1969.

25. Patel, D.J., Janicki, J.S., and Carew, T.E.: Static
     anisotropic elastic properties of the aorta in living
     dogs. Circ. Res. 25: 765-780, 1969.

26. Patel, D.J., Janicki, J.S., Vaishnav, R.N., and Young, J.T.:
     Dynamic anisotropic viscoelastic properties of the
     aorta in living dogs. Circ. Res. 32: 93-107, 1973.

27. Vaishnav, R.N., Young, J.T., Patel, D.J.: Nonlinear
     viscoelastic theory for large blood vessels.
     Proceedings of the International Congress on
     System Dynamics, Valley Forge, Pa., 1975.

28. Patel, D.J., and Vaishnav, R.N.: Rheology of large blood
     vessels. In Bergel, D.H. (Ed.): Cardiovascular
     Fluid Dynamics. Academic Press, Inc., London, 1-64,
     1972.

29. Patel, D.J., and Vaishnav, R.N.: Mechanical properties of
     arteries. Proceedings of the NATO-Advance Study
     Institute in Cardiovascular Fluid Dynamics,

30. Lind, N.C.: An elastic analysis of the stress concentration
     of a pressurized T-branch pipe connection, in First
     Int'l Conf. Pressure Vessel Technology, Part 1, ASME,
     269-275, 1969. Approximate stress-concentration
     analysis for pressurized branch pipe connections, in
     Pressure Vessels and Piping: Design and Analysis
     Part 2, ASME, 952-958.

31. Peterson, L.H., Jensen, R.E., and Parnell, J., Mechanical
     properties of arteries in vivo. Circ. Res. 8: 622, 1960.

32. Leitz, K.H., and Arndt, J.O.: Die Durchmesser-Druck-
     Beziehung des intakten Gefassebietes der A. carotis
     communis von Katzen. Pflugers Archiv. 301-50, 1968.

Chapter 2   FLUID MECHANICS OF ARTERIAL FLOW

DR. DEWEY: The primary objective of my talk* today is
to summarize those aspects of fluid mechanics that relate to
arterial disease.   Some simple quantitative estimates of
fluid shear stress will be made and the effects of flow
pulsatility and vessel geometry will be noted.   I hope
specific topics that warrant additional research will be
suggested.

In viewing the great body of literature that exists on
arterial hemodynamics, one comes face to face with the fact
that a large fraction of the existing literature is specifically
limited to either a particular artery or a particular experiment
in vitro for which the fluid dynamicist has some hope of
making theoretical interpretation. I emphasize this because,
if we are really serious about understanding arteriosclerosis
and possible exacerbating effects arising from hemodynamics,
we have to talk about complex arterial geometries for which
accurate theoretical calculations are nearly impossible. We
have to be, I think, more sensitive than we have collectively
been in the past to the full complexity of the problem that
faces us.

For this reason, I have chosen as Figure 2-1 an x-ray
angiogram of the coronary circulation. Understanding this
                              complicated flow network is
The Coronary Circulation   the real problem we are trying
                              to solve. The coronary circulation
is a very tenuous delivery system. Compromise of one or
more of the small arteries which feed the myocardium can
lead to death. We are talking about a very detailed tree, with
many bends, bifurcations, and collateral branches; if we are
going to make any sense out of this problem, this is the
situation we have to address.

Most quantitative hemodynamic information that is
available refers to the larger isolated vessels such as the
aorta and the femoral arteries. I would like to take the
point of view that such information is useful insofar as it
helps us to understand more complicated problems such as the
coronaries.

_____

*The research reported in this talk was sponsored by
the National Heart, Lung, and Blood Institute, Grants HL14209
and HL21859.
                              55

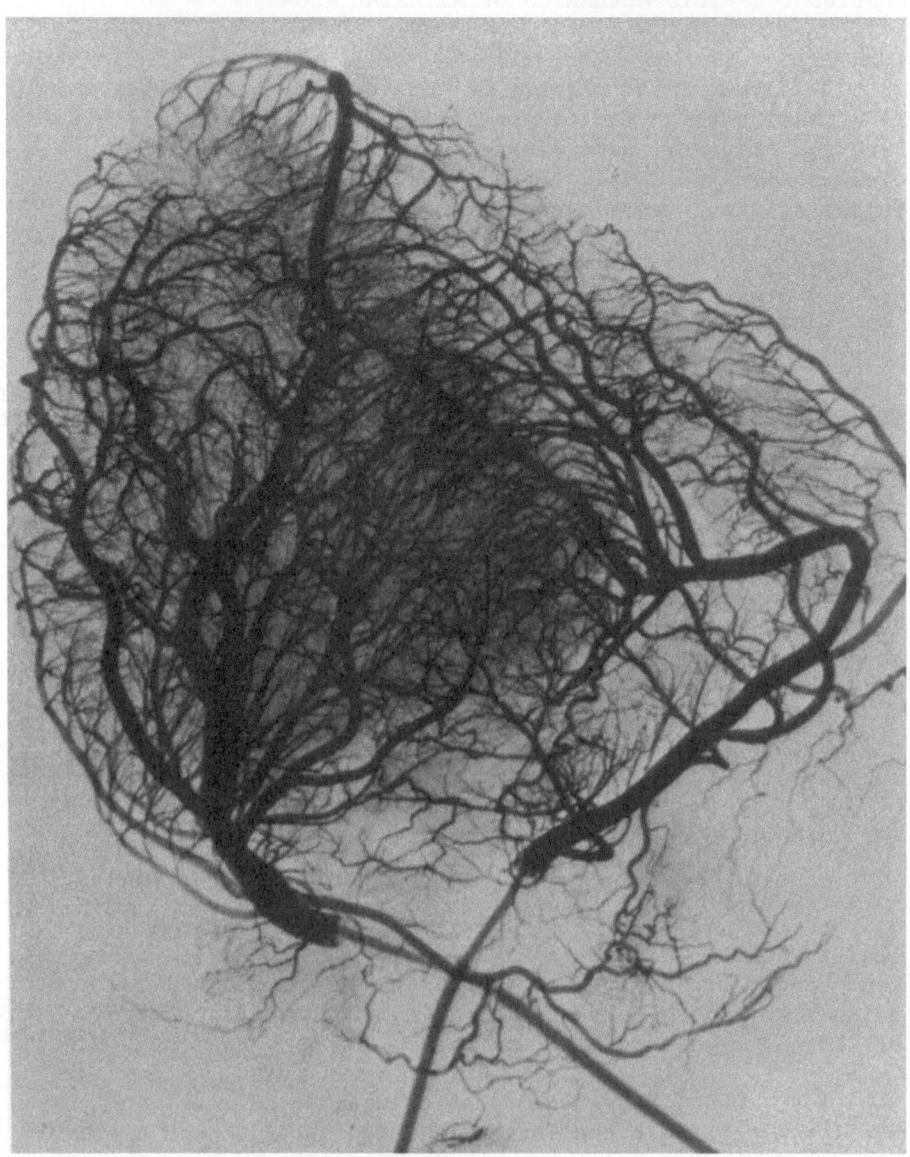

Fig. 2-1: X-Ray angiographic picture of the human coronary circulation. The angiogram was taken using an excised human heart (from Fulton (52) p. 164).

In spite of these pejorative statements, of necessity one must refer to experiments in the large isolated arteries simply because the amount of data available on the coronary circulation is woefully inadequate to the tasks that one would like to confront as a fluid dynamicist.

One encouraging fact is that Drs. Caro, Schwartz, Nerem and others have been sensitive to this problem and have been looking at coronary circulation with more than just a passing glance. One of the things we will talk about later is the problem of modeling; ways in which information gleaned from one artery may be used to estimate the flow parameters in a different artery. In particular, I would like you to be conscious of the differences
In Vitro Modeling   between animal models and the human circulation. These differences are often larger than the variations that exist between animal species or between the human circulation and a well-designed in vitro model. We are really interested in the human condition and have to be realistic with regard to whether or not the animal experiments we are doing are in elucidation of the human condition or simply of the particular test animal.

Figure 2-2 was borrowed from McDonald's book (1); it gives you a simplified overview of the variety of velocities and pressure waveforms that
Velocities and Pressure   one finds in the systemic arteries.
Wave Forms in Systemic   Figure 2-3 comes from Mills and his co-workers (2); it gives a a sequence of waveforms in vivo in a single human male at various locations in the systemic circulation. Similar results have been obtained by other workers, notably Nerem et al., (3) and Clark and Schultz (4). The amount of information that could potentially be generated in experiments of cardiac output and vessel tone is enormous. When one is trying to measure a particular physical quantity (for example the wall shear stress or the relation between velocity waveforms and local pressure waveforms), one is forced to concentrate on a small fraction of the total available information and then work very hard to acheive a consistent physical interpretation of the data obtained. Examples of such careful work are two papers by Ling, Atabek and co-workers (5,6) reporting blood velocity measurements at the aorto-iliac trifurcation in dogs. Their results are applicable to the particular state of cardiac output and muscle tone existing in an anesthetized animal.

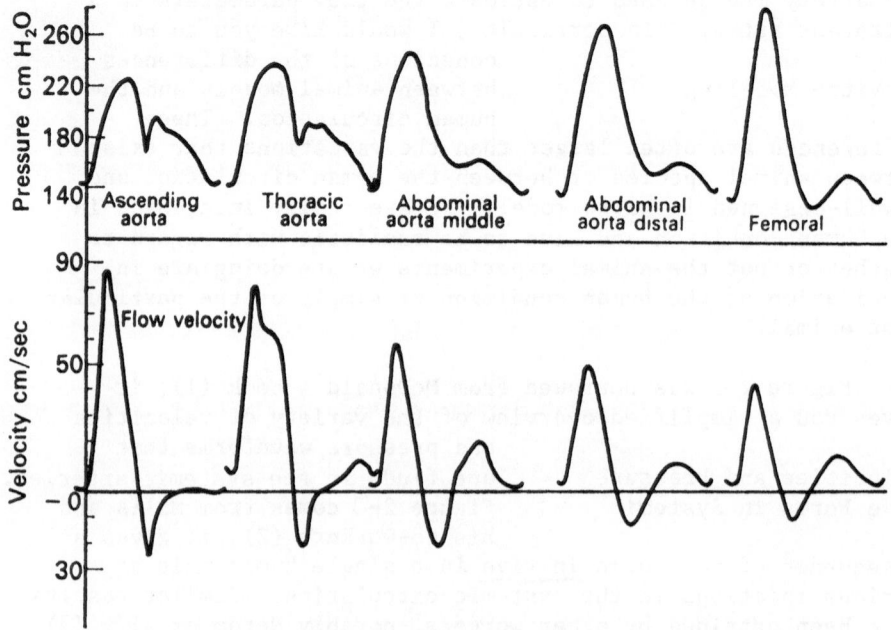

Fig. 2-2: Representative waveforms in the major human
arteries (from McDonald (1) p. 356).

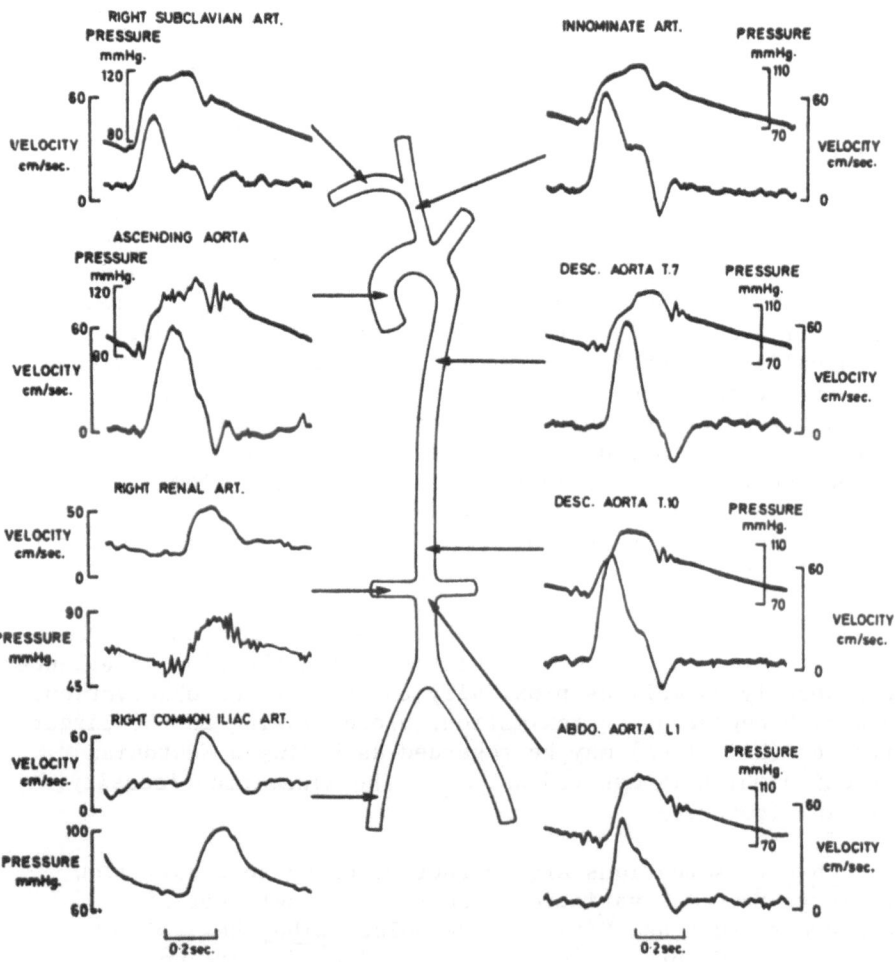

Fig. 2-3: <u>In Vivo</u> pressure and velocity waveforms in a
human male (from Mills et al. (2)).

How do we generalize these results to the aorto-iliac
bifurcation of man, or to different states of cardiac output
and flow division between the distal vessels? The velocity
waveforms in these latter instances will have different
harmonic contents and different ratios between maximum and
minimum flow; there may even be retrograde flow in some
circumstances and not in others. In the ensuing portions of
this presentation, I will attempt to illustrate some simple
methods of fluid dynamic scaling and assess their accuracy.

Many investigators, including Dr. Fry and others attending
this Conference, have suggested that fluid shear stresses
acting on the artery
Estimates of Wall   wall may participate in the
Shear Stress   physical processes which lead to
atherosclerosis. This particular
fluid dynamic parameter has been implicated by in vivo measurements, (7) where very large wall shearing stresses were
chronically or acutely induced and degradation of the arterial
wall structure ensued. The wall shear stress, τ_w , is
simply the force per unit area exerted on the artery surface
by the motion of blood adjacent to the surface. This force
on the endothelium acts in the direction of the flow.

Physiological values of τ_w (dynes/cm ^{2}) are determined
primarily by the time-varying volumetric mean velocity, $\bar{U}$ (t)
(cm/sec), the tube radius R (cm),
In Vivo   and the geometrical and temporal
history which the flow experiences
both locally as well as proximally to the site of observation.
To a high degree of approximation, blood flowing in the larger
arteries (D > 1 cm) may be regarded as having a Newtonian
viscosity which is denoted as μ . The kinematic viscosity,
μ/ρ is ν(cm^2/sec).

In vivo situations are characterized by secondary flow
and large temporal variations, so that a single set of
parameters, such as $\bar{U}$(t), the Reynolds number Re $\equiv \bar{U}D/\nu$,
unsteady, or Womersley, parameter $\alpha \equiv R\sqrt{\omega/\nu}$ are not
sufficient to characterize the local flow dynamics without a
detailed geometrical description of the arterial lumen and a
specification of the flow variation during the cardiac
cycle. Aortic flow is dominated by a primary systolic flow
pulse containing some 60-90% of the total stroke volume;
coronary flow, on the other hand peaks during diastole and
is strongly influenced by myocardial contractility during
systole.

Available evidence (8) (9) (10) suggests that the harmonic
content of coronary flow is at least as high as that of the
major systemic arteries, with significant content in the
first 5 or 6 harmonics of the heart period.

In spite of these regional differences there are many
useful conclusions regarding flow in human arteries that may
be drawn from animal and
Turbulent Flow   laboratory experiments. We
                                       may examine possible velocity
profiles and scaling laws for wall shear stress induced by
flow. We may estimate conditions under which disturbed flow,
including turbulent flow, can be produced. And we can suggest
the effects which flow separation may have on fluid properties
at the endothelial surface.

In arriving at predictions of wall shear in various
human arteries, I would like to begin with two very simple
estimates. The first is steady flow in a long straight tube
(Poiseuille flow) for which

$$\underline{\text{Poiseuille}} \qquad \tau_w = 4\left(\frac{\mu \overline{U}}{R}\right) \ .$$

Here $\overline{U}$ is the volumetric mean velocity (i.e., half the
centerline velocity in Poiseuille flow). This result under-
estimates the shear in regions of reattachment of a separated
flow, on a surface where the adjacent velocity is high
because of a skewing of the velocity profile (i.e., strong
secondary flow), in pulsatile flow, and near the entrance of
a vessel.

A better estimate for oscillating flow (again, a long
tube is assumed) is the Womersley result for flow sinusoidally
modulated at a frequency $f \equiv \omega/2\pi$. The parameter α ,
which is the ratio of the unsteady acceleration of the fluid
to the viscous forces acting on the fluid, is $\alpha \equiv R\sqrt{\omega/\upsilon}$.
If one chooses ω to be equal to 2π times the basic
heart frequency f_H, typical values of α for the major
human arteries range from 3 to 15. A more appropriate value
of α for the strongly-peaked waveforms such as those seen
in the aorta would be based on (approximately) the third
harmonic of the heart frequency, and we shall denote this
value of $\alpha*$ which is equal to $\sqrt{3} \ \alpha$.

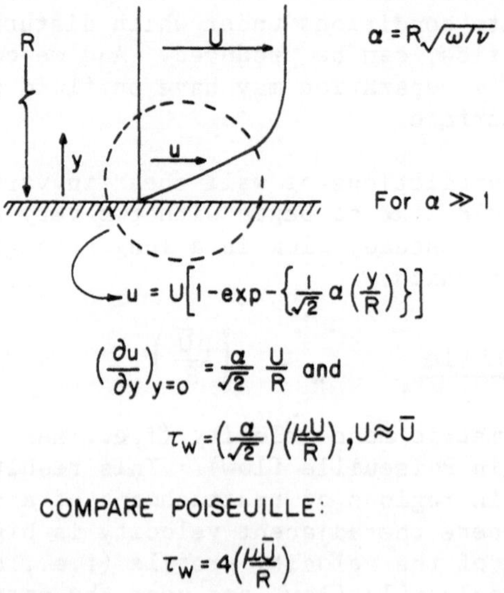
R
U
$\alpha = R\sqrt{\omega/\nu}$
y
u
For $\alpha \gg 1$
$u = U\left[1-\exp-\left\{\frac{1}{\sqrt{2}}\alpha\left(\frac{y}{R}\right)\right\}\right]$
$\left(\frac{\partial u}{\partial y}\right)_{y=o} = \frac{\alpha}{\sqrt{2}}\frac{U}{R}$ and
$\tau_w = \left(\frac{\alpha}{\sqrt{2}}\right)\left(\frac{\mu U}{R}\right), U \approx \bar{U}$
COMPARE POISEUILLE:
$\tau_w = 4\left(\frac{\mu \bar{U}}{R}\right)$

Fig. 2-4: Diagram illustrating the velocity profile near the arterial wall in pulsatile flow.

For large α , the flow near the wall at peak systole is described by the equation shown in Figure 2-4, and the wall shear stress is given by

$$\underline{\text{Womersley}} \qquad \tau_w = \frac{\alpha}{\sqrt{2}} \left(\mu \frac{U}{R} \right) \, .$$

The appropriate value of U to be used in this relation is the volumetric mean velocity. For $\alpha \gg 1$, the Womersley relation predicts a larger shear stress than Poiseuille flow; the numerical factor is $(\alpha/\sqrt{2})$ rather than 4. In the aorta, where values of $\alpha*$ are less than 20, the shear stress in pulsatile flow would exceed the instantaneous value given by Poiseuille flow by a factor less than 5. For the arteries of interest, the coronaries and the carotids, the effects of pulsatility are much less dramatic because, in those arteries, an appropriate value of α is 3 to 10 and Poiseuille flow provides a useful estimate of τ_w . The effects of a distensible arterial wall on the estimated velocity $\overline{U}$ (t) and τ_w, at least at peak flow velocity, can be shown to be on the order of the arterial distensibility, $\Delta R/R$, during the pulse.

Except for the pulmonary artery, this effect is unimportant.

Serious errors would result from applying the Womersley and Poiseuille flow estimates to entrance regions of arteries and to bifurcations. Distal to rapid changes in cross-sectional area or changes in flow direction, strong secondary flows and regions of flow reversal may be produced, yielding wall shears which exceed the previous estimates by factors exceeding 5. Further consideration will be given to these effects shortly.

On the basis of the previous discussion, it is useful to estimate the limits of τ_w which might be encountered in human and animal arteries, and to compare these values with the critical shear stress that was found, by Fry [7] and Carew [11], to produce significant changes in the endothelial surface of dog aortas. This shear stress, approximately 400 dynes/cm ^{2}, has been referred to as a "critical" stress, although subtle endothelial changes were observable at much lower values of shear. Don Fry has commented upon the effects of long-term "sub-critical" shear in previous publications, and his observations are most valuable [11,12].

Typical peak systolic velocities in the aorta of a resting man or dog is about $\bar{U}$ = 100 cm/sec, and in the carotids and femorals it is about $\bar{U}$ = 60 cm/sec.* The radii of these vessels vary substantially, and typicall values are as follows:

RADIUS (cm)

	Aorta	Femoral	Carotid
Man	1.25	0.5	0.4
Dog	0.50	0.3	0.2

For the larger arteries, such as the human aorta, Womersley's estimate yields (assuming μ = 0.04 poise, f_H = 1 Hz, $\bar{U}$ = 100 cm/sec, and α = α*):

$$\tau_w \approx \frac{\alpha_3}{\sqrt{2}} \frac{\mu\bar{U}}{R} \cong 61 \text{ dynes/cm}^2 .$$

For the small arteries, such as the femoral, the flow at peak systole more nearly resembles a Poiseuille velocity profile as you can see in Figure 2-5. Hence the Poiseuille estimate is appropriate:

$$\tau_w \approx 4 \frac{\mu\bar{U}}{R} \cong 19 \text{ dynes/cm}^2 .$$

---

*The estimate of 60 cm/sec for the human carotids and femorals is based on experiments by several authors and summarized by McDonald (1974). This velocity is larger than some ultrasound measurements would suggest. (See, for example, Fronek et al. 13)) as contrasted to the results of Hisland et al. (14) and Fronek et al. (15). The large discrepancy between various ultrasound measurements and previous data (1) remains unresolved.

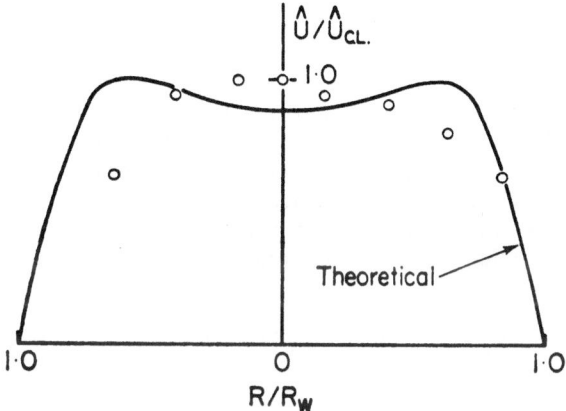

Fig. 2-5: Predicted and measured velocity profiles in the
femoral artery of a man (from Schultz (53)). The solid line
is calculated from Womersley's theory.

Both of these estimates of τ_w are less than the so-
called critical shear stress by a factor of more than 6.
The estimates are for resting subjects, and an increase of a
factor of 2-4 is not unrealistic at peak cardiac output.
(But note that carotid flow remains essentially constant,
irrespective of cardiac output or flow distribution to the
abdominal organs.) And the estimates themselves are most
certainly not accurate to better than a factor of 2. But
taking all of these considerations into account, one is
forced to conclude that the only fluid-mechanical mechanisms
available to increase local shear rates to the "critical"
value suggested by Fry are <u>very</u> strong secondary flows, as
in the vicinity of bifurcations, or in flow profiles modified
by atherosclerotic narrowing or separation phenomena.

DOG   By way of comparing these crude estimates to actual
<u>in vivo</u> data, I'd like to refer to the experiments of S. C.
Ling (5) in which shear stress measurements were made in the
descending aorta of a dog. Although the details <u>o</u>f the
experiment are lacking, we estimate R = 0.5 cm, $\overline{U}$ = 150
cm/sec, υ = 0.04 poise and f_H = 3 Hz. Again, using $\alpha*$ in
place of α for the aorta, the Womersley model gives

$$\tau_w = 160 \text{ dynes/cm}^2 \quad ,$$

which is in fortuitous agreement with the measured shear
stress of 160 dynes/cm^2.

Clearly, the higher linear velocity and heart rate of
these dog experiments by Ling et al. (5) yield shear stresses
                                    which are larger than one
DOG Shear Rates   would expect in humans. These
                                    measurements made with a hot
film probe, bear on an important point and deserve to be
repeated. Perroneau et al. (16) have used Doppler ultrasound
to measure maximum velocity gradients in the aortic arches
of anesthetized and implanted conscious dogs. Peak shear
rates did not exceed values corresponding to τ_w = 10 dynes/cm^2
 Atherosclerosis is observed in the abdominal aorta where
strong secondary flows and flow separation would not be
expected. And yet in some regions where the shear is known
to be high, such as the carina (or flow divider) side of a
bifurcation, the presence of atherosclerosis is not common
(12).

The original in vivo measurements of "critical" stress
by Fry, and the subsequent experimental results of Carew

"Critical" Stress

(11) on excised dogs' aortas,   DOG
were obtained under conditions
producing laminar flow. No
analogous experiments have been performed to determine if an
equivalent "critical" stress exists for human endothelium,
or if the "critical" value is influenced by the presence of
substantial turbulence or other disturbed character of the
flow.

To conclude this discussion of shear stress estimates,
let's return to the major coronary vessels and estimate the

Shear Stress in
Coronary Vessels

shear stresses there. Figure
2-6, taken from Gregg's useful
book (8), illustrates   the type
of flow rate variation one
may expect in the coronaries during the cardiac cycle. Taking
R = 2.5 mm, a peak velocity of 50 cm/sec, and an effective
value of α of 5 (10) we conclude from either the Poiseuille
or Womersley formulas that the wall shear stress is on the
order of 30 dynes/cm ^{3}. This is some 10 times smaller than
the "critical" shear. Even during extreme exercise, critical
values would not be approached. However, in Figure 2-1, you
will recognize that the major coronary arteries twist, turn,
and branch profusely in their course over the myocardium. Clearly,
the peak shear stress will be strongly increased by secondary
flows and may exceed these simple estimates by a substantial
amount.

I want to proceed now to a discussion of flow separation
and secondary flow. Frequently the two effects occur at the

Significance of
Bifurcations

same location, as has been
observed at bifurcations. Because
of the importance which has been
attached to atherosclerosis
occurring near bifurcations, many in vivo and in vitro
experiments have been performed on bifurcation geometries.
Some of the particular experiments which come to mind are
those of Gutstein and Schneck (17), Ferguson and Roach (18),
Attinger (19), Rodkiewicz and Roussell (20), Fuerestein et
(21), Freedman (22), and Ling et al. (5). There are other
data and calculations which will be mentioned later during
the talk. But to fix some of our quantitative ideas, let's
look at Figure 2-7 which contains data from Brech and Bellhouse
(23). The model was a symmetric Y-branch with a 90°
included angle between the two branches and an area increase
from parent vessel to two daughter vessels of 1:1.12.

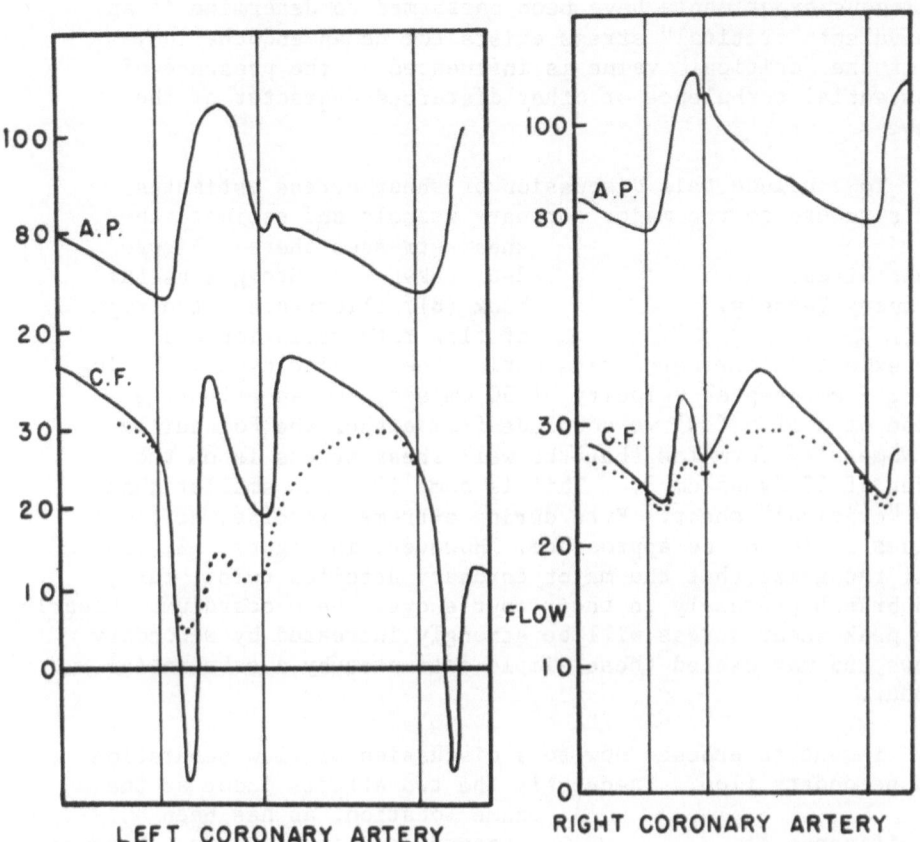

Fig. 2-6: Flow rates in the coronary arteries (from Gregg (8)).
Reconstruction and comparison of typical flow curves obtained with
the orifice meter from the anterior descending branch of the left
coronary artery in a small dog and from the right coronary artery
in a large dog. AP, aortic pressure CF, coronary inflow. Ordi-
nates, upper, mm. Hg; lower, flow in cc. per min. Vertical inter-
cepts demarcate systole and diastole. Dotted lines, predicted
intramural velocity curves.

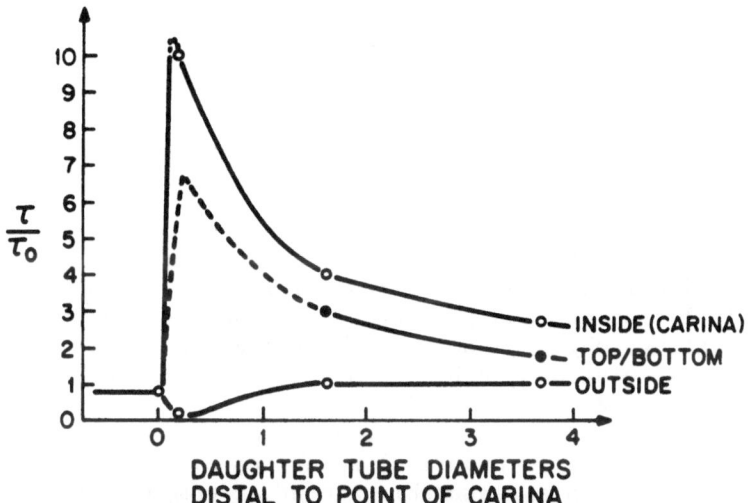

Fig. 2-7: Wall shear stress distribution in a 90° Y- tube
with equal branches (from Brech and Bellhouse (22)). Cross-
sectional area increases (1:1.12) at bifurcation.

The abscissa is distance along the daughter vessel, measured in
daughter diameters, and the ordinate is local wall shear stress
τ normalized to the upstream (parent) shear stress τ_0.

    The shear stress on the flow divider or carina side of this
bifurcation is substantially elevated -- by factors in the
vicinity of 10. On the other hand, on the outside surface of
this region you see a dramatic drop in the wall shear stress,
and studies that have been done with appropriate instrumentation
have actually demonstrated a reverse flow and the shear stress
in the opposite direction from the main flow.

In these bifurcations, we find substantial secondary flows,
portions of the wall that experience very high shear rates
(factors anywhere from three to ten higher than you would
estimate on the basis of a simple undisturbed axial-flow
model), and the potential for separation and substantial
oscillation of the local shear as a function of the cardiac
cycle.

    Let me take a moment to discuss the difficulty of
obtaining results similar to those shown in Figure 2-7 from
a theoretical calculation. In a branching vessel with real
physiological contours and pulsatile flow, you have all of
the complications which a theorist would like to avoid.
Even recent calculations such as those of Kandarpa and
Davids (24) and O'Brien et al. (25) have, of necessity, made
dramatic simplifications of the actual geometry and flow
characteristics to allow numerical solutions of the Navier-
Stokes equations with a reasonable amount of computer time.
To obtain accurate values for velocity profiles and wall
shear, it is necessary to take very closely-spaced grid
points in the numerical calculations, both in space and
time, and also to extend the physical domain covered by the
calculation to include substantial distances both proximal
and distal to the site of interest. These calculation are
very expensive to program and debug, and are also expensive
to run on a computer. An
Reynold's Number   additional limitation of substantial
Calculations   importance is that the calculations
                            become geometrically more difficult
as the Reynolds number $R = 2\bar{U}R/\nu$ increases.   Perhaps
for the coronary arteries where the Reynolds numbers are on
the order of 100-300, such calculations might be constructive.
But for these calculations to be meaningful, the complicated
geometries which we saw in Figure 2-6 would necessitate very
small calculation steps in time.

As an experimentalist, I find in vitro model studies much more exciting and efficient, and an absolute necessity for high Reynolds numbers and complicated geometries. In a sense, you can view in vitro models as analog computers which have substantial flexibility and the important advantage of being able to reproduce turbulence when and if it occurs. The experimentalist must defend his in vitro models against a number of criticisms if he purports his data to be representative of in vivo conditions. Figure 2-6 indicates that coronary artery flow is not in phase with aortic pressure, and a substantial contribution to this behavior is the change in coronary artery cross-section caused by contraction of the myocardium. A laboratory model with rigid walls will not model this situation.

But available evidence indicates that the carotid and aorto-iliac bifurcations do not change shape appreciably during the cardiac cycle, and rigid models should be reasonably accurate representations of in vivo conditions. Theoretical calculations (and I include here dimensional analysis) are invaluable in estimating the quantitative values of the parameters to be measured, in assessing potential systematic experimental errors (including the effects of unsteady flow and wall distension), and in scaling experimental results to conditions that differ from those used to obtain the experimental data.

Let's return to Figure 2-7 to examine the details of the flow in bifurcations and the complicated patterns which arise in realistic geometries. For purposes of our discussion I'm going to limit my presentation to in vitro data obtained in our laboratory by Scott Smith (26), even though a number of the phenomena he observed have been described by previous authors (17, 18, 20, 21, 23, 27, 28, 29, 30).

First, let me describe the experimental techniques which were used. Figures 2-8 and 2-9 show, respectively, the overall experimental arrangement and cross-section of the glass model bifurcation which was used. The experimental protocol is as follows: first, the flow is clamped off and a fluorescent dye is injected into the model and mixed with the working fluid. A laser beam is spread out into a thin sheet of light by a cylindrical lens and passed through the center of the model so that the laser-induced dye fluorescence, as seen from above, gives a clear cross-section of the model (31).

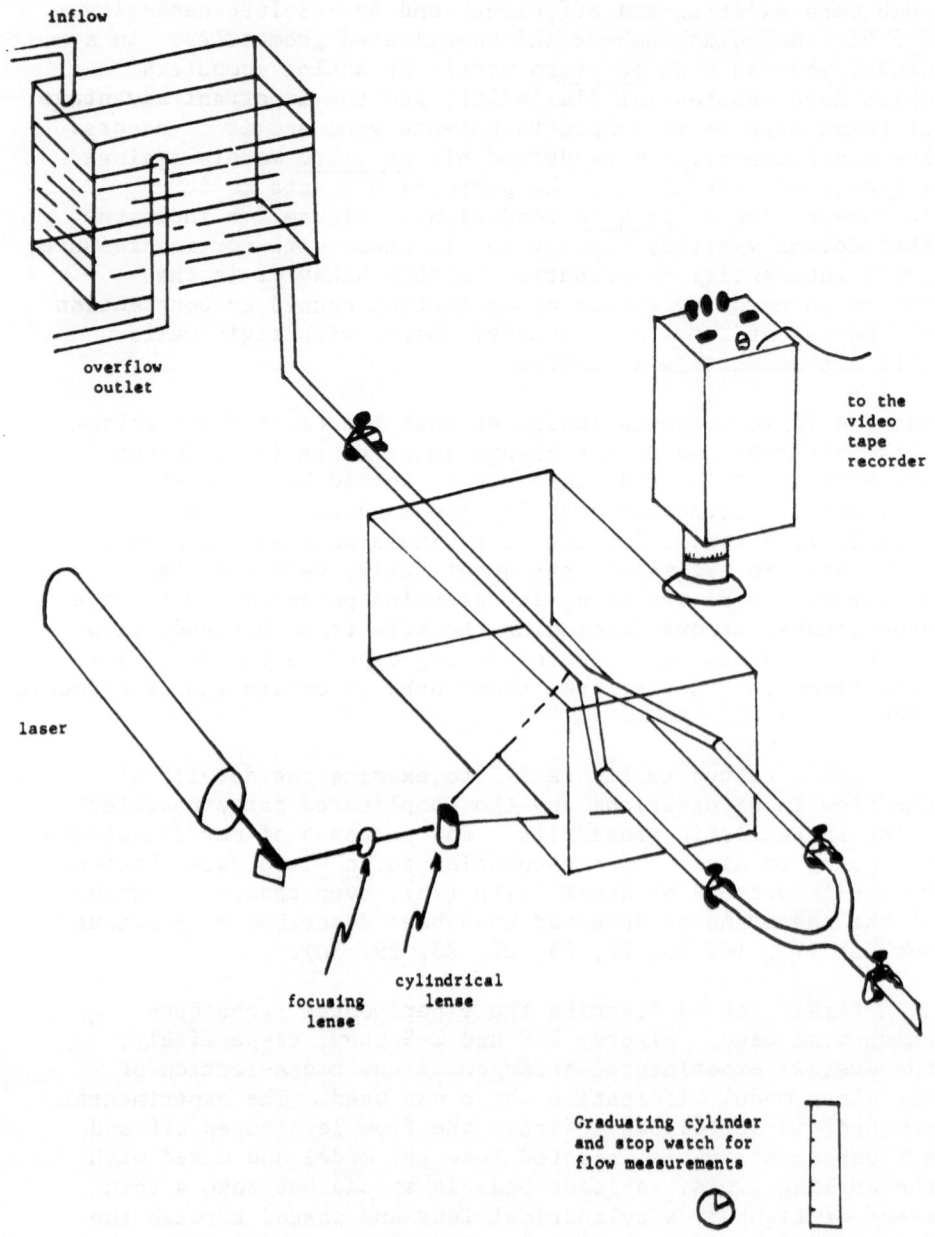

inflow

overflow
outlet

to the
video
tape
recorder

laser

focusing
lense

cylindrical
lense

Graduating cylinder
and stop watch for
flow measurements

Fig. 2-8: Facility for laser fluorescence visualization of
flow in a model carotid bifurcation (Smith (25)).

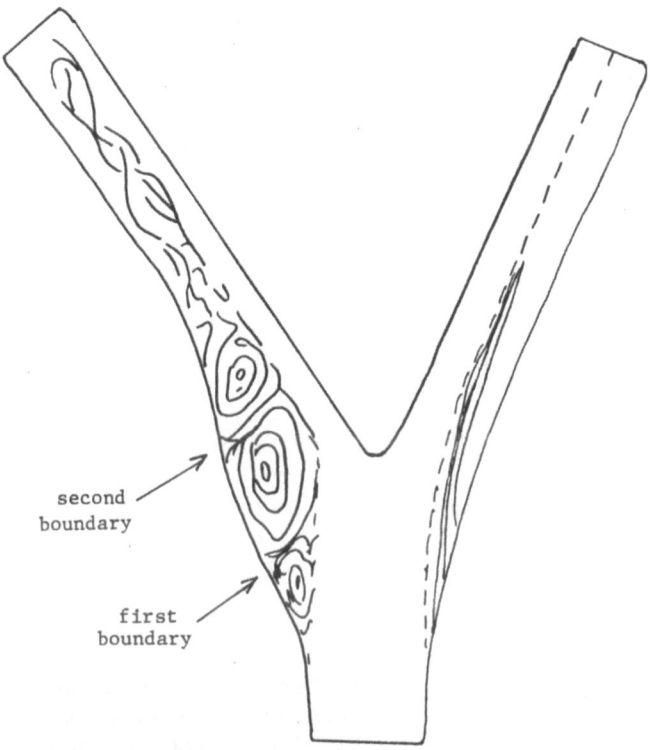

Fig. 2-9: Outline drawing of the glass model bifurcation,
illustrating the observed secondary flow patterns (Smith (25)).

Now we start the flow; as fresh fluid enters the model,
the fluid containing fluorescent dye is washed out, first
in the regions where the velocity
Steady Flow   is highest and later in regions
where the velocity is low. So
in the first instant, what one sees is essentially equivalent
to a cross-section of the model artery just as one would
obtain with an x-ray angiogram (32) and as the flow continues
streaks of dye will be formed which will move with the fluid
and describe the complicated motions across the entire
vessel section. The flow pictures in the next 5 figures
were taken with a camera photographing the plane of fluorescence
from above, although we have also used a TV camera to record
the flow with excellent results.

Figures 2-10a, 2-10b, 2-10c, and 10d, in chronological
order, show how the flow starts from rest and washes out the
dye. The first is with no flow. We now start the fluid
motion; the Reynolds number is 1000, characteristic
of peak systolic flow in the carotids, and the flow branching
ratio at the bifurcation is ($Q_{external}/Q_{internal} = 1.3$,
which is the physiological ratio for an undiseased artery.
By the time the fluid has moved 10 or so diameters along the
artery, the flow field has settled down to a quasi-steady
state and subsequent motion of the dyed fluid presents a
very useful picture of the dynamics of the fluid motion.

In Figure 2-11, we have another picture at Re = 1000
and $Q_E/Q_I = 1.3$, selected to most clearly illustrate the
complicated patterns we see.
Separation of Flow   There are several features
that I want you to focus on.
First, separation occurs on the outise of both branches, not
just the internal carotid branch. The second remarkable
feature is that the separation regions extend a long way
down the daughter vessels, which was indeed a surprise to us
when we first observed this. A third feature, which was
anticipated from the detailed velocity profiles obtained by
Brech and Bellhouse (23), is the very high-velocity flow on
the carina (bifurcation) side of each branch. The dye is
very rapidly washed away from this region, and the resulting
shear stresses are extremely high as we observed in the
previous Figure 2-7.

Our conclusion from these preliminary studies (and I
want to emphasize that much work remains to be done) is that
the detailed geometry, branching ratio, and Reynolds number
are very important to the local shear stresses along the
external sides of the bifurcation in both branches.

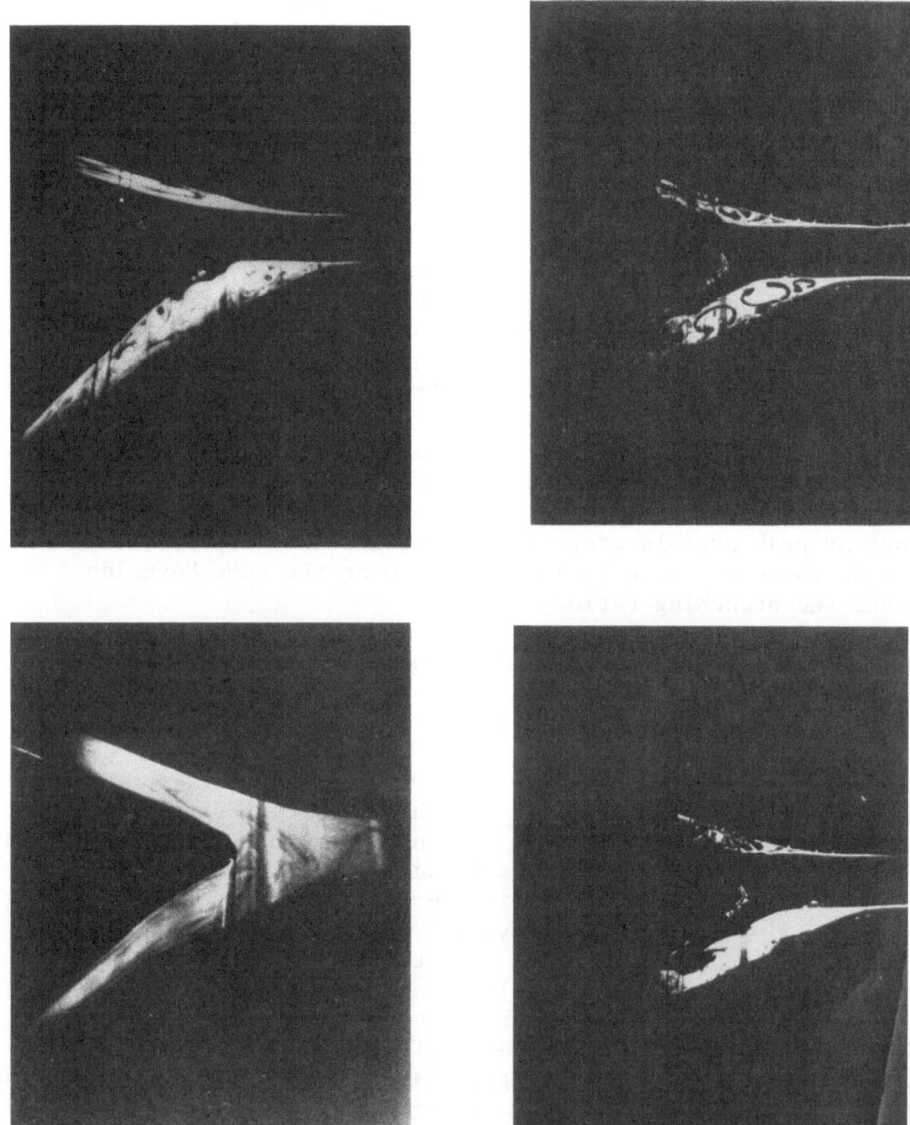

Fig. 2-10: A sequence of laser fluorescence pictures showing
washout of dyed fluid in the carotid bifurcation model
(Smith (25)).

I emphasize particularly the geometry because the complicated vorticity pattern you see in the carotid sinus (in Figure 2-11) would be entirely different, both qualitatively and quantitatively, if we had a straight tube without a sinus.

Now all of the fluorescence pictures I've shown you so far have been for steady flow. Scott Smith (26) a preliminary study of the vorticity patterns in the sinus with a pulsatile flow. The technique was to use

Pulsatile Flow

a peristaltic pump instead of a constant-head gravity feed as the flow source. The temporal waveform was far from physiological for the carotids (it looked, in fact, more like the coronary waveforms we saw earlier in Figure 2-6, but the qualitative results are interesting nonetheless).

Without going into a lot of detail, Scott's conclusion was that the flow near peak systole was quasi-steady; by that, I mean that the vorticity patterns in the carotid sinus at peak systole are, for all intents and purposes, the same as those one sees in a steady flow at the same Reynolds number and branching ratio.

DR: WEINBAUM: Let me understand your use of the term "unsteady" here. The whole experiment is based on a transient effect, and you have used the term quasi-steady in two different contexts.

DR. DEWEY: I apologize if this has been confusing. When the flow starts from rest and instantaneously rises to a steady value, this produces in the first instant, a starting vortex phenomenon which rapidly

Steady vs. Unsteady Flow

washes downstream. It is analogous to the old aerodynamics problem where an airplane accelerating off the runway leaves behind a trailing vortex but very rapidly this vortex becomes unimportant to the steady lift on the plane. The flow field in the vicinity of the plane is then considered steady. By analogy, after the starting vortex has passed through the model artery, the remaining dye is set into motion in a manner which, for steady inlet flow, persists in time. Eventually, the dyed fluid washes out and is replaced by undyed fluid, but the detailed fluid motion persists and is unchanging in time. Even though the experimental technique is based on a transient phenomenon, the flow patterns are essentially steady, hence the use of the term quasi-steady.

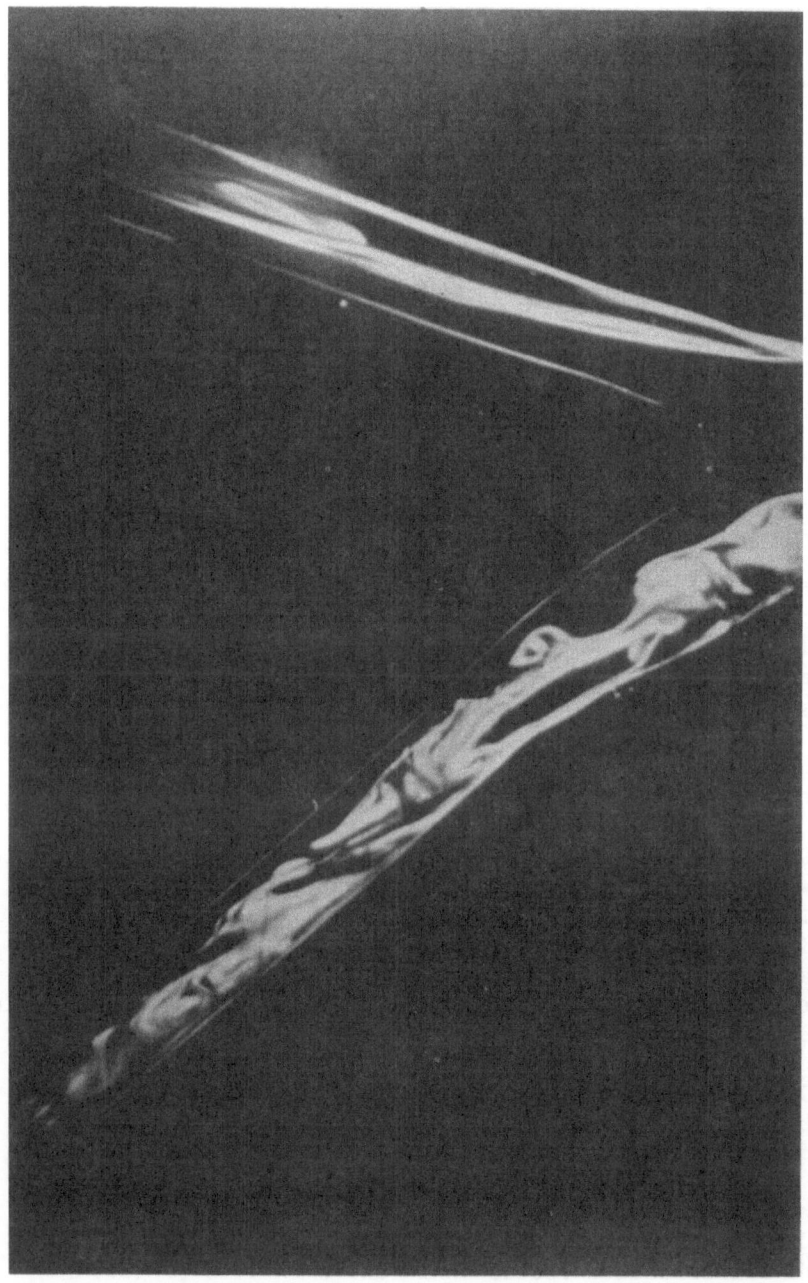

Fig. 2-11: Flow in the model carotid bifurcation at a proximal Reynolds number of 1000 and a branching ratio ($Q_{external}/Q_{internal}$) of 1.3 (Smith (25)).

     With cyclic unsteady inlet flow, the fluid motions
within the model artery go through cyclic variations. The
detailed flow field at any instant depends on the instantaneous
value of volumetric flow as well as the previous time history
of the fluid oscillation. The term quasi-steady in this
instance refers to the fact that the instantaneous flow
patterns quantitatively resemble a steady flow with the same
volumetric flow existing at that instant. We observe this
quasi-steady behavior near peak systole in our models of
bifurcations, as well as our models of stenosed arteries:

     DR. COLTON: Dr. Dewey, isn't the tracer dye subject
to dispersion with time, so that the dye doesn't really
follow the fluid streamlines?

     DR. DEWEY: That's correct. The saving grace is that
the dye molecular weight is large, on the order of 500, and
diffuses across streamlines only very slowly.

In a steady separated region, for example, some small diffusion
takes place from the flow within the cavity to the external
fluid, and the dye concentration decreases with time. But
this process is quite slow; and, furthermore, we can follow
the dye patterns over several decades of concentration.

     DR. CARO: You haven't told us what the waveform was
for the unsteady tests.

     DR. DEWEY: The unsteady flow was created by a peristaltic
pump which produced flow rate variations ranging between 0.5
and 1.5 of the mean during each cycle. The detailed waveform
contained significant harmonics up to about the third. But
the waveform was not modeled after the human circulation and
so these tests were only suggestive of the unsteady contribution
to flow dynamics.

     DR. CARO: Why I raised the question was because two
possibly relevant studies have been undertaken: One is by
Howard Lyne (33) and the other is by Peter Blennerhasset
(34) which may still be in thesis form. Howard Lyne looked
at the secondary flow due to sinusoidal oscillations in a
curved pipe and found essentially that this is directed
inwards rather than outwards as in the work of Dean (35)
with steady flow. Blennerhasset studied the secondary flows
due to a combination of steady and non-steady pressure
gradients.

     DR. COLTON: Our experiments show very clearly separation
in the internal carotid as you go around the bend.

DR. DEWEY: In all of the steady-flow models of bifurcations which we have studied, separation occurs on the outside of the branch just distal to the bifurcation. All of the high Reynolds number numerical calculations I have seen support this view.

DR. CARO: In fact a very crude experiment was done. Lyne injected a dye stream and under appropriate conditions found the secondary flow to be directed inwards, i.e., towards the inner wall of curvature of the tube.

DR. DEWEY: I think it's clear that we need more definitive data to resolve some of these questions. And it is especially imperative that the geometry of the bifurcation or branch or aortic arch be modeled accurately.

But let me return to a review of the phenomena we have observed in our model studies, because there is still one important point I want to make.

Let's get back to Figure 2-11 which illustrates the flow patterns we see when the ratio of flows in the external and internal carotids is 1.3. We're now going to decrease the branching ratio to 0.73 and then again to 0.40, simulating what would happen with substantial obstruction of the external carotid.

Figure 2-12 is for branching ratio of 0.73, and you can see that the flow patterns have changed dramatically. With the largest amount of flow going through the external carotid, we saw very little detailed vorticity in the external branch. The flow hugged the carina side of the tube but the streamlines emanating from the point of separation at the junction were smooth and laminar. Now we see substantial vortex shedding and vortex formation at the mouth of the vessel. We even notice that some of these disturbances propagate upstream and lift dye filaments off the proximal tube wall.

Flow Patterns with Simulated Obstruction

Figure 2-13 indicates where the external flow has been further reduced, the branching ratio being 0.4. The unsteady disturbances produced near the mouth of the external branch are so strong that they seriously affect the flow patterns in the internal branch.

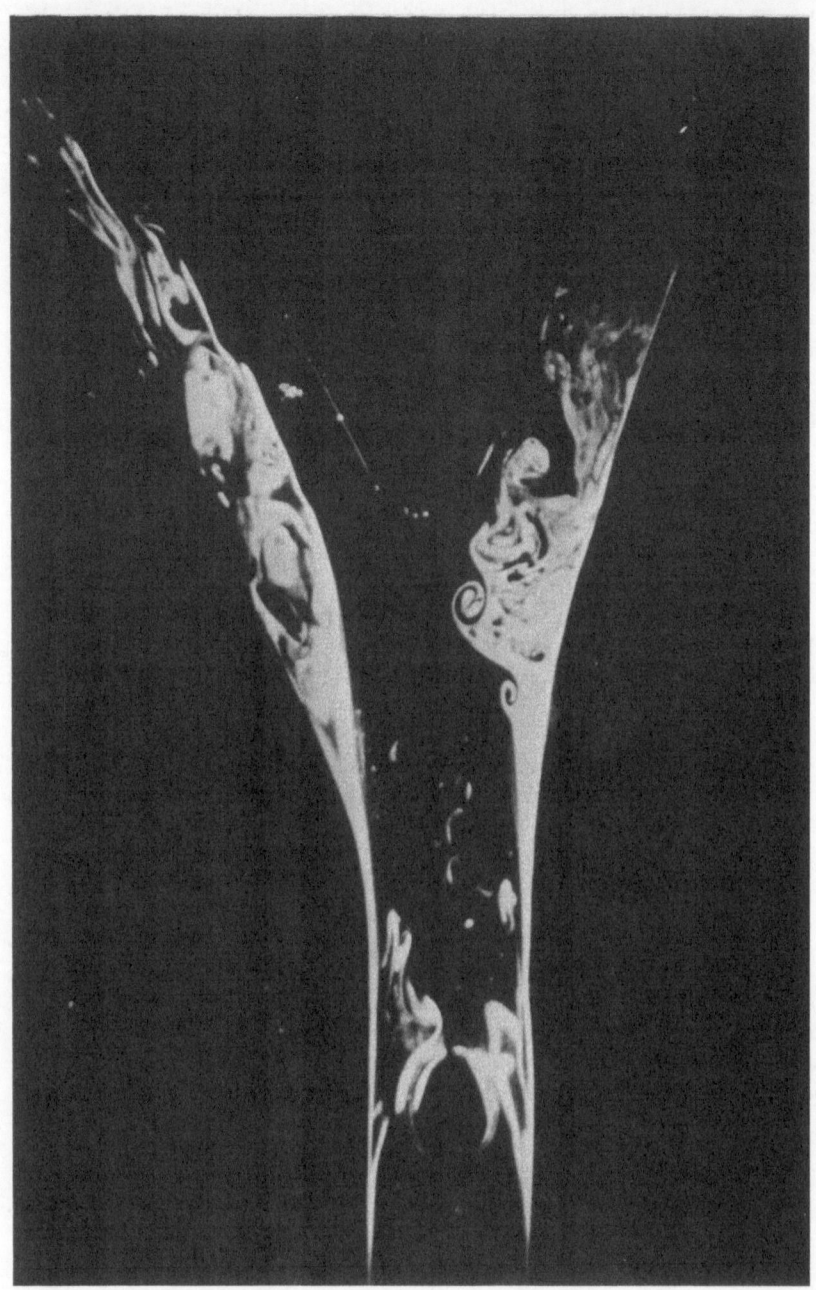

Fig. 2-12: Carotid flow as in Fig. 2-11, but with a
branching ratio of 0.73.

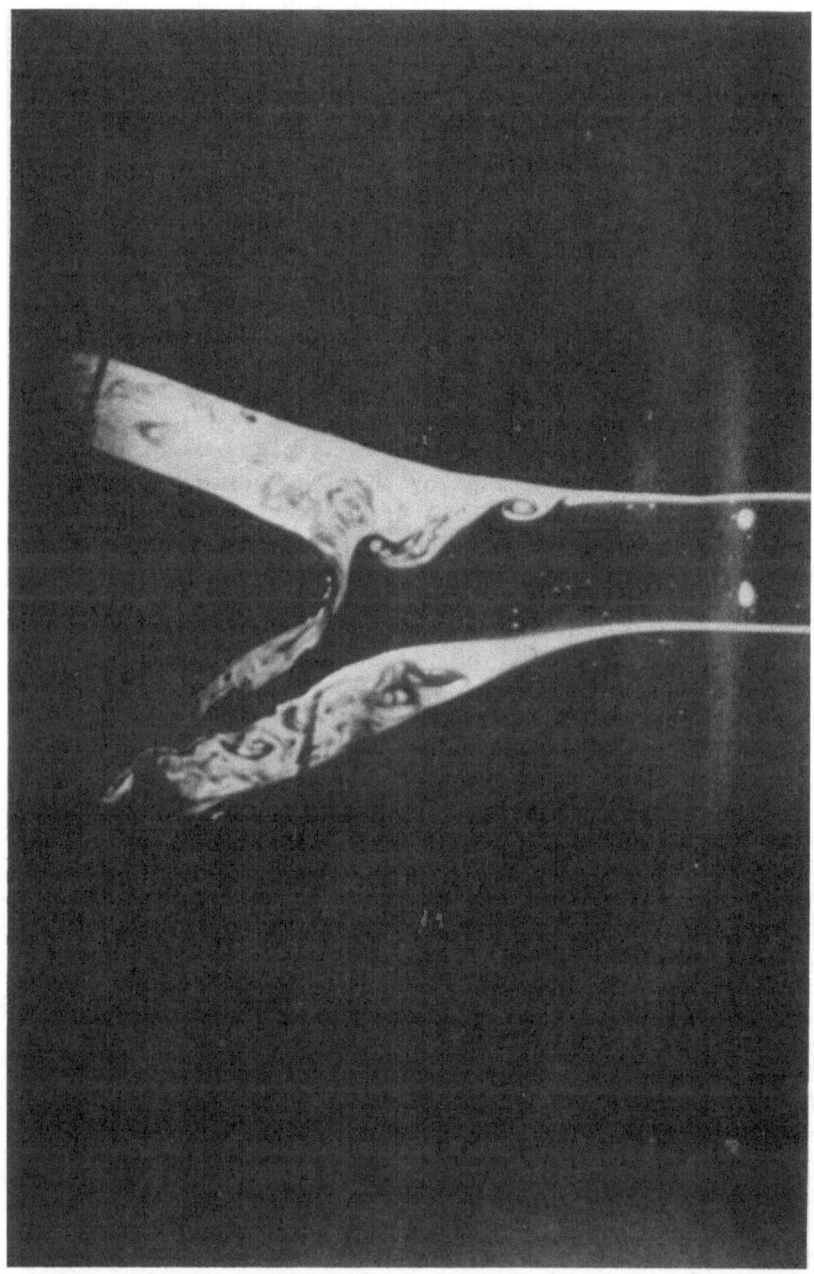

Fig. 2-13: Carotid flow as in Fig. 2-11, but with a branching
ratio of 0.4.

In this figure, we even see what appears to be a small
separation bubble on the carina side of the internal branch,
with a high-velocity jet-like flow near the carina side of
the lumen and adjacent to this region of separation. A
large separation region persists in the sinus of the internal
branch, and the overall sinus flow pattern resembles that
found at equivalent internal branch velocities but with
physiological branching ratios.

These florescence pictures dramatize what I believe to
be a most important parameter in characterizing flows through
physiologically-dimensional
Scale of Vorticity   vessels: that is the scale
of vorticity. In several of the
figures, you saw vorticities whose dimensions were some
substantial fraction of the vessel diameter. This is what I
would call large-scale vorticity. Many authors such as Dr.
Nerem, have referred to these patterns as disturbed flow,
and I think that their terminology is also very appropriate.
It is <u>not</u> turbulence in the ordinary sense because the
small-scale vorticity and accompanying high-frequency fluctuations
in wall pressure and wall shear are absent.

The presence of large-scale vorticity in the carotid
sinus is very evident in all of the measurements which O'Brien
Erlich and Friedman (25) have made. They observed that as
the flow velocity was increased and decreased, either with a
slow variation or with the unsteady waveforms produced by
the peristaltic pump, the large-scale vortex pattern in the
sinus expanded and contracted. So if I were an endothelial
cell sitting on the surface of the carotid sinus, I would
see first flow in one direction and then, as the vorticities
within the sinus expanded and contracted, flow in the other
direction, scrubbing first in one direction and then in the
other during the cardiac cycle.

We have no idea what this oscillatory shear stress does to
the endothelium.

In this connection, it is interesting to note that we
have examined some 200 x-ray angiograms of atherosclerotic
carotid bifurcations in
Atherosclerotic Carotid   connection with our work on
phanoangiography (36) and in a
substantial majority of these cases we find the focal point
of lesions to be in the sinus area. The plaques build up from
the external sinus wall toward the interior lumen.

In many advanced cases, the only open area is a small orifice
on the carina side located where we observe high-velocity
flow in models of the patent artery. I think it is provocative
that the carina side, the region of very high shear stress,
is spared whereas the sinus area, which contains large-scale
vorticities which scrub back and forth during each heartbeat,
exhibits a propensity for lesion formation.

Let me digress for a moment to discuss a method we have
developed for modeling unsteady flows. Figure 2-14a is a
photograph of our pulsatile
flow source which we have used
for several investigations (37).
Our objective was to develop a
system which could be programmed to deliver flow pulses containing
up to 8 harmonics of the fundamental period and could be
easily reset to any desired Reynolds number and waveform.
The system contains a 16-segment diode function generator to
provide the programmed waveform. The resulting electrical
signal drives a servo-controlled piston which delivers a
pulsatile flow component; this is superimposed on a steady
flow to achieve the desired waveform. Figure 2-14b, you see
that the results are quite good; we can simulate all types
of waveforms, all the way from aortic flows to coronary
flows.

**Method for Modeling
Unsteady Flow**

There are two final topics which I wish to cover briefly
before concluding the formal portion of my remarks. The
first has to do with flow instabilities which may lead to
disturbed flow and turbulence; and the second deals with the
effects of arterial stretch.

I mentioned previously that we must be careful to
distinguish between highly-disturbed flows, with discrete
large-scale vorticity, and
turbulence, which exhibits a
wide frequency spectrum. One
question many of you may ask is, "what causes the instabilities
which lead to these disturbed conditions?"

Highly Disturbed Flows

One very common source of large-scale vorticity in the
cardiovascular system is curvature of the axis of the vessels
as, for example, in the aortic
arch. A centrifugal force is
generated when the flow goes
around a bend and one expects the
velocity to be highest on the
inside of the bend, with secondary flow around the circumference
from the outside to the inside.

**Curvature of Axis of
Vessels. A Source of
Vorticity**

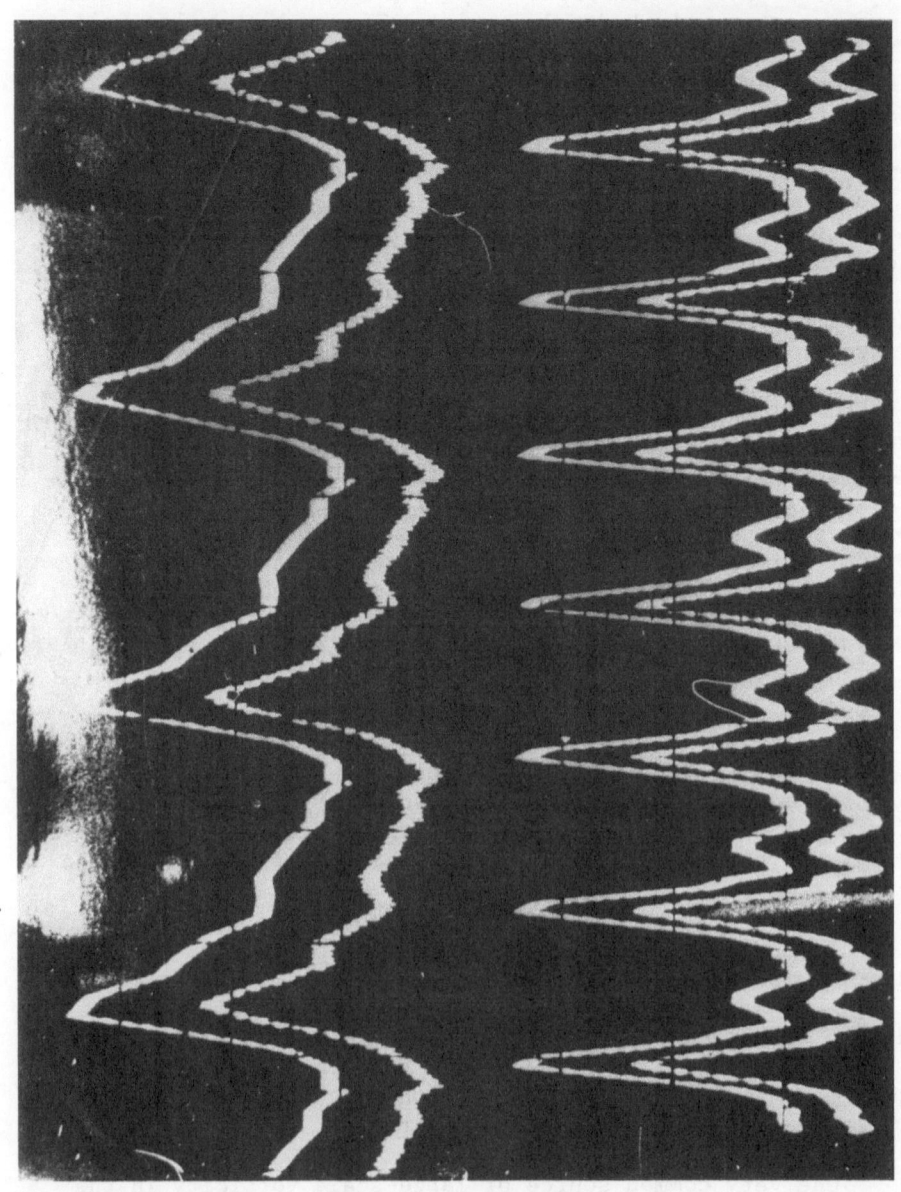

a.   b.

Fig. 2-14a & 14b: Pulsatile flow system (Pitts and Dewey (54)).
    a. Photograph of system
    b. Oscilloscope record of command signal (upper trace)
        and instantaneous test section flow rate (lower trace).

Dye tracer studies, such as those of Stehbens (27) and
Brech and Bellhouse (23) show that at the bifurcations, this
pattern is more complicated; helical motion is set up which
transports fluid from the carina side (internal side) of the
bifurcation to the external side along the circumference, with
a return flow from outside to inside along the mid-plane.
Thus, a double helix pattern of secondary flow is established.
This secondary flow can become unstable with appropriate
geometric and temporal perturbations, and can break down
into highly-disturbed and even turbulent motion.

And Lowell Stone has some data which suggest that vessels in
the heart and brain can change dramatically in caliber on the
basis of both nervous and
pharmacological stimulus. So
again we have a very important
coupling between the arterial
mechanics and the fluid flow:
endothelial response to fluid stresses may depend strongly
upon the state of arterial stretch.

**Endothelial Response to
Fluid Stress Depends on
State of Arterial Stretch**

Dr. Cox will present data on arterial properties, the
numbers you see on Figure 2-15 are simply a small representation
of the data which are available in the literature. This table,
compiled from citations in McDonald's book, (1) lists the
changes in radius which one would expect in several major   DOG
arteries during the cardiac cycle for humans and for dogs and
cats. The column labeled Δ R/R (calc.) is the percentage   CAT
change in radius one would calculate from elastic moduli,
arterial radii, and systolic-diastolic pressure changes which
have been reported in the literature. The predications are
in reasonable agreement with those measurements which have
been made.

From these data, there are two conclusions one can draw,
and I invite your comments on them. The first is that there
are very substantial differences between the distensibility of
human arteries and those of common test animals upon which we
lavish so much experimental attention.

    DR. WOLF: All animals are not alike!

    DR. DEWEY: Precisely. If you take the human carotid and
the dog carotid artery, for example, the value of ΔR/R for the   DOG
human artery is 17% whereas it is only 4.5% for the dog.

Vessel		Static E_p ($\times 10^{-6}$) (dynes/cm²)	Resting ΔP (mm Hg)	$\left(\dfrac{\Delta R}{R}\right) \times 100$	
				Calc	Expt'l
Human	Carotid	0.4	50	17	14.3
Dog	"	2.0	67	4.5	—
Human	Asc. Aorta	0.47	45	11.3	12.0
Dog	" "	0.8	40	7.5	5.0
Cat	" "	—	—	—	18.5
Dog	Femoral	3	90	4	
Human	Pulmonary	—	20		64

NOTE: τ_w SHOULD BE SIMILAR IN THE PULMONARY ARTERY
AND THE AORTA.

Fig. 2-15: A table of arterial distensibilities compiled from data in McDonald (1).

Be very cautious in Inferences Regarding Human Atherosclerosis from Results of Animal Tests

What I would conclude from this is that, if arterial stretch is really important in determining trans-endothelial flux into the artery, then there is a factor of about 3 or 4 differences between the experimental animal you are testing and the human situation you are really interested in. If a facotr of 3 or 4 is important, then you better be very cautious about what you infer about human atherosclerosis from the results of animal tests.

There appear to be less dramatic differences between the dog and human descending aorta. But the only piece of data I have been able to find on the pulmonary artery, quoted in McDonald's book, is quite dramatic. This experiment, based on serial x-ray angiograms, concludes that $\Delta R/R$ is 64% for this vessel. This occurs in spite of the fact that the internal pressure change between systole and diastole is half that in the systematic circulation. If one takes the flow rates and vessel diameters of the aorta and pulmonary artery, you estimate that the wall shear stresses in the two vessels are quite comparable, give or take a factor of 2.

DOG

Yet the pulmonary artery does not exhibit atherosclerosis.

DR. MANSFIELD: We do find arteriosclerosis in the pulmonary arteries of patients with pulmonary vascular hypertension.

DR. DEWEY: That implies that it is not only the delta P but also the absolute value of the internal pressure which is important.

DR. CARO: There could of course be quite different explanations. For example it might be that thrombosis has a more important role in the development of atherosclerosis in the pulmonary system than in the systemic arterial system.

DR. MANSFIELD: Yes, but you see arteriosclerotic disease in the major branches of the pulmonary vessel under circumstances of high pulmonary flow (such as left to right intra cardiac shunts) with only modest elevations in pulmonary artery pressures.

DR. CARO: Well another difference is, of course, that in the presence of pulmonary hypertension the pulmonary artery is stretched, and if the cardiac output is unchanged the mean wall shear stress will be reduced. Some of us have suggested that that would favor the development of atheroma.

DR. DEWEY: One of the things I want to suggest here is that wall stretch and shear stress are both important to the properties of the endothelial layer and the uptake of labeled materials. In the pulmonary arteries under normal circumstances there is approximately the same shear as in the aorta; there is also an enormous amount of stretch, but no disease.

Approximately same Shear Pulmondary Arteries as in Aorta

I have a number of additional comments concerning uptake and transport, as well as further remarks to make concerning the character of vascular turbulence and the importance of proper scaling in experiments. I think I will save those for Dr. Nerem when he presents some of his information on Wednesday morning.

To conclude, let me identify several specific examples of arterial fluid dynamics which are of particular interest for future research. The first is suggested by an experiment performed by Flaherty et al. (38) in which they produced arterio-venous shunts both in the carotids and the iliac arteries of the dogs. They found that substantial disease developed in the iliacs but not in the carotids. Yet the shear stresses produced in the two regions were very similar and, in both instances, were factors of 8-10 below the so-called critical shear stress. I have reread this paper several times, and each time I find the results to be most provocative. An adequate explanation of this experiment, and perhaps additional confirmatory data, would be a very important contribution to our understanding of endothelial integrity.

Examples of Arterial Fluid Dynamics for Future Research

Several times in this meeting we have touched upon the topic of arterial distensibility and its potential importance to the properties of the endothelium. Let me reiterate a statement by Dr. Kenyon this morning: when the coronary arteries pass underneath bridges of myocardial tissue they are free from disease; but both proximal and distal to the bridges, one can find substantial atherosclerotic deposits.

The minute the artery dives underneath the myocardium and is
supported on both sides, there is no disease. I find this
to be another very provocative result. One may speculate
about wall vibrations and the lack of damping, or possibly a
dramatic change in distensibility between the tethered and
untethered artery. If Professor Stehbens were here, I'm
sure he would have addressed this subject. I don't have the
answer to this problem; but inasmuch as the coronaries and
carotids are our preeminent targets, these facts demand
attention.

There are, of course, many more questions which we
would like to have answered. We need additional data on the
scale and the power and
spectral density of unsteady and
turbulent vascular flows. In
particular, we need to determine
the effects of unsteady shear
stress on endothelial integrity.

**Unsteady and Turbulent
Vascular Flows and Effects
Unsteady Shear Stress
on Endothelial Integrity**

We are beginning a series of experiments in this direction in
the Fluid Mechanics Laboratory at MIT. At present, there
are only two important experiments--one by Fry (7) and the
other by Carew (11) upon which all of our concepts of "critical
shear" are based. All of our speculations about what happens
to the endothelial cell under stress are based on these two
sets of data. The implications of this concept are sufficiently
powerful to motivate much additional research in this area.

DR. MALLIANI: Do you think that important differences
may exist between your experimental preparation and a normal
in vivo situation where the elastic vessels undergo relevant
movements?

DR. DEWEY: I would like to answer that in two different
ways. Basically it means are you going to sit on an erythrocyte
and move through the fluid and
try to figure out things that are
going on in the fluid side, that

Importance of Tethering

is one answer. And the second one is if you are sitting on an
endothelial cell in the wall, you want to understand what is
going to happen to you. From the point of view of understanding
fluid mechanics it is not, in my opinion, essential that the
wall move. If you go through any reasonable estimate of
secondary flows and so forth, the maximum extent of the
secondary flow is roughly on the order of magnitude of
delta R over R, in fact it is usually substantially less.

What this means is that if you are talking about shear
stress on the wall, for example, trying to estimate what
shear stress exists in the carotid bifurcation, you can do
an experiment in vitro with a solid wall and expect to get a
number which is clinically significant in terms of predicting
what it would be in vivo. On the other hand, the response
of the endothelial cell can vary dramatically if the wall is
tethered or untethered. For example, in the external carotid
artery and probably the coronary which are free on the
outside, tethering is all important.

DR. SMITH: I would just like to present one figure
that seems to be relevant both to Dr. Dewey's last figure
and to Dr. Schwartz's first
group of figures. This is some
Developing Arteries   work from the Chicago group (39)
Before and After Birth   who looked at the developing
RABBIT arteries in young rabbits and examined the ascending aorta and
adjacent-pulmonary artery segment before birth and during
the period after birth. In the neonatal period these are,
of course, joined at the ductus arteriosus and they are both
at the same pressure and in the rabbit they are similar in
size and structure. The ductus closes over the first two
months after birth, and the pressure in the ascending aorta
rises from about 30 mm up to about 90 mm of mercury whereas
the pressure in the pulmonary trunk falls from about 30 to
15 mm. There was, of course, rapid growth; DNA and the
number of cells in the segments increased greatly and at the
same rate in both vessels, but the ratios of collagen to DNA
and of elastin to DNA, showed marked changes as in Figure 2-16.
In the ascending aorta, the elastin to DNA ratio increased
ten fold, whereas in the pulmonary artery it remained almost
constant and again for collagen there was a ten fold increase
in aorta and for the pulmonary artery it remained almost
constant. Either the pressure or the stretch is having an
enormous influence on connective tissue production and
obviously on the whole rheological properties of the vessels.

DR. NEREM: I believe your flow visualization studies
are particularly useful to this group because too often when
physiologists hear fluid
Flow Visualization Studies   mechanics people talk, they
actually think that we know what
is going on. When you look at those flow visualization studies,
you realize that we have a long way to go in our understanding.

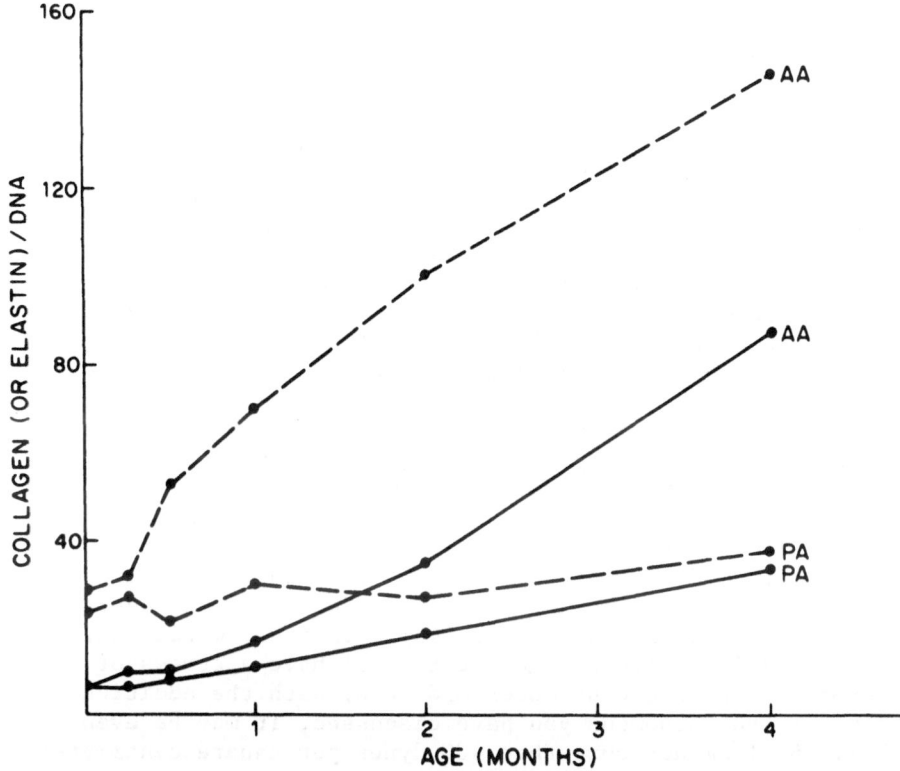

Fig. 2-16: (Smith) The ratio of collagen/DNA and elastin/DNA in ascending aorta (AA) and pulmonary artery (PA). Collagen (———) and elastin (------) contents of rabbit arteries during early growth. (From Leung et al., ref. Reproduced by permission of Academic Press.)

As you know, we have been doing some studies on the coronary
system and we don't have quite as vivid pictures to show,
but we feel the complexities there are similar. One of the
things that complicates the coronary system, forgetting
about your first figure, if one wants to take a simple
minded view of the extramural vessels, is the fact that the
major coronary bifurcations are essentially in a plane which
is in itself curving as the vessels move distally over the
heart. You have the curve of the bifurcation together with
the curve of the entire plane turning as they move around
the heart, thus the secondary flows have to be extremely
complex and important to what is going on. I did want to
come back to the question of shear stress in the arterial
system. You mentioned Peronneau's data which he reported at
our Ohio State meeting (16). In fact, from his numbers for
shear rate, one does compute a shear stress of 10 dynes per
square centimeter. However, I find it hard to place much
faith in a shear stress which is deduced from a velocity
profile. As a fluid mechanics person, I have had little
success in the past trying to make that kind of an estimate.

I would rather turn to the type of analysis of Ling and his
co-workers (40,41). They have developed a mathematical
model into which experimental waveform and pressure information
is entered; the details of the flow are then calculated.
Pedley (42) has carried out a similar type of calculation
for the aorta and both of those give values which are more
in line with the measurement, albeit crude, that was reported
in the 1968 paper of Ling et al. (43). In other words, without
other mitigating factors, one might still have a stress of
100 dynes per square centimeter and then, with the addition
of some of the phenomena you have discussed, it may be even
higher. So I am not sure that 400 dynes per square centimeter
is out of the question in some locations. Furthermore, and
I am sure Dr. Fry will agree, these critical values that are
often quoted could be considerably altered by various biochemical
influences that might affect the endothelial cells.

        DR. DEWEY: To respond to the last statement first. I
emphasize first of all I could not agree with you more that
                              the "critical" shear stress is
Critical Shear Stress   simply a suggestion of the level
                              at which substantial rapid changes
take place. They are quantifiable in some systematic statistical
way.

There are potentially other things that happen at lower
shear levels which, over a long period of time, may be
equally as important to the survival of the vasculature as
we know it in a young person. But in addition to that I find
it interesting that the critical shear stress is available
only for dog aortic endothelium and not for man, or for   DOG
other arteries. In view of the other differences between
the animal models and human models I would suggest that this
is a potential contribution that somebody can make in giving
us equivalent data, hopefully on a human endothelium. I
think you made the point about the coronary arteries and so
I have nothing to add.

   DR. NEREM: You mentioned turbulence and either I misheard
you or else I would like to discuss this further. You talked
about these flow disturbances essentially being initiated, I
thought you said during the diastolic portion of the beat.
Did you mean systolic, or did I hear you wrong?

   DR. DEWEY: What I meant to say was in the diastolic
side of the systolic beat. On the backside of the systole.

   DR. STONE: Yes, conceptually, Dr. Dewey, in your
models of coronary vessels what would be the changes if the
coronaries were highly tethered?

   DR. DEWEY: I can only suggest one thing. I am very
slow when it comes to this kind of speculation. There is
                              only one thing that has occurred
Tethering   to me and that is that an
                              untethered artery, or a potentially
untethered artery is subject to a substantial wave propagation
phenomenon and potential resonances which are not present in
a tethered artery.

This has been true in many experiments where people have
exposed, for example, femoral and carotid arteries and we
have done it too in dogs and got absolutely erroneous results
with respect to the paraspectral density of the unsteady
flow. They have been absolutely and totally wrong and
people still do that with unsupported tubes of latex to get
these absolutely wrong results with respect to tethered
arteries in the circulation. There is a long standing
controversy about this in which I have a very strong opinion.
Arteries like femoral and carotids in vivo are well tethered
and they don't resonate.

However, we have seen resonant spectra obtained from the external carotid artery. I would expect that the same kind of resonance phenomena could occur in the coronary arteries on the upper cardiac surface.

DR. SCHWARTZ: I have two questions. One relates specifically to the concept of critical shear. My understanding is that it is associated with significant endothelial injury. Is this correct?

Critical Shear Assoicated with Significant Endothelial Injury

DR. FRY: Correct. The definition of the acute critical yield stress (t_c) implies detection of identifiable structural changes in certain members of the endothelial cell population (44,45). This is not to be confused with the shear stress dependent increase in endothelial permeability which occurs at much lower levels of stress and is not associated with any detectable structural changes either by light or by electron microscopy (46).

DR. SCHWARTZ: Is it possible that much lower shear stresses modify, for example, the process of vesicular transport?

DR. DEWEY: I would suggest that either you or Dr. Fry make a comment about your critical shear.

DR. FRY: The experimentally observed relationship among hemodynamic stresses amd altered endothelial surface permeability with and without associated structural changes recently have been reviewed elsewhere (46). Turning specifically to the question of "acute critical yield stress" (t_c), this quantity represents the stress at which there is the greatest conversion of structurally normal cells to structurally abnormal cells. Thus t_c represents the rheologic behavior of a population of endothelial cells, not of an individual. Very roughly speaking, t_c is the stress at which half of the endothelial cells in a given population will show structural changes. It follows that many endothelial cells in this individual's population have yielded at stresses below t_c and the hardier members won't yield until exposed to stresses above t_c. The value of t_c appears to be relatively insensitive to the duration of stress exposure; however, this should be studied further. Although the group mean value of t_c for the canine ventral thoracic aorta (23 animals) is around

400 dynes cm $^{-2}$, it is important to note that the range of these values was from less than 200 to 990 dynes cm $^{-2}$ (44,45). Thus it appears that the (rheologic) strength of the endothelial surface may vary widely even in normal animals and at the same site. Moreover, subsequent studies, summarized elsewhere (46), suggest that t_c may vary considerably from site to site in a given animal and may also vary significantly with the metabolic state of the animal.

The acute critical shear stress is a term that refers specifically to a level of stress that produces overt structural changes in the endothelial
Acute Critical Shear Stress   surface. As might be expected, a massive increase in endothelial permeability is associated with these structural changes. However, at considerably lower levels of stress exposure that are unassociated with any detectable histologic or ultrastructural changes in the endothelial cells, one also sees a stress dependent increase in permeability (45,47). In studies specifically designed to study this shear dependent increase in permeability, e.g., in an arteriovenous shunt preparation, transmission electron microscopy suggests occasional changes in the subendothelial region consistent with mild edema. However, these observations are highly variable. In the inverse situation, i.e., if transmission and scanning electron microscopy are done at sites in the vascular system that are normally more permeable to plasma substances, one commonly finds subendothelial edema and also occasional small patches of endothelial cell erosion. These structural changes are never seen in regions of low or "normal" permeability. One wonders if subendothelial edema associated with increased permeability might not be one of the common mechanisms of lowering the critical yield stress and promoting endothelial erosion (46).

DR. SCHWARTZ: I wasn't questioning that Dr. Fry. I was trying to suggest that perhaps critical shear could be very much lower in terms of, say modification of transport by some process other than endothelial injury.

DR. NEREM: Dr. Fry, relative to your studies...correct me if I am wrong, I believe the yield stress is 400 dynes per square centimeter. Was that the stress above which you observed cell abnormality and was actual cell erosion associated with a stress of about 1000 dynes per square centimeter?

DR. FRY: Not quite. Any stress equal to or in excess of the t_c for that animal would be associated with significant cellular structural changes. These altered cells will finally erode, provided the stress exposure is maintained for a sufficient duration, say 2 hours. Studies in which the stress was considerably in excess of t_c , of course, would show erosion in a shorter period of time.

DR. NEREM: What was the lowest stress at which you observed erosion?

DOG   DR. FRY: The lowest value of t_c in the 23 dogs was less than 200 dynes cm^{-2}.

DR. DEWEY: May I make a comment? With all due respect to the concept of critical shear, I think one of the reasons I brought it up was to promote discussion about it, because in trying to estimate shear stresses particularly in coronary arteries and the carotid arteries, really the ones that kill us, you may get very high values from time to time. But it seems to me that a concept like critical shear is not necessarily the kind of thing we are looking for.

DR. FRY: I agree.

DR. CAREW: I believe both in the studies that I did, which Dr. Dewey alluded to, and also in Dr. Nerem's and Caro's studies, which bear the albumin transport across either the aortic endothelium or, in the case of Nerem and Caro the carotid endothelium, and in another study I did with Cronwright on vessels in situ, there was no evidence that there was a distinct threshold of shear stress below which permeability was not a function of shear stress. There seemed to be a fairly smooth continuation with increasing shear stress from the very lowest levels. That could be very important.

DR. GREENE: Concerning the idea of a critical shear stress at the wall, there are a great deal of data of critical shear stresses for human
Critical Shear Stress   erythrocytes, even if there are
for Erythrocytes   little for human aorta. The data
                           have been summarized by Leverett
(48), and show that there is no such thing as a single critical shear stress for an erythrocyte. Instead, there is a time-shear stress domain such that cell rupture occurs rapidly at exposures to 1500 dynes/cm^2, but much more slowly when stress level is in the region of 100 dynes/cm^2.

In the absence of sufficient data, one might hypothesize that aortic tissue responds similarly and that the 400 dynes/cm^2 value turns out to be critical only in the context of the time frame of current experimentation.

DR. DEWEY: There is another type of instability mechanism which may be operative here, but not, to my knowledge, invoked previously in describing cardiovascular flows. It is called a "Gortler Instability."
"Gortler Instability"
As you can see in Figure 2-17, a steady laminar viscous flow over a curved wall can generate a series of longitudinally-oriented vortex cells within the viscous boundary layer next to the surface. One can calculate (49) the conditions under which these vortex cells will become unstable and cause turbulence in the boundary layer. My calculations suggest that this type of instability should be generated in the major arteries, and it would be interesting to set up some experiments which are specifically designed to demonstrate this effect.

The final topic I will cover returns to the problem of arterial distensibility, a phenomenon which couples the flow dynamics and the solid mechanics of the arterial wall.
Problems of Arterial
Distensibility
As Dr. Kenyon pointed out so clearly this morning, the stretch of the artery depends on its geometry, tethering, and elastic properties; and how these mechanical properties are acted upon by the internal pressure and fluid shear stress. But the internal fluid pressure and motion depend intimately upon the stretch of the artery, so the whole problem is strongly coupled. Several theoretical models have been developed to represent the aorta and other major vessels with axially varying compliance, and references to this work can be found in McDonald's book (1) the two volumes edited by Bergel (50) and the book edited by Attinger (29). One may briefly summarize these results as follows: it is necessary to model the taper and axial variation of compliance of the arterial tree if one wishes to predict the temporal variations of flow and pressure at each point along the arterial tree. But once the flow and pressure are known, the velocity profile across the lumen, the wall shear stress, and other flow parameters are the same as those which would be observed in a rigid tube with the same temporal variations of flow and pressure.

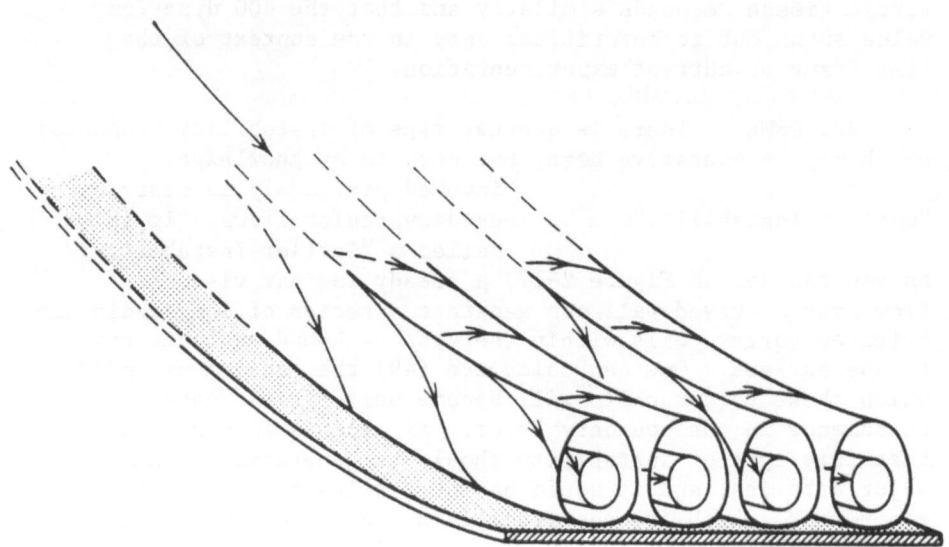

Fig. 2-17: Gortler instabilities in a viscous shear flow on a
curved wall.

        But such a simplistic summary ignores one potentially
important variable, namely the effect of arterial distensibility
on the integrity of the endothelial layer. Circumferential
stretch clearly alters the morphology of the endothelial
cell, just as Fry (12) has shown that stretch alters the
cell permeability. Several years ago, Bergel (51) pointed
out that we know very little about the distensibility in and
around arterial bifurcations, and suggested that deformation
would be a maximum on the outside of the branch (i.e. the
side with the smallest radius of curvature). This was
emphasized by Dr. Kenyon this morning when he established
quantitative estimates for this effect.

BIBLIOGRAPHY

1. McDonald, D.A.: Blood Flow in Arteries. 2nd Ed.,
        Williams and Wilkins, Baltimore, esp. pp. 92-95, 1974.

2. Mills, C.J., Gabe, I.T., Gault, J.H., Mason, D.T.,
        Ross, J., Braunwall, E., and Shilling, J.P.: Pressure-
        flow relationships and vascular impedance in man.
        Cardiovascular Research 4, 405-417, 1970.

3. Nerem, R.M., Seed, W.A., and Wood, N.B.:   An experimental
        study of the velocity distribution and transition
        to turbulence in the aorta. J. Fluid Mech., 52,
        137-160, 1972.

4. Clark, C., and Schultz, D.L.: Velocity distribution in
        aortic flow. Cardiovascular Research 7, 601-613, 1973.

5. Ling, S.C., Atabek, H.B., Fry, D.L., Patel, D.J., and
        Janicki, J.S.: Application of heated-film velocity
        and shear probes to hemodynamic studies. Circulation
        Research 23, 789-801, 1968.

6. Ling, S.C., Atabek, H.B., and Carmody, J.J.: Pulsatile
        flow in arteries. In Proc. XII Int. Appl. Mech.
        (Me, He te nyi and Vincenti, W.G., Eds.) Springer-
        Verlag, Berlin, pp. 277-291, 1969.

7. Fry, D.L.: Acute vascular endothelial changes associated
        with increased blood velocity gradients. Circulation
        Research 22, 165-197, 1968.

8. Gregg, D.E.: The Coronary Arteries, Charles C. Thomas,
        Publ., Springfield, Ill., 1965.

9. Nerem, R.M., Rumburger, J.A., Jr., Gross, D.R., Jamlin, R.L.,
        and Geiger, G.L.: Hot-film measurements of coronary
        blood flow in horses. Proc. Specialists Conf. on Fluid
        Dynamic Aspects of Arterial Disease (R.M. Nerem, Ed.)
        Ohio State University, pp. 28-31, 1974.

10. Wells, M.K., Winter, D.C., Nelson, A.W., and McCarthy, T.C.:
        Estimated blood velocity profiles in the coronary
        artery. Proc. 27th ACEMB, Philadelphia, 282, 1974.

11. Carew, T.E. III: Mechano-chemical response of canine
        aortic endothelium to elevated shear stress in vitro.
        Ph.D. Thesis, Catholic University of America,
        Washington, D.C., 1971

12. Fry, D.L.: Responses of the arterial wall to certain
     physical factors. In Atherosclerosis: Initiating
     Factors, CIBA Foundation Symposium 12 (New Series)
     Elsevier, Amsterdam, pp. 93-125, 1973.

13. Fronek, A., Johansen, K.H., Dilley, R.B., and Bernstein, E.F.:
     Noninvasive physiologic tests in the diagnosis and
     characterization of peripheral arterial occlusive
     disease. Am. J. Surgery, 126, 205-214, 1973.

14. Hisland, M.B., Miller, C.W., McLeod, F.D., Jr.: Trans-
     cutaneous measurement of blood velocity profiles and
     flow. Cardiovascular Research, 7, 703-712, 1973.

15. Fronek, A., Coel, M., and Bernstein, E.F.: Quantitative
     ultrasonographic studies of lower extremity flow
     velocities in health and disease. Circulation, 6,
     957-960, 1976.

16. Perroneau, P., Gisbertz, K.H., Steckmeier, B., Xhaard, M.,
     Dalbera, A., and Bournat, J.P: In vitro and in vivo
     experimental studies of pulsatile flow patterns in
     curved and stenotic vessels. Proc. of Specialists
     Meeting on Fluid Dynamic Aspects of Arterial Disease
     (R.M. Nerem, Ed.) Ohio State University, pp. 5-8, 1974.

17. Gutstein, W.H., and Schneck, D.J.: In vitro boundary layer
     studies of blood flow in branched tubes. J. Athero. Res.
     7, 295-299, 1967.

18. Ferguson, G.G., and Roach, M.R.: Flow conditions at
     bifurcations as determined in glass models, with
     reference to the focal distribution of vascular
     lesions. In Cardiovascular Fluid Dynamics, Vol. 2
     (D.H. Bergel, Ed.), Academic Press, N.Y. pp. 141-156,
     1972.

19. Attinger, E.O.: Flow patterns and vascular geometry.
     In Pulsatile Blood Flow (E.O. Attinger, Ed.),
     McGraw-Hill, N.Y. pp. 179-198, 1964.

20. Rodkiewicz, C.M., and Roussel, C.L.: Fluid mechanics in
     a large arterial bifurcation. Trans. ASME, Series I
     (Fluid Engineering), 95, 108-112, 1973.

21. Feuerstein, I.A., Elmasry, O.A., and Round, C.F.: Flow
     pattersn and wall shear rates in a series of symmetric
     bifurcations. (Abstract), Proc. 27th ACEMB, Philadelphia
     Oct. 6-10, 278, 1974.

22. Freedman, R.W.: The measurement of wall shear rate in a model of the human aorto-iliac bifurcation using an electro-chemical technique. Ph.D. Thesis, M.I.T., 1976,

23. Brech, R., and Bellhouse, B.J.: Flow in branching vessels. Cardiovascular Research, 7, 593-600, 1973.

24. Kandarpa, K., and Davis, N.: Analysis of the fluid dynamic effects on atherogenesis at branching sites. J. Biomechanics, 9, 735-741, 1976.

25. O'Brien, V., Erlich, L.W., and Friedman, M.H.: Nonlinear simulation of unsteady arterial flows in a branch. Paper presented at the A.I.Ch.E. Annual Meeting, Philadelphia, 1973.

26. Smith, C.S.: Flow studies in a model arterial bifurcation. 1st Prize Student Paper, presented at the 29th Annual Conference on Engineering and Medicine and Biology, Nov. 6-10, Boston, 1976.

27. Stehbens, W.E.: Turbulence of blood flow. Quart. J. Exper. Path., 44, 110-117, 1959.

28. Stehbens, W.E.: Flow in glass models of arterial bifurcations and berry aneurysms at low Reynolds numbers. Quart. J. Exper. Physiol., 60, 181-192, 1975.

29. Attinger, E.O. (Ed.): Pulsatile Blood Flow, Mc-Graw-Hill, N.Y., 1964.

30. Fox, J.A., and Hugh A.E.: Static zones in the internal carotid artery: correlation with boundary layer separation and stasis in model flows. Br. Jour. Rad. 43, 370-376, 1970.

31. Dewey, C.F., Jr.: Qualitative and quantitative flow field visualization utilizing laser-induced fluorescence. AGARD Conference Proceedings No. 193 on Applications of Non-Intrusive Instrumentation in Fluid Flow Research, St. Louis, France, pp. 17-1 to 17-7, 1976.

32. Hugh, A.E., and Fox, J.A.: Precise localization of atheroma and its association with stasis at the origin of the interval carotid artery -- a radiographic investigation. Br. Jour. Rad., 43, 377-383, 1970.

33. Lyne, W.H.: Ph.D. Thesis, University of London, 1970.

34. Blennerhasset, P.: Ph.D. Thesis, University of
     London, 1970.

35. Dean, W.R.: Philosophical Mag. Series 7, $\underline{5}$ 673,
     1928.

36. Duncan, G.W., Gruber, J.O., Dewey, C.F., Jr.,
     Meyers, G.S., and Lees, R.S.: Evaluation of carotid
     stenosis of phanoangiography. New Engl. J. Med.,
     293, 1124-1128, 1975.

37. Pitts, W.H. III, and Dewey, C.F., Jr.,: Spectral
     and temporal characteristics of post-stenotic
     turbulent wall pressure fluctuations. Trans. ASME
     J. Biomech. Eng'g, 1976.

38. Flaherty, J.T., Ferrans, V.J., Pierce, J.E., Carew, T.E.,
     and Fry, D.L.: Localizing factors in experimental
     atherosclerosis. Atherosclerosis and Coronary Heart
     Disease. (W. Likoff, B.L. Segal, W. Insull, Jr.,
     and J.H. Moyer, Eds.) Grune and Stratton, N.Y.,
     pp. 40-84, 1972.

39. Leung, D.Y.M., Glagov, S., Clark, J.M., and Mathews, M.D.:
     Mechanical influences on the biosynthesis of extra-
     cellular macromolecules by aortic cells. In:
     Extracellular Matrix Influences on Gene Expression.
     (H.C. Slavkin and R.C. Greulich, Eds.) Academic
     Press, 633, 1975.

40. Ling, S.C., Atabek, H.B., Letzing, W.G., and Patel, D.J.:
     Nonlinear analysis of aortic flow in living
     dogs. Circulation Research, 33:198-212, 1973.

41. Atabek, H.B., Ling, S.C., Patel, D.J.: Analysis of
     coronary flow fields in thoracotomized dogs.
     Circulation Research, 37:752-761, 1975.

42. Pedley, T.J.: Flow in the entrance of the aorta.
     Proceedings from a Specialists Meeting on Fluid
     Dynamics of Arterial Disease, R.M. Nerem, (Ed.)
     Ohio, pp. 20-23, 1974.

43. Ling, S.C., Atabek, H.B., Fry, D.L., Patel, D.J., and
     Janicki, J.S.: Application of heated-film velocity
     and shear probes to hemodynamic studies. Circulation
     Research, 23:789-801, 1968.

44. Fry, D.L.: Acute vascular endothelial changes associated
     with increased blood velocity gradients. Circulation
     Research, Vol. XII, Feb., 1968.

45. Fry, D.L.: Certain histological and chemical responses
     of the vascular interface to acutely induced
     mechanical stress in the aorta of the dog.
     Circulation Research, Vol. XIV, Jan., 1969.

46. Fry, D.L.: Hemodynamic forces in atherogenesis.
     Cerebrovascular Disease, Raven Press, N.Y., 1976.

47. Carew, T.D.: Mechano-chemical response of canine aortic
     endothelium to elevated shear stress In Vitro., Ph.D.
     Thesis, The Catholic University of American,
     Washington, D.C., 1971.

48. Leverett, L.B., Hellums, J.D., Alfrey, C.P., Lynch, E.C.:
     Red blood cell damage by shear stress. 72nd National
     Meeting, American Institutes of Chemical Engineers
     St. Louis, May, 1972.

49. Lin, C.C.,: The Theory of Hydrodynamic Stability,
     Cambridge U. Press, Cambridge, pp. 96-98. See
     also papers by H. Gortler and G. Hammerlin,
     50 Jahre Grenzschictforshung (H. Gortler and W.
     Tollmein, Eds.). Freidr. Vieweg & Sohn, Braunschweig,
     1955.

50. Bergel, D.H.: (Ed.): Cardiovascular Fluid Dynamics.,
     Vols. I and II, Academic Press, N.Y., 1972.

51. Bergel, D.H.: Comments on unpublished work by C. Mellon
     and D.H. Bergel, Appearing in Atherosclerosis:
     Initiating Factors, CIBA Foundation Symposium 12
     (New Series), Elsevier, Amsterdam, pp. 159-161, 1973.

52. Fulton, W.M.F.: The Coronary Arteries, Charles C. Thomas,
     Springfield, Ill., 1965.

53. Schultz, D.L.: Pressure and flow in large arteries. In
     Cardiovascular Fluid Dynamics, Vol. 1 (D.H. Bergel, Ed.)
     Academic Press, pp. 287-314, 1972.

54. Pitts, W.H. III, and Dewey, C.F., Jr.: Programmable
     pulsatile flow apparatus for simulation of arterial
     hemodynamics. Proc. San Diego Biomedical Symposium,
     14, 119-124, 1975.

Chapter 3   CONTROL OF VASOMOTOR FUNCTION AND THE HEMODYNAMIC
CONSEQUENCES OF THE CONTRACTILE BEHAVIOR OF
ARTERIES

DR. COX: In the mammalian organism, a complex array of
control mechanisms exists to fulfill the temporal and spatial
demands of the body for the
Complex Array of   transport services of the
Control Mechanisms   circulatory system. These
control mechanisms appear to
involve almost all of the various elements of the cardiovascular
system: the heart, the microcirculation and the veins.

What about the large so-called conduit or elastic
arteries. Do they play any role in neural reflex mechanisms?
These are the vessels with which we are primarily concerned
at this workshop in relation to their role in atherogenesis.
Are they indeed passive conduits which simply respond to
hemodynamic events in a "programmed" manner or are they
actively involved in the control and regulation of cardiovascular
function?

The view has long been held that neural reflexes produced
at best only modest effects on large arteries (1).   They
were not considered to be involved
Neural Reflexes   in the control of peripheral
resistance and, therefore, to be
of no significance in the scheme of neural control. Yet,
the walls of larger arteries contain an abundant amount of
smooth muscle from 25 to 35% of wall volume. There is also
a significant amount of contractile protein present and
indeed larger arteries of some species are used as tissue
for pharmacological assay of vasoactive substances (2).
Teleologically, this contractile structure (the smooth
muscle cell) must serve some physiological purpose other
than being simply a synthetic structure for other wall
precursors (3).

We are now somewhat more sophisticated and realize
that there is more to neural control than the control of
peripheral resistance and
Control of Smooth   cardiac output. There is now
Muscle Tone   sufficient evidence to suggest
important physiological role (s)
for the control of smooth muscle tone in larger arteries (4,5,6).

My plan for this presentation is to review current knowledge
of neural control mechanisms including the regional differentiation of control as well as the control of both large and
small arteries, primarily under normal conditions but also for
some other physiological and pathophysiological conditions.
Finally, the possible significance of this control in light of
the objectives of this meeting will be discussed.

EFFECTOR MECHANISMS IN ARTERIES

1. Passive Mechanical Properties

Studies on the passive mechanical properties of arteries
(i.e., negligible smooth muscle tone) have been performed on
a variety of preparations
Arteries are Nonlinear   including strips and intact
Viscoelastic Nonuniform   segments. In general, the results
and Anisotropic   of these studies are qualitatively,
                                 if not always quanititatively
similar. Measurements of pressure-volume, pressure-diameter
and force-length relations on arterial samples show that
arteries are nonlinear, viscoelastic nonuniform and anisotropic.
Arteries are nonlinear because they do not obey Hooke's law.
They are viscoelastic because their responses are time
dependent. They are nonuniform because their properties are
different in different parts of the arterial system. They
are anisotropic because their properties are different in
different directions within the wall.

Tangential stress-strain relations from five arterial
sites are summarized in Fig. 3-1 and demonstrate the nonlinear
and nonuniform nature of arterial wall properties. The
nonlinear natures of these curves have been explained on the
basis of a nonuniform contribution of wall elements to load
bearing at different values of wall strain (7), (8), (9).
Wall stress is thought to be supported by elastin in the low
strain range, by elastin and collagen at intermediate strains
and by collagen alone at high strain.

The nonuniform nature of arterial wall properties is
also indicated in Fig. 3-1 by the wide variation in stress-
strain relations at different anatomical sites. One of the
principal contributors to this regional nonuniformity is the
anatomical variation in collagen and elastin content.

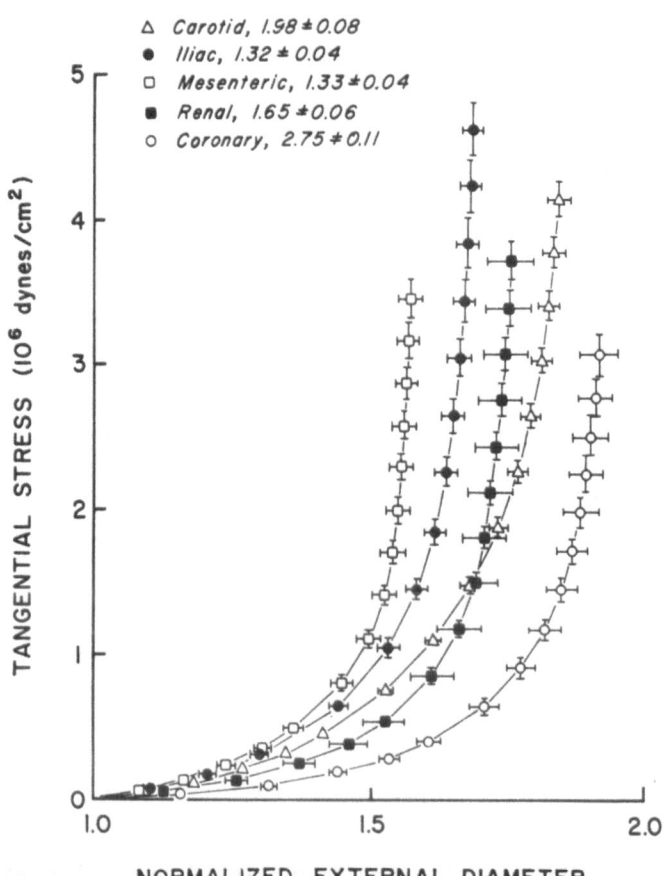

Fig. 3-1: Passive tangential stress-stain relations of isolated
canine arterial segments in vitro. Abscissa is the diameter of
the segment normalized by dividing by the value of external
diameter at zero pressure. Smooth muscle in the arteries was
treated with cyanide, iodacetate and dinitrophenol to inhibit
active force development. Symbols are means and bars ± 1 SEM of
data averaged in transmural pressure steps of lo mmHg from 0 to
250. Data at the top with symbols are the average values of ± 1
SEM of the ratio of collagen to elastin contents determined using
the same segments by chemical means. (Fisher and Llaurado, 1966).

Since collagen fibers are stiffer than elastin, the ratio of collagen to elastin content (C/E) has been suggested as an empirical index of wall stiffness (10). While this relation generally holds along the aorta (11), it is not valid in its daughter branches as shown in Fig. 3-1. Obviously, other factors must be of importance in determining arterial wall mechanics, including, for example, the architectural coupling and distriubtion of connective tissue elements as well as the detailed recruitment of collagen fibers with increasing wall strain (8).

The anisotropic nature of arterial wall properties are the result of the ordered structure of the arterial wall at the microscopic level. The various wall constituents are not homogenously distributed but are structurally oriented. Numerous morphological studies have described the organization of arterial wall elements (12). Fig. 3-2 summarizes values of anisotropic elastic moduli and Poisson ratios obtained from a group of carotid arteries measured at in vivo length (13). At low values of tangetial strain (actually extension ratio, $\lambda_0 = \frac{D}{DO}$ values of tangetial (E_0) and radial (E_r) elastic moduli are nearly equal and both are smaller than the axial modulus (Ex). At higher values of tangetial wall strain, E_0 becomes larger than E_r and E_x while the latter two are nearly equal. The Poisson ratios which relate deformation in one direction to that in another show considerable variatio.i, with $u_{r\theta}$ and $u_{\theta r}$ being nearly identical especially in the low strain range.

The anisotropic elastic properties depend upon values of wall strain in the various directions. The exact manner in which the various wall strains interact to influence anisotropic properties is not completely known, however. The manner in which the various wall constituents contribute to the various anisotropic sontants is also now known.

Viscoelasticity is manifest in arteries as a dependence of the arterial wall response to a deformation upon both the magnitude of the deformation Viscoelasticity and the time course over which it is applied. Viscoelasticity has been studied using time domain transient responses or steady-state frequency domain responses. Fig. 3-3 summarizes data from Bergel (14) on the frequency dependence of the dynamic modulus of several arterial sites studied in vitro at a mean transmural pressure of 100 mmHg with a superimposed sinusoidal pressure variation of different frequencies.

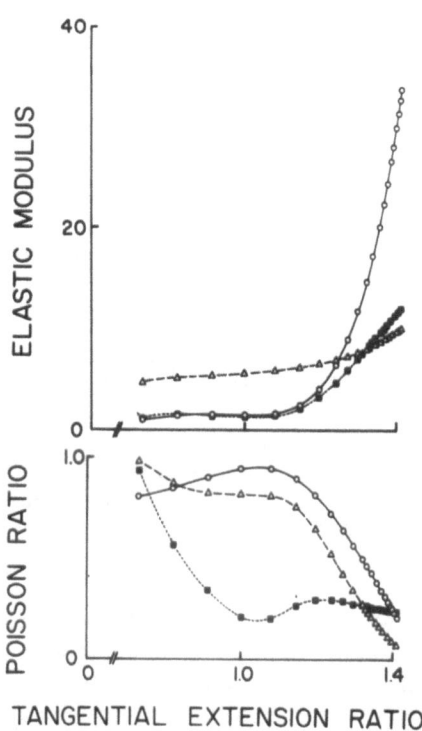

Fig. 3-2: Variation of passive anisotropic elastic constants of a canine carotid artery with tangential extension ratio <u>in vitro</u>. Elastic moduli are tangential (open circles), radial (closed squares) and axial (open triangles). Poisson ratios are $u_{r\theta}$ (open circles), $u_{\theta r}$ (open triangles) and $u_{\theta x}$ (closed squares). Units of elastic modulus are 10^6 dynes/cm^2. Tangential extension ratio is the ratio of mid-wall diameter or a given pressure divided by the unstressed value.

The value of dynamic modulus increases in magnitude between
0 and 2 Hz and remains essentially constant up to 20 Hz.
The dynamic modulus ratio varies considerably at different
arterial sites as seen in Fig. 3-3. This regional variation of
viscoelasticity is thought to be related to the regional
variations in composition. The contribution of the various
wall components to arterial viscoelasticity is not completely
known at this time.

The viscous properties of the arterial wall arise from
at least two sources: inter - and intra-molecular cross-
linking of wall components and the interaction of contractile
proteins. The detailed deformation response of a coiled,
cross-linked macromolecular matrix to the application of a
strain and its removal are bound to be different, producing
a strain rate dependent trajectory in the stress-strain
plan.

The resistance to stretch in non-contracting smooth
muscle has recently been shown to be calcium dependent but
not dependent upon membrane
Calcium Dependence   depolarization of intracellular
release of calcium. This has
been interpreted to suggest that most, if not all, crossbridges
are normally attached in smooth muscle and thus able to
resist deformation. When the muscle is stretched, the
breaking and subsequent reformation of cross-links is the
source of viscoelasticity. Such responses would be strain
rate dependent, i.e., amplitude and frequency of the strain.

The effects of the activation of smooth muscle on
arterial wall properties can be represented in two general
ways. One way is to consider
Effects of Smooth   the artery to be an elastomer
Muscle Activation   and describe the effects of
activation on its mechanical
properties. The other way is to consider the artery to be a
muscle and then describe the effects of activation of force
development and shortening. Both of these approaches have
been utilized in the determination of the contribution of
smooth muscle to arterial wall properties and behavior.

In general, activation of smooth muscle shifts the
tangential stress-strain curve of an artery to the left.
The magnitude of this effect varies with anatomical location
in the arterial system and depends upon a large variety of
factors too numerous to list here.

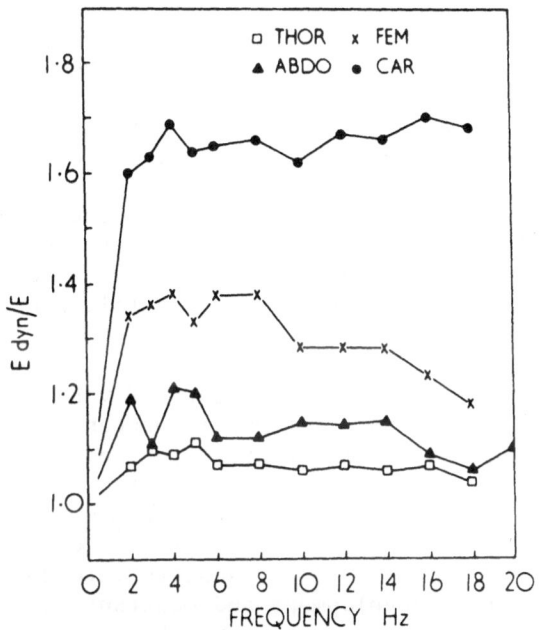

Fig. 3-3: Frequency dependence of the passive dynamic modulus
ratio of several isolated canine artery segments in vitro.
Ordinate is the dynamic modulus divided by the static modulus.
A sinusoidal pressure of variable frequency was imposed with an
amplitude of 5-10 mmHg at a mean pressure of 100 mmHg (Bergel,
1961).

The data in Fig. 3-4 show the effects of maximum activation by norepinephrine on the tangential stress-strain relations of iliac arteries in vitro. At specific values of wall strain, activation of smooth muscles produces an increase in wall stress which is a strong function of strain.

As would be predicted from these results, substantial effects on arterial wall elasticity are produced by smooth muscle activation. For a number of years, a controversy existed in the literature as to whether smooth muscle activation produced an increase or decrease in elastic modulus (1). The reason for this controversy was explained by Dobrin and Rovick (16) who noted that the change in elastic modulus of arteries following smooth muscle activation depended on whether strain or pressure was the independent variable. As shown in Fig. 3-5, the elastic modulus is increased at all values of wall strain when the latter is the independent variable. When plotted as a function of transmural pressure, however, the elastic modulus is increased at low and decreased at moderate to high values of pressure following maximal activation.

In order to describe the effects of vascular smooth muscle activation in terms of muscle mechanics, it is necessary to determine both isometric contraction and isotonic shortening.

Isometric Contraction and Isotonic Shortening

For intact arterial segments in the form of cylinders, these characteristics of muscle mechanics translate into constant radius (isometric) stress development and constant pressure (isobaric constriction). These responses are shown diagrammatically in Fig. 3-6. The steady state pressure-diameter points to the right correspond to passive muscle while the points to the left correspond to fully activated muscle. The region between these two curves delineates the range of control of arterial wall properties by the smooth muscle. Qualitatively similar relations exist at all arterial sites studied to date.

As would be predicted from Fig. 3-6, these two forms of FROG active response depend strongly upon the initial pressure or diameter. The variation of the diameter response of vessels in the frog mesentery to maximal norepinephrine activation with the initial value of tangential wall stress (i.e., pressure) is shown in Fig. 3-7. (17). Stress is used in this diagram to allow a more meaningful comparison among different vessels from which these measurements were made.

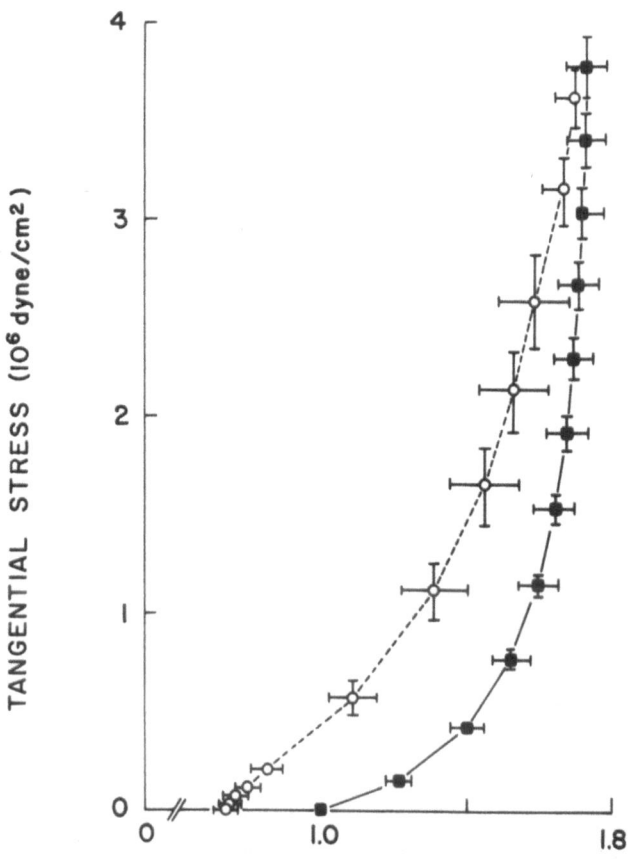

Fig. 3-4: Relation of tangential wall stress and normalized external diameter for passive conditions (closed squares) and for maximal norepinephrine activation (open circles). Symbols are means and bars ± 1 SEM of data averaged in 20 mmHg steps. Data were obtained from isolated intact segments of canine iliac artery (N-12) and averaged at specific values of transmural pressure.

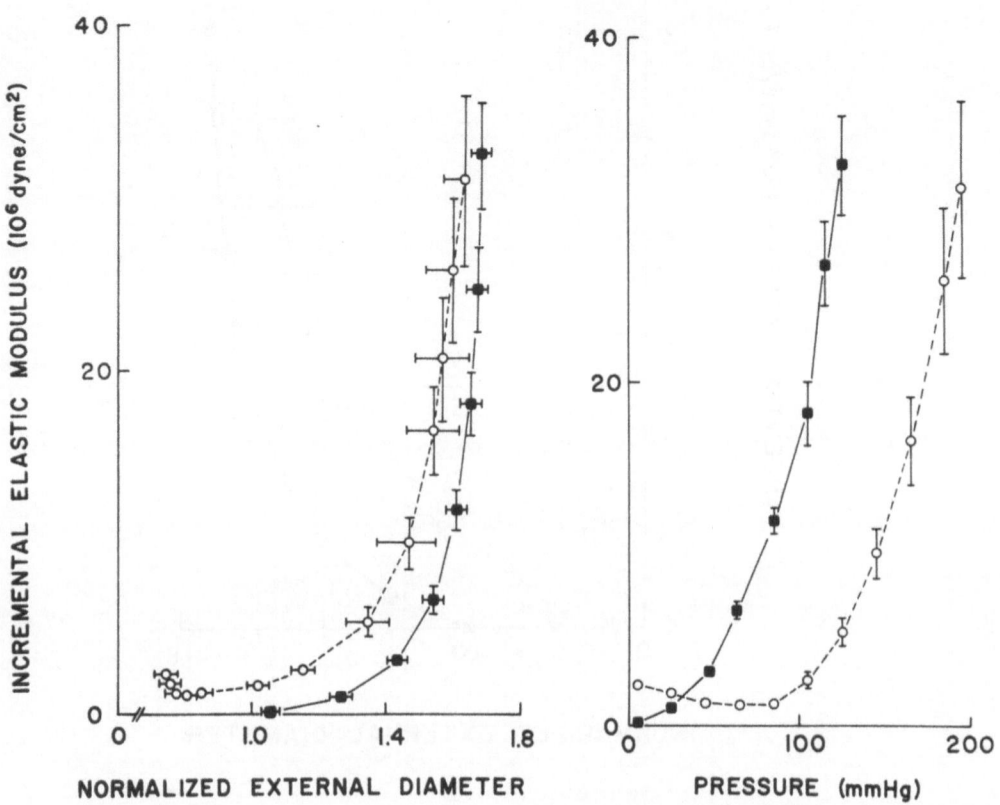

Fig. 3-5: Effects of smooth muscle activation by norepinephrine on the static incremental elastic modulus of canine iliac arteries. The panel at the left shows elastic modulus as a function of normalized external diameter while the panel at the right its variation with transmural pressure. Data are for active (open circles) and passive (closed squares) conditons.

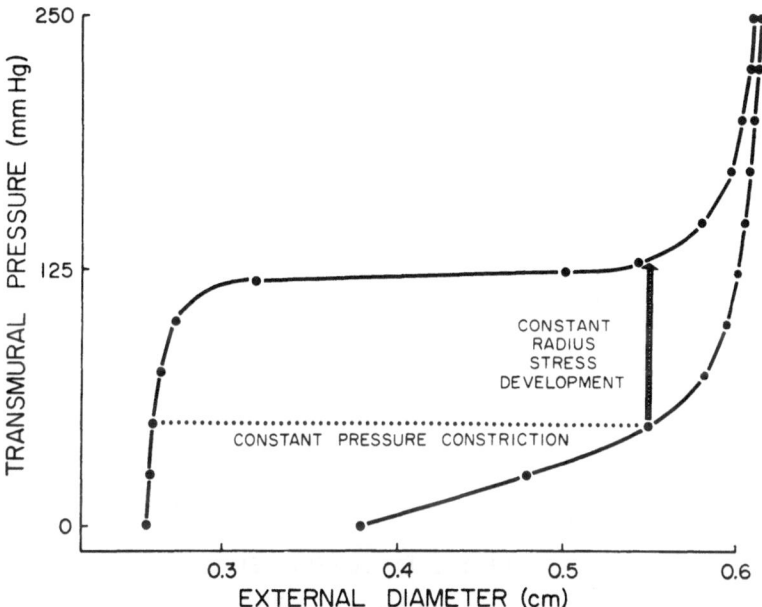

Fig. 3-6: Schematic representation of the mechanics of arterial smooth muscle. Curve and points to the right represent the pressure-diameter relation for passive muscle while the points to the right are data for active muscle. The mechanics of arterial smooth muscle can be represented in terms of constant radius (isometric) stress development or constant pressure (isobaric) constriction responses to smooth muscle activation.

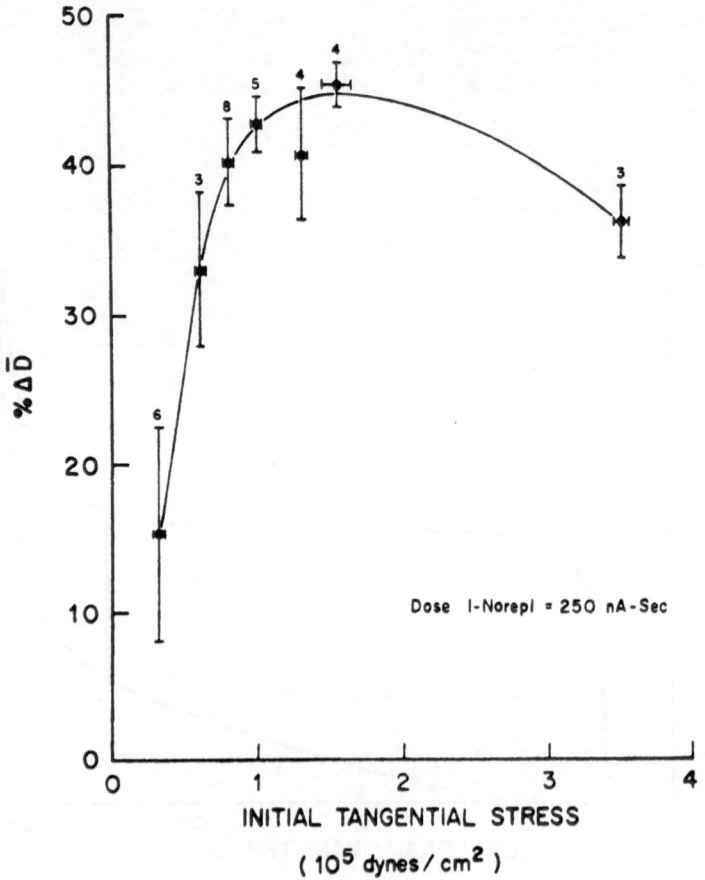

Fig. 3-7: Dependence of diameter responses to norepinephrine activation on initial tangential stress for arterial vessels in the frog mesentery. The diameter response is normalized by dividing by the initial control value of diameter. Norepinephrine was applied topically by an iontophoretic method. The numbers over the data points represent the number of observations per data point (17).

The diameter response is expressed as a percentage of the initial diameter. The diameter response is a strong function of the initial stress exhibiting a maximal response between 1 and 2 X 10^5 dynes/cm^2 for this preparation. Rather similar results have also been reported by a number of investigators for mammalian arterial smooth muscle preparations (18,19,20).

Values of tangential wall stress developed in response to smooth muscle activation show a strong dependence on wall strain as shown for iliac arteries in Fig. 3-8. For all arterial sites, an optimum strain exists at which the stress response to maximal activation is largest. Both above and below this value of strain the stress response decreases. The general characteristics of this relation are qualitatively similar at all arterial sites which have been studied to date (19,20,21). Both of these two manifestations of arterial smooth muscle activation are consistent with a sliding filament model of muscle function.

DOG

The results described in the previous section delineate the limits of control of arterial wall properties by smooth muscle. In vivo a number of factors will affect this relationship in such a manner as to decrease the effective range over which smooth muscle can exert control of arterial wall properties. Of these factors, probably the most important is the density and distribution of the post ganglionic sympathetic nerve fibers.

Density and Distribution
of Post Ganglionic
Sympathetic Nerve Fibers

Not only is there a nonuniform distribution of nerve fibers as well as nerve activity to different vascular beds within the body but also to the various series coupled vascular elements in a particular vascular bed. Fig. 3-9 shows a diagrammatic representation of the density of innervation of mesenteric blood vessels in the rat (22). The distribution of nerve fibers is particularly dense to the small and medium sized arteries in the mesenteric circulation as well as to the terminal arterioles. Beyond the terminal arterioles adrenergic innervation to precapillary arterioles has not been observed (22). An analogous nonuniform distribution of innervation density is also observed on the venous side as well.

RAT

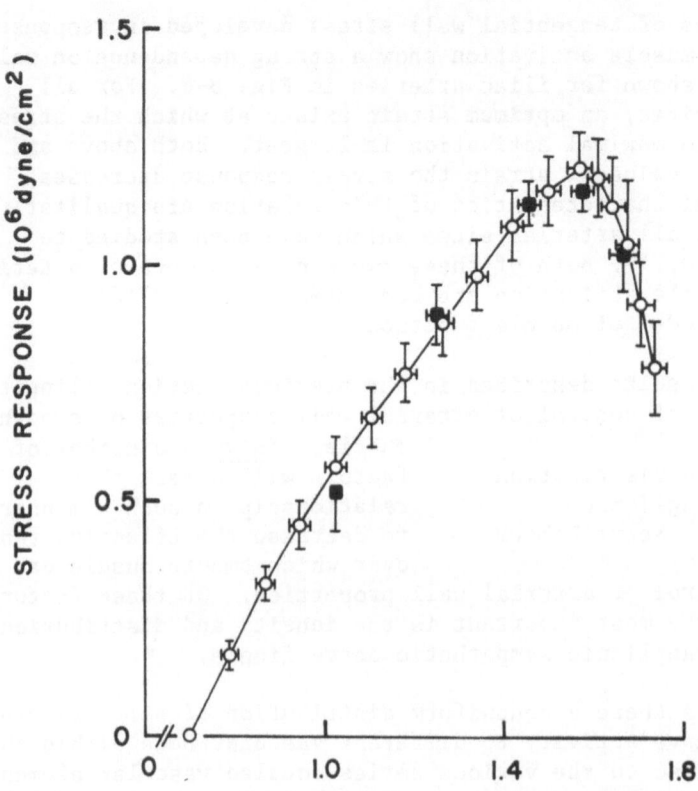

Fig. 3-8: Active tangential stress response to norepinephrine
for canine iliac artery segments as a function of normalized
external diameter. Symbols are mean and bars $\pm$ SEM (20).

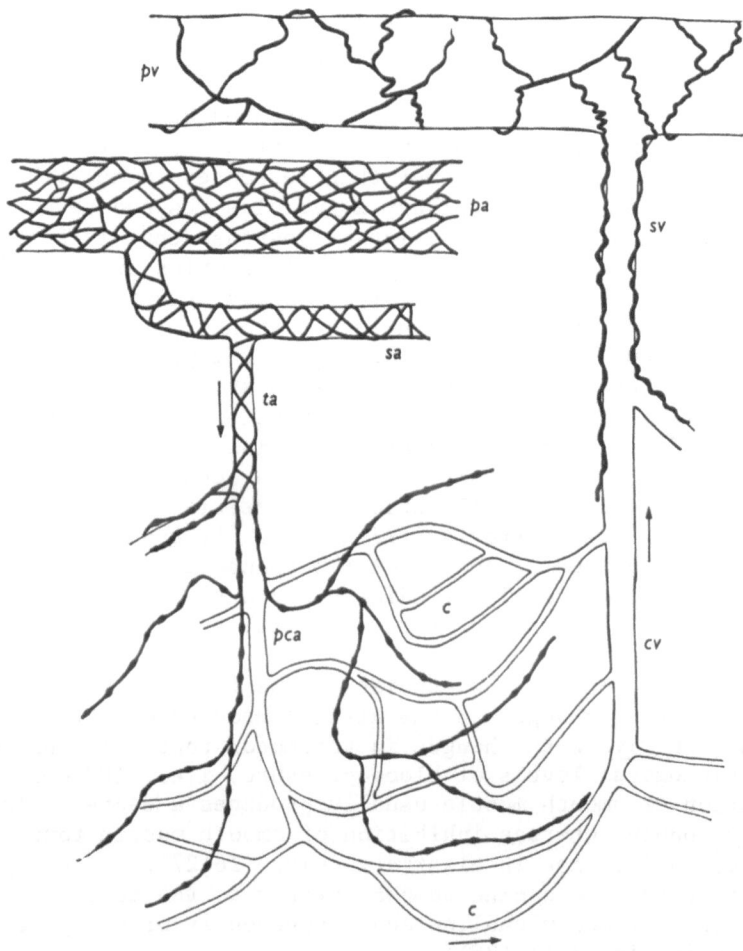

Fig. 3-9: Diagrammatic representation of the distribution of sympathetic nerves to the various vessels in the mesenteric circulation of the cat. Vessels are pa, principal artery, sa, small artery, ta, terminal artery; pca, precapillary arteriole; c, capillary; cv, collecting venule; sv, small vein, pv, principal vein (22).

As would be anticipated from this functional distribution
of sympathetic nerves there are considerable differences in
                                the response of various elements
Range of Control In Vivo   within the mesenteric circulation
                                to both sympathetic nerve
stimulation and the intraarterial infusion of norepinephrine.
A comparison of such responses is shown in Fig. 3-10 (22).
While only minor differences exist in the maximum constrictor
response to nerve stimulation in innervated arterial segments,
responses to norepinephrine in larger arteries of the mesenteric
circulation are somewhat lower than responses in the other
arterial vessels. Precapillary arterioles respond to norepinephrine infusion with a constriction response that is equal
in magnitude to that produced in small arteries and terminal
arterioles. Therefore, while precapillary arterioles are
not innervated they are nonetheless responsive to circulating
plasma neurohumoral agents. The relative magnitude of these
constrictor responses (40-60% for nerve stimulation) are
qualitatively similar to those constriction responses which
have been determined for isolated arterial segments in vitro.
Responses of similar magnitude have also been recorded on
perfused segments of small metacarpal arteries, dorsalpedal
and anterior tibial arteries (23,24,25). It appears, therefore,
that this magnitude of constrictor response is a general
characteristic of small to medium sized arteries and terminal
arterioles in all regions of the arterial tree.

There are only a few studies in the literature that
have documented changes in the elastic modulus of arterial
segments in vivo with changes in vasomotor tone. In general,
at physiological levels of blood pressure, i.e., 100 mmHg,
activation of smooth muscle usually produces a decrease in
elastic modulus whereas inhibition of smooth muscle tone
produces an increase in elastic modulus (26,27). An example
DOG of a response of a canine femoral artery to the topical
application of acetylcholine and subsequently of norepinephrine
is shown in Fig. 3-11 (26).

Under normal circumstances, a tonic level of sympathetic
nerve activity exists to vascular smooth muscle. Vasoconstrictor
responses involve a further increase in vascular smooth
muscle tone and vasodilatation is produced by a withdrawal
of sympathetic tone. This is also illustrated in Fig. 3-11.

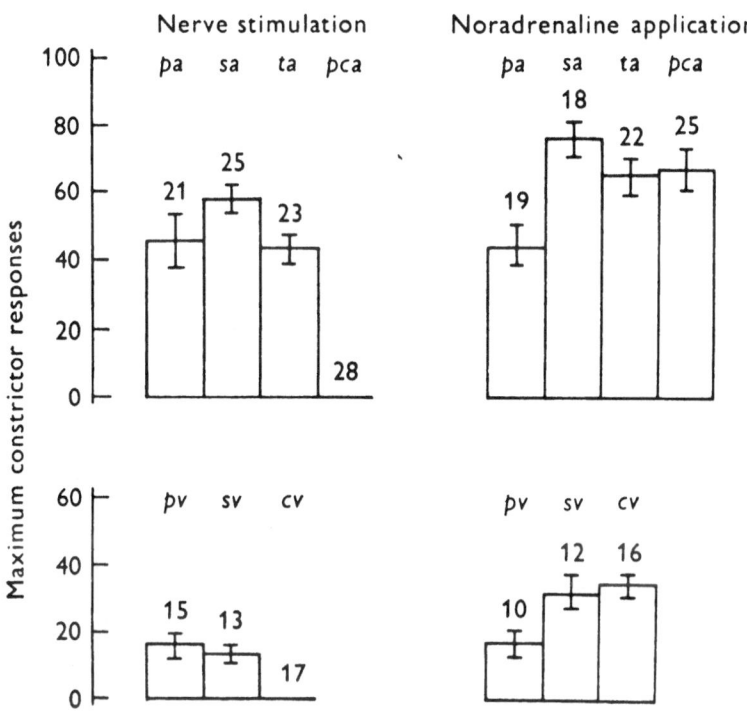

Fig. 3-10: Maximum constrictor responses to perivascular nerve stimulation (1 to 6 Hz) and to topical norepinephrine (10^{-10} to 10^{-5} g/ml). Bars represent $\pm$ 1 SEM. Letters refer to vessel types in Fig. 3-9. Numbers above bars represent the number of vessels of each type studied. Constrictor response was normalized by dividing by the initial control value of diameter (22).

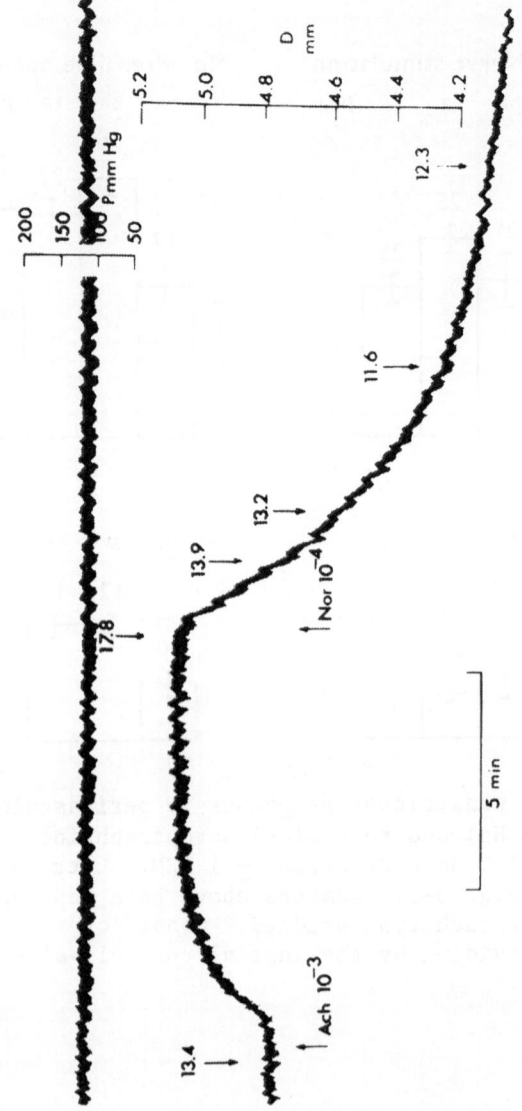

Fig. 3-11: The effects of the topical application of acetylcholine (10^{-3} g/ml) and of norepinephrine (10^{-4}) on the diameter of a canine femoral artery in vivo. Numbers along the diameter response represent values of dynamic elastic modulus in 10^6 dynes/cm^2 (26).

The characteristics described above are generally properties of all arteries in the vascular system.   Quantitative differences may exist between

Properties of   different anatomical locations but
Receptor Sites   the general characteristics are
                                      similar.   This includes sites
within the arterial system which contain specialized receptors that provide afferent information to the central nervous system, i.e., the baroreceptors.   In general, a complex but direct relationship exists between the transmural pressure to which these receptor sites are exposed and the activity of these afferent nerves.   The two principal sites of arterial baroreceptors are the carotid sinus and the aortic arch. These are the sites that have been studied in the most detail as well.   It should be recognized that many other sites exist within the chambers of the heart and the vascular system which contain receptors sensitive to hemodynamic variables (28).

Morphological studies have shown that the receptors in the wall of the carotid sinus and aortic arch are primarily located in the adventitial and medial adventitial border region of the blood vessels. As the blood vessel wall deforms in response to changes in transmural pressure, the receptors respond with a qualitatively equivalent deformation.   The deformation of these receptors is responsible for the production of generator potentials which then summated in the individual axons generates action potentials (29).   It is presumed that a direct relation exists between the deformation of receptors and the deformation of the wall of the blood vessel in which they are situated.   This relationship has not been clearly demonstrated to date experimentally.   As we shall see subsequently there is some question about the nature of this relationship.

Changes in transmural pressure at these baroreceptor sites usually produce changes in nerve activity.   A considerable amount of information exists describing the relationship between receptor site pressure and nerve activity both in individual nerve fibers and in whole nerve bundles.   There are some limitations in evaluating data from whole nerve recordings, however, such as the contribution of individual nerve fibers within a bundle.

Nevertheless, the relationship between nerve activity and
pressure is reasonably well established. An example of the
relationship between pressure
Threshold Pressure and   within the aortic arch and carotid
Saturation Pressure   sinus, and integrated whole nerve
activity is given in Fig. 3-12 (30).
The relationship between nerve activity and pressure has the
following general characteristics: There is a threshold
pressure below which no nerve activity exists. As pressure
is raised above threshold there is a nearly linear relationship
between frequency of nerve activity and transmural pressure.
There is a high pressure value at which nerve activity
saturates at a maximum level. Differences in the threshold
and saturation pressure of different individual receptors
produces a sigmoid curve such as shown in Fig. 3-12 rather
than a curve having distinct sharp changes in nerve activity/
pressure relations. The results shown in Fig. 3-12 indicate
that the threshold pressure for the aortic arch receptors is
higher than that for carotid sinus receptors and that both
receptors appear to saturate at about the same level of
transmural pressure.

The relationship between nerve activity and mean transmural
pressure at the receptor site is a strong function of the
presence of a pulsatile pressure component as shown in Fig. 3-13
(31,32). In general, the nerve activity at a particular
value of pressure above threshold increases monotonically
with the amplitude of a pulsatile pressure component. The
magnitude of the increase, however, decreases with increasing
sinus pressure. At an above saturation pressure there is,
of course, no effect of pulse pressure on nerve activity.
As a consequence of this relationship, an increase in mean
arterial pressure and pulse pressure which often occur
simultaneously produce a more effective reduction of efferent
sympathetic nerve activity.

On the other hand, the aortic arch baroreceptors have
been shown to be essentially unresponsive to pulsatile
pressure (33,34). It is
Baroreceptors Unresponsive   not clear, at the present time,
to Pulsatile Pressure   why the carotid sinus receptors
should be sensitive to pulse
pressure and the aortic arch receptors not. Clearly the
carotid sinus receptors are responding to wall deformation.

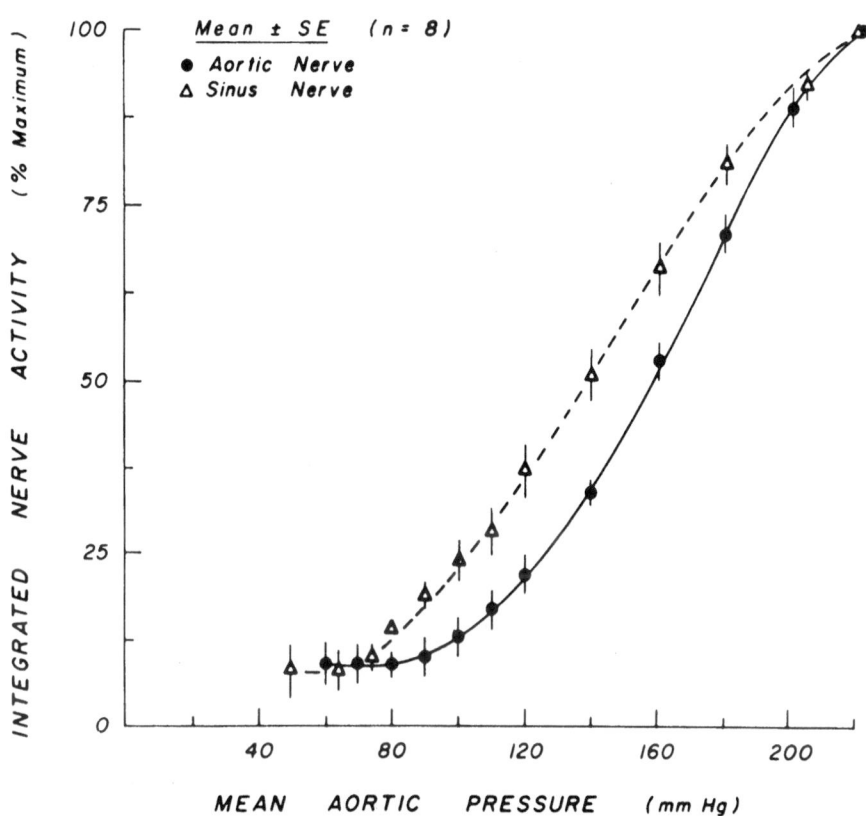

Fig. 3-12: Comparison of integrated nerve activity as a function of arterial pressure from carotid sinus and aortic nerves in the dog (N=8). Threshold pressure was 70 mmHg for the carotid sinus and 100 mmHg for the aortic arch. (30).

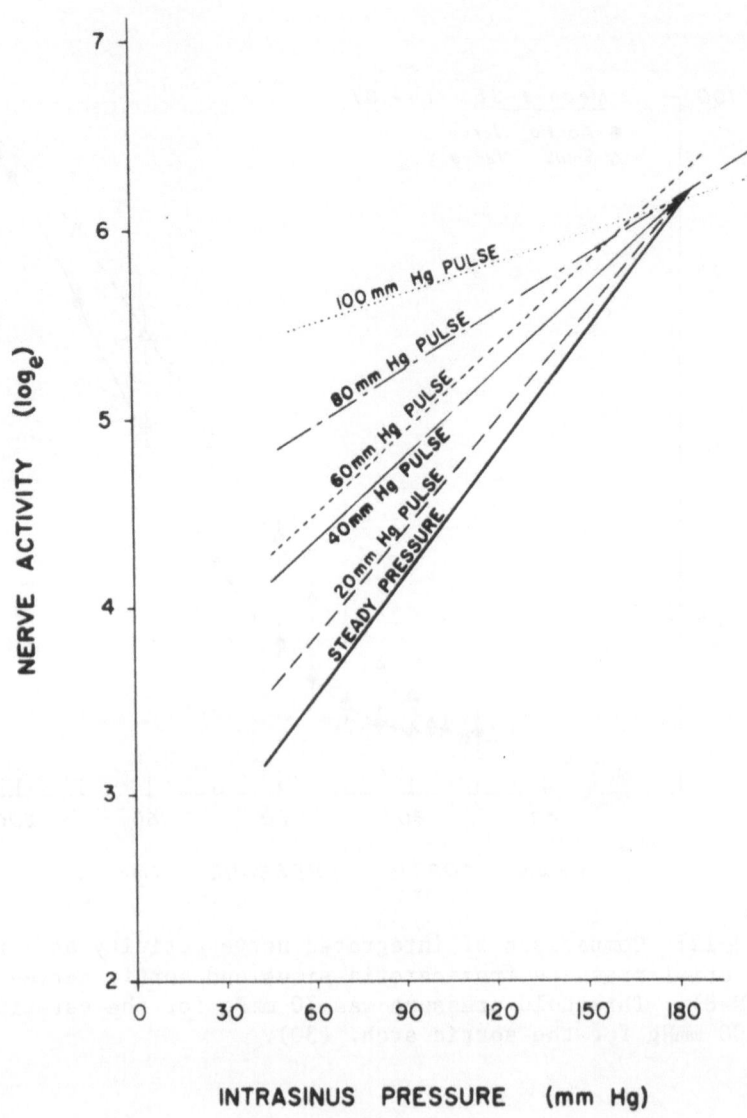

INTRASINUS   PRESSURE   (mm Hg)

Fig. 3-13: Comparison of the response of integrated carotid sinus whole nerve activity to static and dynamic carotid sinus pressure variations. Curves are plotted versus mean intrasinus pressure at a variety of superimposed pulse pressures. (32).

Therefore, the presence of a pulsatile component of pressure should produce an equivalent pulsatile deformation of both the sinus or the aortic arch wall. One would expect both receptor sites to respond in a qualitatively similar fashion to pulsatile pressure variations. This is an area that requires further research to elucidate the reason for this difference if, in fact, one exists.

The response of the carotid sinus wall to mean pressure and to pulse pressure can be explained in terms of the mechanical properties of the carotid sinus or aortic arch per se. The mechanical properties of these two sites possess the same characteristic as arterial sites, i.e., a nonlinear relationship between pressure and diameter (4,35). With increasing transmural pressure, the elastic modulus of the carotid sinus increases as shown in Fig. 3-14 (35). Associated with the increased elastic modulus, a reduction of wall strain occurs associated with a pulsatile pressure of given amplitude. Since nerve activity is directly related to wall strain, the nerve activity associated with a given level of pulse pressure would produce a smaller increment in afferent nerve activity as mean sinus pressure increases. This is, in effect, the result shown in Fig. 3-13. One finds, therefore, that with increasing mean pressure, pulsatile pressure becomes a less effective stimulus of baroreceptor nerve activity.

Responses of Carotid Sinus

DOG

As with other anatomical sites in the arterial system, the carotid sinus and aortic arch also respond to variations in activation of their smooth muscle. The walls of these baroreceptor sites contain postganglionic sympathetic nerve fibers with numerous norepinephrine containing vesicles. It has been shown that in response to efferent sympathetic nerve stimulation and local perfusion with norepinephrine or relaxing agents such as phenoxybenzamine that baroreceptor sites are normally tonically activated and respond to smooth muscle activation (4). At physiological levels of arterial pressure, activation of postganglionic sympathetic nerve fibers to the carotid sinus produces a reduction in carotid sinus diameter and a reduction in dynamic elastic modulus of the carotid sinus (36). Similarly, perfusion of the aortic arch with norepinephrine produces a vasoconstriction in the aortic arch smooth muscle and a reduction in diameter. The infusion of penoxybenzamine produces a relaxation of the smooth muscle and an increase in aortic diameter (4).

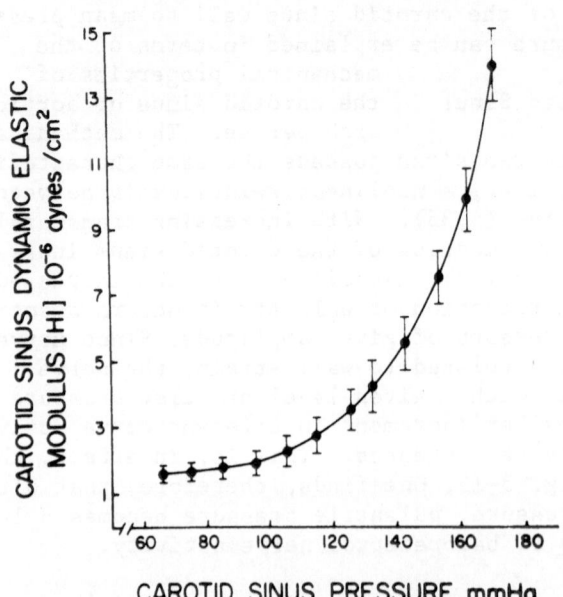

Fig. 3-14: Variation of the dynamic elastic modulus of the canine carotid sinus with carotid sinus perfusion pressure. Points are means and bars ± 1 SEM (N=7) of data averaged at specific values of pressure (35).

Changes in the degree of activation of carotid sinus smooth muscle has significant effects on its reflex responses. The effects of the introduction of norepinephrine into the isolated perfused carotid sinus changes the relationship between mean sinus perfusion pressure and arterial blood pressure as illustrated in Fig. 3-15. This effect is manifest as a shift of this curve downward and to the left with increasing concentration of norepinephrine in the perfusate (37). Since no pressure pulsations were present, the activation of smooth muscle simply reduced the diameter of the carotid sinus. If the receptors in the sinus wall were functionally connected in parallel with connective tissue and smooth muscle elements, a reduction in diameter should have produced a reduction in receptor deformation.

This would have produced a decrease in afferent nerve activity and an increase in arterial pressure. To the contrary, norepinephrine produced a

Norepinephrine Effect   decrease in systemic pressure. This would suggest that afferent nerve activity was increased by the norepinephrine. If the receptors are functionally connected in series with the smooth muscle cells an increased contractile force by smooth muscle in response to norepinephrine could increase receptor deformation and could, therefore increase afferent nerve activity. However, morphological studies indicate that the receptors exist in the adventitia and not in the media of the carotid sinus. One possible explanation is that in addition to its affect of smooth muscle on carotid sinus, norepinephrine may have a direct action on the receptors themselves. This area requires further research in order to elucidate the mechanisms involved in the action of norepinephrine on the carotid sinus wall and on afferent receptor mechanisms.

There are studies in the literature that suggest a physiological role for these properties of receptor site smooth muscle activation. It has been demonstrated that the pressor response to carotid occlusion in the cat is decreased   CAT
if the postganglionic sympathetic fibers to the carotid sinus are stimulated during the occlusion (38). Release of norepinephrine from sympathetic nerve endings activating carotid sinus smooth muscle would decrease both diameter and elastic modulus of the sinus wall (Bagshaw and Peterson, 1972) (36). The pulse pressure in the carotid sinus would then produce an increase in wall strain thereby increasing afferent nerve activity.

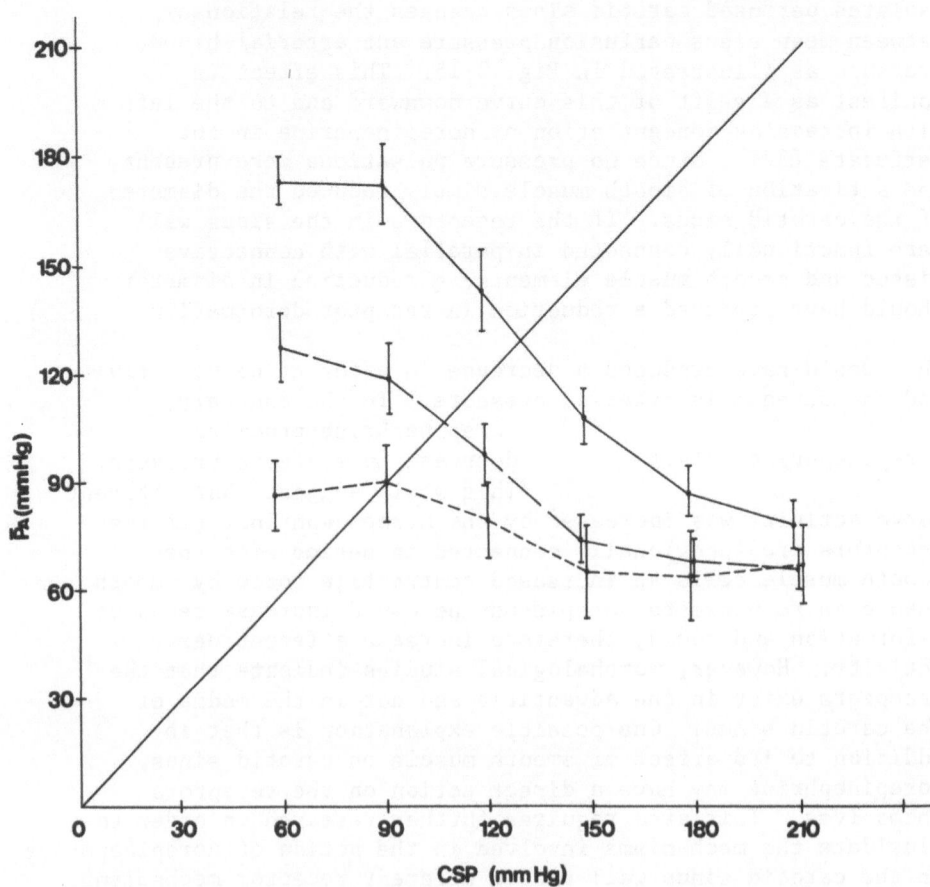

Fig. 3-15: Variation of mean aortic blood pressure (P_a) with
mean carotid sinus perfusion pressure (CSP). The right carotid
sinus was perfused while the left was denervated. The upper
curve shows data for controlled perfusion, the middle curve for
perfusion with 1 u g/ml norepinephrine added and the lower curve
with 5 u g/ml added. The points and bars are means and ± 1 SEM
of data averaged at specific values of carotid sinus perfusion
pressure. The solid line through the origin is the line of
identify, i.e., P_A = CSP.

If norepinephrine also affects the receptors per se, this
sympathetic release of norepinephrine will also directly
activate these receptors and also contribute to an increased
afferent nerve activity. The role played by the sympathetic
innervation of the carotid sinus and aortic arch is not
completely clear at this time but it is possible that this
mechanism acts to increase the sensitivity of these receptor
sites, making them more effective in opposing changes in
arterial pressure.

NEURAL REFLEX CONTROL MECAHNISMS

The reflex responses produced by the carotid sinus
baroreceptor mechanism have been studied using a variety of
direct and indirect techniques.
Carotid Sinus Reflex   These techniques include
Responses   carotid artery occlusion (39)
                            carotid sinus nerve stimulation
(40) carotid or neck counterpressure (41), and perfusion of
the isolated carotid sinuses (42). Obviously, these various
preparations are limited in terms of the information they
provide as well as in their applicability to different
animals including man. I will restrict my comments to
studies made on isolated perfused carotid sinuses in anesthetized
animals.

The isolated perfused carotid sinus preparation originally
developed by Moissejeff (1926) (42) allows for the quantitative
description of the control of systemic hemodynamics by the
carotid sinus in a preparation where changes in systemic
hemodynamics do not affect the carotid sinus pressure, that
is, an open loop preparation. When perfusion pressure in
the isolated carotid sinus is increased, afferent nerve
activity increases. This results in an inhibition of efferent
nerve activity to the various elements of the cardiovascular
system which is nonuniform in terms of its spatial or anatomical
distribution. The net effect is that increasing carotid
sinus perfusion pressure produces a reduction in systemic
arterial pressure. The response of systemic circulation to
increased carotid sinus perfusion pressure is strongly
dependent upon the presence and magnitude of pulsatile
perfusion component increases. Around a given mean carotid
sinus perfusion pressure there is generally a decrease in
systemic resistance as illustrated by the results in Fig. 3-16
(43). That is, carotid sinus perfusion pressure is more
effective in producing systemic hypotension when the amplitude
of pulsatile variation is increased.

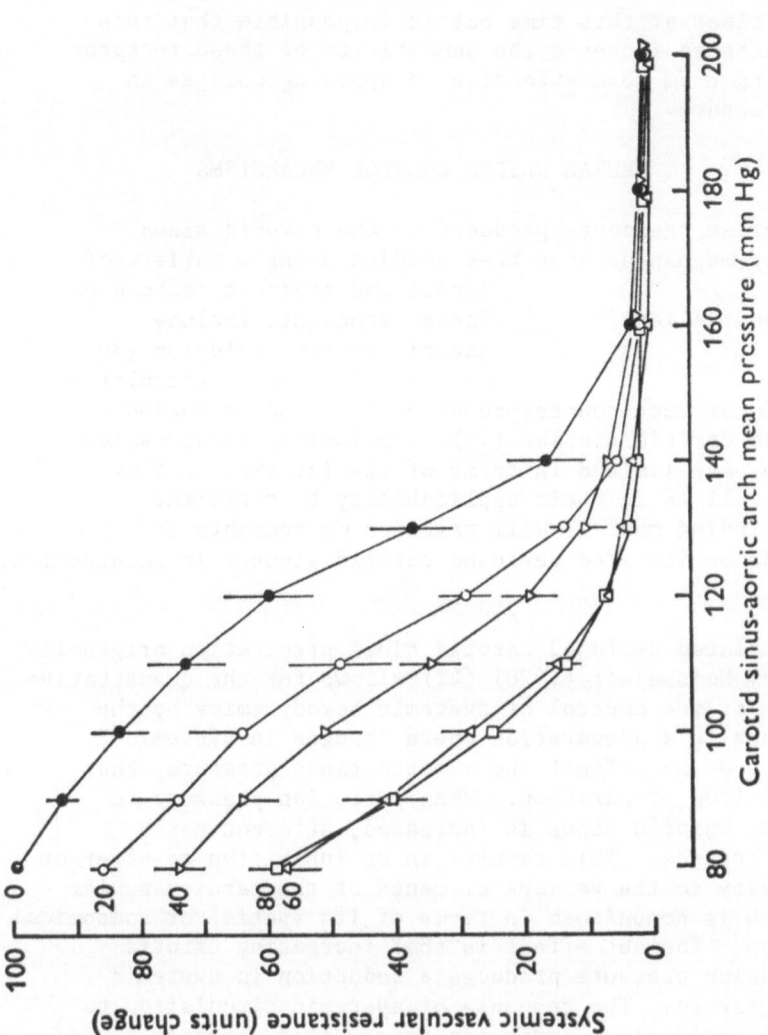

Fig. 3-16: Effects of pulsatile perfusion pressure amplitude on the variation of systemic vascular resistance and pressure in the combined carotid sinus – aortic arch areas. Values of pulse pressure are given along the ordinate axis along each curve. (43).

The relative contribution of the various elements of the cardiovascular system to the reflex control of arterial pressure is extremely nonuniform. The changes in arterial pressure that occur with changes in carotid sinus perfusion pressure are the result of changes in both peripheral resistance and cardiac output as shown in Fig. 3-17. (44,45). With the vagi intact, the aortic arch mechanoreceptors buffer the reflex effects of changes in carotid sinus pressure to some degree. Prior to vagotomy approximately 75% of the change in arterial pressure is the result of changes in peripheral resistance, with the other 25% resulting from changes in cardiac output. Following vagotomy, the contribution of changes in cardiac ouput increases to approximately 35% of the change in arterial pressure. These changes in cardiac output are the result of changes in myocardial contractility as well as changes in preload (left atrial pressure) and afterload (aortic blood pressure) subsequent to changes in carotid sinus perfusion pressure. The results in this figure also illustrate the nonuniform effect of the aortic arch mechanoreceptors on the system circulation. This nonuniform contribution is indicated by the differences in these two curves at given values of carotid sinus pressure. At high carotid sinus pressure the aortic arch afferents have a minor effect. At low values of carotid sinus pressure their effect, on the other hand, is much larger.

The variation in peripheral resistance with carotid sinus pressure is nonuniformly distributed throughout the various vascular beds (45).

Variation in Peripheral Resistance with Carotid Sinus Pressure

A summary of variation of blood flow resistance in the celiac, superior mesenteric, renal and femoral arteries is shown in Fig. 3-18. Following vagotomy, the unmasked effects of carotid sinus baroreceptors is indicated by the closed symbols. The largest variation of regional resistance with carotid sinus perfusion pressure occurs in skeletal muscle (femoral artery). Resistance in the splanchnic circulation and primarily in the celiac artery, on the other hand, is much less sensitive to changes in carotid sinus pressure than the changes in peripheral resistance. This diagram also illustrates the nonuniform contribution of aortic arch baroreceptors to regional resistance control, both at various values of carotid perfusion pressure and in the different vascular beds. The effects of the aortic arch are largest in the mesenteric circulation and smallest in the skeletal muscle. Reasonably large effects also occur in the celiac and renal circulation.

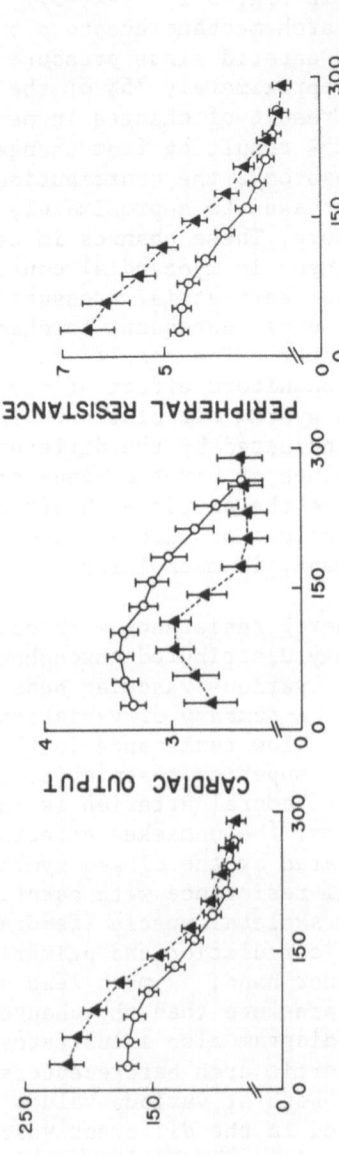

CAROTID SINUS PRESSURE

Fig. 3-17: Variation of mean arterial pressure, cardiac output and peripheral resistance with (mean) perfusion pressure in the isolated perfused carotid sinuses before (open circles) and after (closed triangles) bilateral cervical vagotomy in dogs (N=11). Symbols are means and bars ± 1 SEM of data averaged at specific values of carotid sinus pressure.

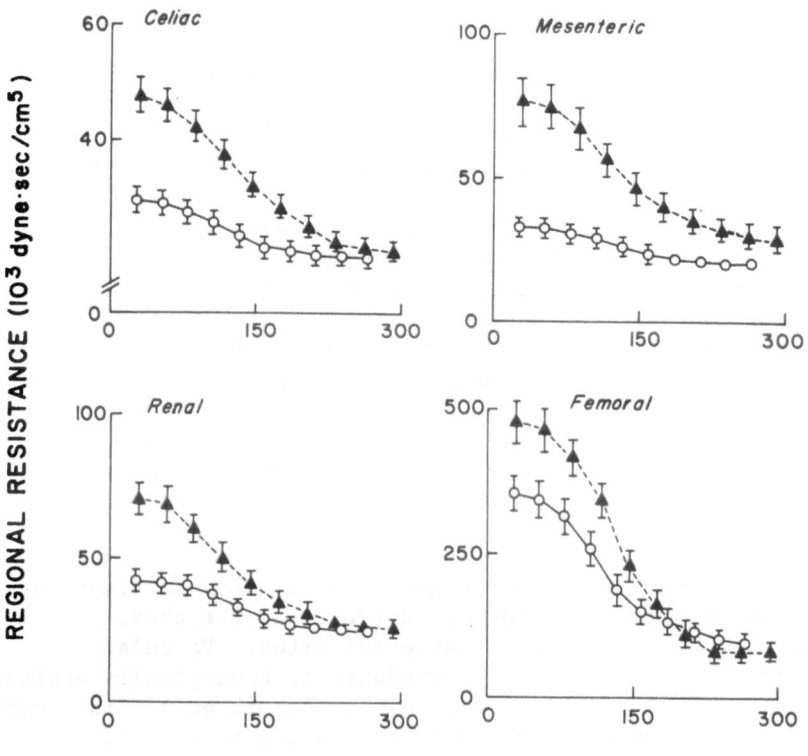

CAROTID SINUS PRESSURE (mmHg)

Fig. 3-18: Variation of regional resistance with mean carotid
sinus perfusion pressure before (open circles) and after
(closed triangles) bilateral cervical vagotomy.

The effects of baroreceptor reflexes on blood flow in
different vascular beds will be the result of the combined
changes in regional resistance and cardiac ouput. As indicated
by the data summarized in Fig. 3-19, significant differences
exist in the changes of regional blood flow with carotid
sinus perfusion pressure. In general, regional blood flow
in the celiac, mesenteric and renal beds remains reasonably
constant with changes in carotid sinus perfusion pressure
after vagotomy. On the other hand, blood flow in the femoral
artery significantly increases with carotid sinus pressure
both before and after vagotomy.

The relative distribution of cardiac output with activation
of carotid sinus afferents has also been demonstrated in a
slightly different manner by a number of investigators. For
example, with carotid sinus hypotension following carotid
occlusion skeletal muscle blood flow generally declines
while splanchnic and renal flow increase (46). In addition,
in response to stimulation of the carotid sinus nerve,
skeletal muscle blood flow increases while splanchnic and
renal flow decrease (40). These responses with an intact
closed loop function of the carotid sinus reflex support the
validity of these data obtained in this open loop preparation.

In addition to determining the effects of the carotid
sinus on regional resistance, we have also performed studies
to assess the effects of carotid sinus reflex on large
vessels (45).

This has been done by determining values of vascular impedance
from pulsatile pressure/flow measurements at the above
arterial sites. Vascular
Impedance   impedance is conceptually analogous
to electrical impedance in a circuit
and represents the ratio of an a.c. pressure to an a.c.
flow. Values of vascular impedance can be determined from
pulsatile pressure and flow using either Fourier series or
time series analysis (47). By such techniques, pulsatile
pressure and flow are resolved into a number of harmonic
components at different frequencies. In this way, a frequency
spectrum of impedance can be determined It has been demonstrated
that the mechanical properties of large arteries close to
the measurement site of pulsatile pressure and flow primarily
contribute to the determination of the high frequency values
of impedance at that site (48). Accordingly, we have used
measurements of vascular impedance to determine the properties
of large vessels from the high frequency portion of the
impedance spectrum.

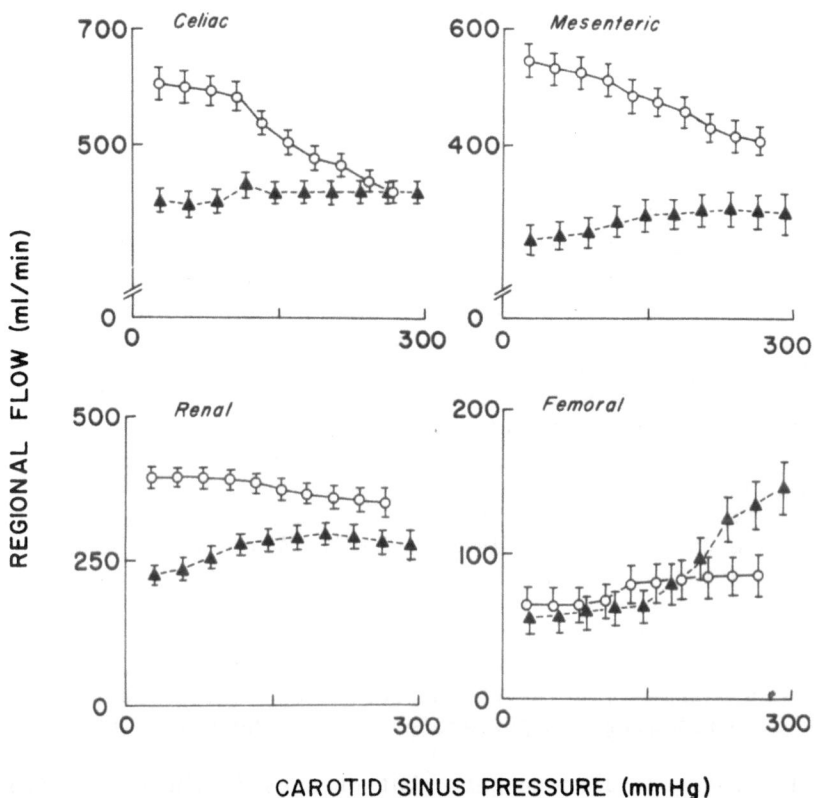

Fig. 3-19: Variation of regional blood flow with carotid sinus perfusion pressure. Symbols are as before.

   The results summarized in Fig. 3-20 (45) show the
variation of impedance spectrum in the ascending aorta,
renal, celiac and femoral arteries at three values of carotid
sinus perfusion pressure before and after vagotomy. At the
more peripheral sites not only is there a downward shift in
the d.c. value of impedance i.e., resistance, with increasing
carotid sinus pressure but also the a.c. portion of the
impedance spectrum is likewise decreased. When high frequency
values of impedance are averaged and plotted as a function
of carotid sinus pressure, results of the form shown in Fig.
3-21 are obtained (45). Associated with the inverse relationship
of regional resistance and carotid sinus pressure is a
similar but quantitatively different variation in regional
impedance. In the femoral artery, the variation of impedance
with carotid sinus pressure is smaller than that of femoral
resistance. On the other hand, the variation in the renal
artery is the same order of magnitude. These results suggest
that values of vascular impedance which once again reflect
the properties and geometry of large vessels are under the
reflex control of the carotid sinus.

   The variations in impedance of the ascending aorta are
considerably different than those of the peripheral vascular
beds. These data are shown in Fig. 3-22. (45). While an
inverse relationship exists between aortic resistance and
carotid sinus pressure, aortic impedance shows a minimum at
normal values of carotid sinus pressure, both before and
after vagotomy. The physiological significance of this
minimum plays some role in the energetics of cardiac contraction,
perhaps by minimizing the pulsatile work of the heart (45).

   While these results suggest that changes in the properties
of large arteries do occur they are certainly not definitive.
However, taken together with the results previously presented
on the effects of efferent sympathetic nerve activity and
catecholamines on the properties of large vessels it seems
reasonable to interpret these results to indicate that
neural reflexes exert a tonic activity on the smooth muscle
in large arteries. Furthermore, this tonic activity does
have a significant hemodynamic effect in large arteries by
virtue of its effect on vascular impedance.

   There have been relatively few studies of the effects
of aortic arch baroreceptors on the reflex control of cardiovascular
                                    function. In general, the results
Aortic Arch Reflexes   have indicated a similar though
                                    quantitatively smaller effect of
aortic arch afferents on the heart and the vascular system.

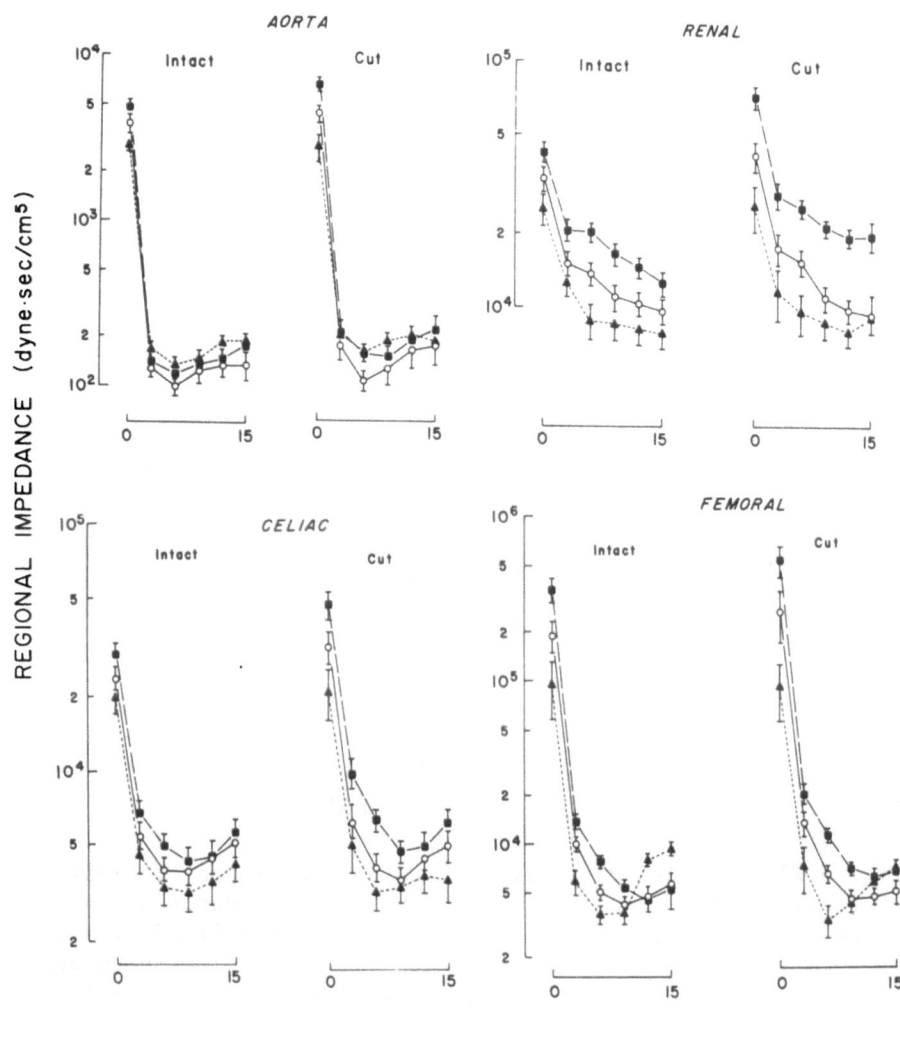

FREQUENCY (Hz)

Fig. 3-20: Regional vascular impedance spectra at four arterial
sites before and after bilateral cervical vagotomy. Data are
given for three values of carotid sinus perfusion pressure:
25 (solid square), 125 (open circles) and 250 mmHg (solid
triangles). Points are means and vertical bars ± 1 SEM. (45).

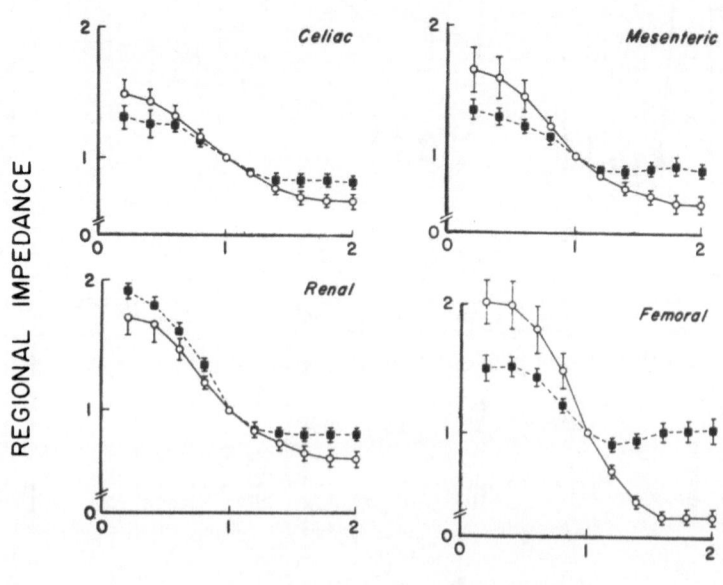

CAROTID SINUS PRESSURE

Fig. 3-21: Variation of regional resistance (open circles) and characteristic impedance (closed squares) with carotid sinus perfusion pressure. The variables are all normalized by dividing by normal control values of each quantity. Vertical bars are ± 1 SEM. Data were obtained after sectioning the cervical vagi. (45).

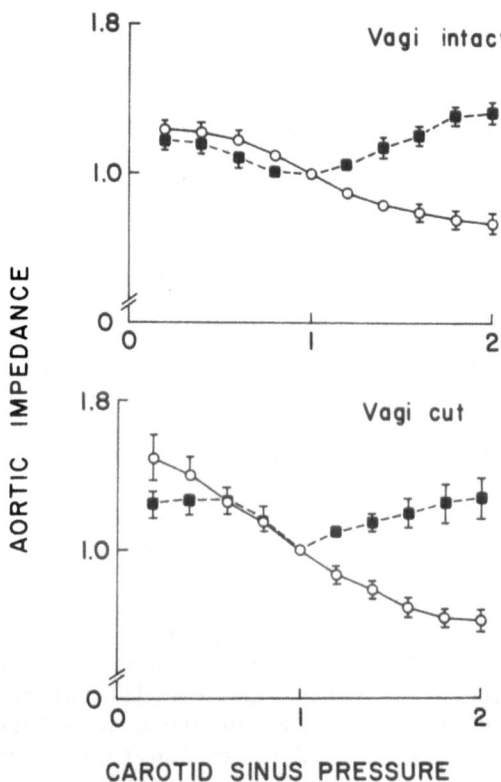

Fig. 3-22: Variation of aortic resistance (open circles) and aortic impedance (closed squares) with carotid sinus perfusion pressure. Variables were normalized as described previously. (45).

As described above in previous sections, there are some
quantitative differences in the afferent characteristics of
aortic arch baroreceptors. Studies using isovolumic contractions
of the isolated left ventricle have demonstrated that the
aortic arch mechanoreceptors do have a significant effect on
the contractility of the left ventricle (49). In addition,
other studies have indicated that the aortic arch receptors
do exert a significant effect on regional resistance at
least in the renal and skeletal muscle circulation (50,51).   In
this control of regional circulations, there is a very
strong interaction between the aortic arch and the carotid
sinus baroreceptor mechanisms. This interaction is exemplified
by the results in Fig. 3-23 (50). This figure compares the
DOG control of the constant flow perfused canine hind limb and
heart rate by these two receptor mechanisms. The effects of
varying aortic arch perfusion pressure on these two variables
is a strong function of the perfusion pressure existing in
the isolated carotid sinuses. When carotid sinus pressure
is high and efferent nerve activity low, limb resistance is
essentially unresponsive to aortic arch perfusion pressure
while heart rate becomes strongly dependent upon the latter.

A number of attempts have also been made to analyze and
represent the interaction between carotid sinus baroreceptors
and other types of receptor mechanisms including chemoreceptors
and cardiopulmonary receptors. Activation of chemoreceptors
by hypoxia and hypercapnia produce an augmentation of vasomotor
reflex responses initiated in the aortic arch, carotid sinus
and cardiopulmonary areas (52,53,54). In addition, changes
in left atrial pressure also produce profound interaction
with carotid sinus induced reflex responses. Increases in
left atrial pressure antagonize the vasodilator response in
the renal and skeletal muscle vasculature associated with
carotid sinus hypertension. Hypotension in the left atrium
considerably augments the reflex vasoconstriction in the
renal and skeletal muscle circulations associated with
carotid hypotension (55). Most of the studies involving the
interaction of baro - and chemoreceptor mechanisms have
involved the constant flow perfusion of isolated vascular
beds such as the limb and the kidney. Such studies are
difficult to interpret because they artificially maintained
regional blood flow at a constant level. In contrast,
reflex alterations in cardiovascular function are associated
with changes in the distribution of cardiac output especially
to skeletal muscle.

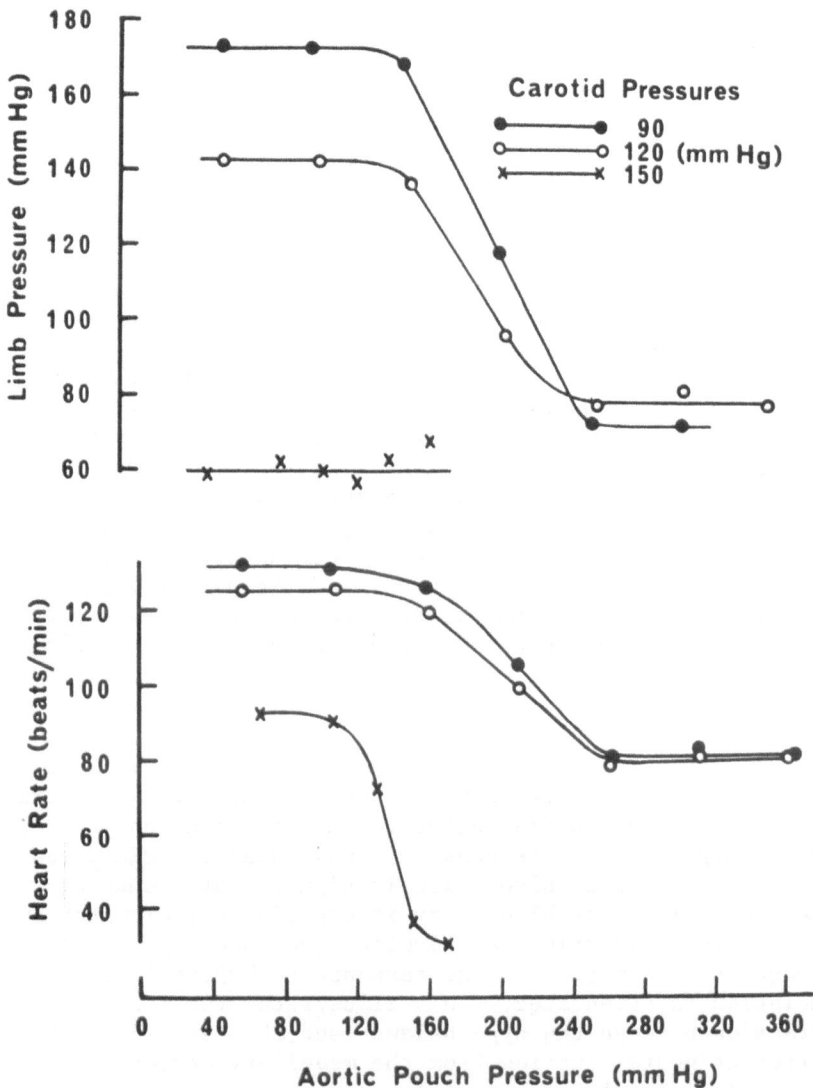

Fig. 3-23: Variation of perfusion pressure in the isolated constant flow perfused canine hindlimb and of heart rate with pressure in the isolated aortic arch at three values of perfusion pressure in the isolated carotid sinus. (50).

The significance and quantitative aspects of the interaction of these reflex mechanisms under conditions in which
blood flow changes occur and are influenced by autoregulatory
responses as well are not clear at this time. This area
certainly represents one in which much more experimental
study is necessary before we understand the physiological
significance and role of these multiple baro- and chemoreceptor reflex mechanisms in the regulation of cardiovascular
function.

It is important to realize that not only does the
function of the carotid sinus baroreceptor mechanisms interact
                                        and depend upon the function
Hypothalamic Interactions   of other peripheral vascular
                                        receptor mechanisms but it is,
in addition, affected by higher central nervous system
structures. One in particular, the so-called hypothalamic
defense response has a significant effect on the regulatory
function of the peripheral circulation produced by the
carotid sinus (56). Stimulation of specific areas in the
hypothalamus produce cardiovascular responses which are
similar to those occuring in stress and exercise (57). It
is for this reason that the interaction between this hypothalamic
defense area and the medullary cardiovascular centers is of
importance. The data in Fig. 3-24 illustrate the cardiovascular
responses to hypothalamic defense area stimulation at different
levels of perfusion pressure in the isolated carotid sinuses
(57). At low levels of carotid sinus pressure in particular,
stimulation of the hypothalamus produces increases in arterial
blood pressure and cardiac output. The distribution of
cardiac output and the response of individual vascular beds
is nonuniform. Renal blood flow is significantly reduced
while skeletal muscle blood flow is considerably elevated by
hypothalamic stimulation. As carotid sinus pressure is
increased the magnitude of the response to hypothalamic
stimulation is attenuated. This illustrates the strong
interaction between the hypothalamus and the carotid sinus
on efferent neural outflow from the medullary centers. At
physiological levels of arterial pressure the responses
produced by hypothalamic stimulation mimic those that occur
in stress and exercise in man and experimental animals.

While the above quantitative description of the carotid
sinus reflex is based primarily upon animal experiments, the
                                        function of this control
Comparative Aspects of   mechanism is at least qualitatively
Neural Control   similar in man. There are very
                                        few quantitative studies in man
that can be used for comparison with experimental animal results

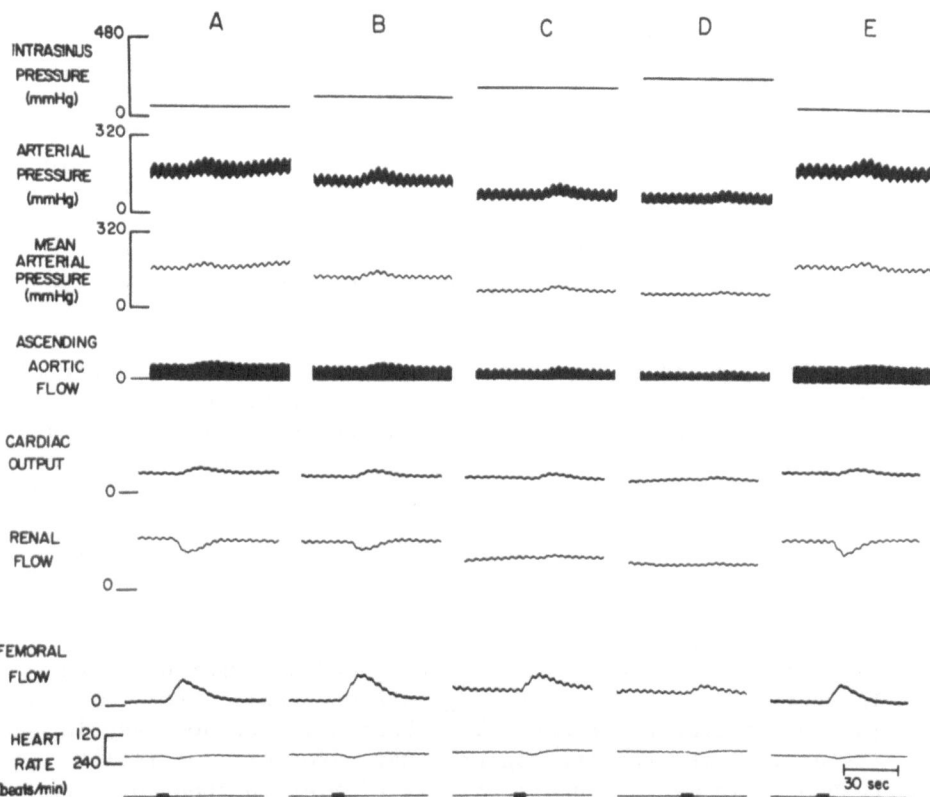

Fig. 3-24: Cardiovascular response to hypothalamic stimulation at four values of carotid sinus perfusion pressure. Duration of stimulation is indicated by the dark bars at the bottom of the figure. Values of carotid sinus pressure were 60 (A and E), 120 (B), 180 (C) and 240 (D) mmHg. (57).

for obvious reasons. There are data from two types of
DOG experiments, however, that can be compared. The first is
the effects of vasoactive drugs on heart period and arterial
pressure, and the second is the effects of carotid sinus
nerve stimulation. Both of these maneuvers have been performed
in unanesthetized dog and man.

The reflex increase in heart period in response to the
hypertension following the intravenous infusion of phenylephrine
has been used as an index of baroreceptor sensitivity (58).
In normal supine humans, Bristow, et al. (59) found the
relation between heart period and diastolic blood pressure
during phenylephrine injection (IV) to be linear with a slope
HUMAN of 16.7 $\pm$ 1.9 msec/mmHg, Higgins, et al. (60) performed
DOG similar studies in conscious dogs and found a slope of 22.4
$\pm$ 2.3 msec/mmHg in normal animals. While the slope for
dogs is higher than for man, the difference is not statistically
significant.

In response to carotid sinus nerve stimulation, arterial
pressure and peripheral resistance both decrease. In man
these decreases averaged 23% and 16% respectively (61). In
the dog, these decreases were similar at 28% and 29%, respectively
HUMAN (40). Cardiac output was decreased significantly in man (by
DOG 8%) but unchanged in the dog. Forearm vascular resistance
decreased by 16% in man during carotid sinus nerve stimulation
as compared to 62% in the canine hindlimb. Heart rate is
significantly reduced in man (9%) but unchanged in dog
following a brief, transient decline. During exercise,
carotid sinus nerve stimulation produced a larger decrease
in arterial pressure in the dog (31% vs. 16%). Skeletal
muscle vascular resistance also shows a larger decrease in
the dog. These results suggest that carotid sinus reflex
responses in man are qualitatively similar to those of the
canine, with some quantitative differences.

The characteristics of the carotid sinus reflex described
above are those of the normal, healthy subject. Pathological
conditions are associated with
Pathological Changes in the   substantial changes in the
Carotid Sinus Reflex   characteristics of this reflex
mechanism. Perhaps the best
known of these changes is the baroreceptor resetting associated
with arterial hypertension (62).

The afferent properties of the baroreceptor areas (carotid sinus and aortic arch) are reset in established hypertension in such a fashion that a higher transmural pressure is necessary to produce a given level of afferent nerve activity (62,63). Resetting usually involves a shift of the nerve activity transmural pressure curve to the right. A decreased receptor sensitivity (i.e., slope) and an increased threshold pressure are usually observed in such conditions.

Similar changes in arterial baroreceptor properties have been reported in experimental atherosclerosis (64) and Vitamin D sclerosis (65). Aortic baroreceptor resetting, decreased sensitivity and increased threshold have all been described. A reduction in the distensibility of the receptor areas has been suggested as at least a primary cause of these observations.

A decrease in the baroreceptor reflex responses in experimental heart failure in the dog has also been reported (60). In this study, baroreceptor sensitivity was determined from the phenylephrine induced heart period-arterial pressure relation, and from bilateral carotid occlusion (carotid sinus hypertension) responses. Similar conclusions have been reached concerning the effects of heart disease in man. The precise mechanism(s) responsible for this observation is not known at this time.

Studies of changes in baroreceptor sensitivity in man and rat have shown a decrease associated with aging. These demonstrations have been made using the heart period-arterial pressure relation following phenylephrine (66,67). We have also compared baroreceptor reflexes in young and old dogs using the isolated perfused carotid sinus preparation. Data showing the variation of mean arterial pressure and peripheral resistance with carotid sinus pressure are shown in Fig. 3-25 (68). These results show that if anything, carotid sinus control of these two variables is more sensitive in the older animals. A question therefore exists concerning the validity of the heart period arterial pressure relation as a general measure of baroreceptor sensitivity.

Changes in Baroreceptor Sensitivity Associated with Aging

HUMAN

RAT

DOG

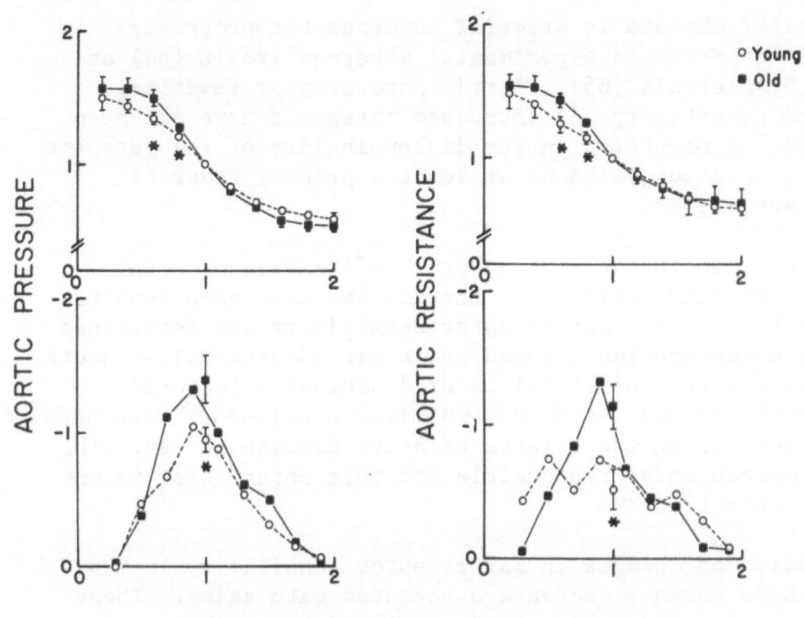

NORMALIZED CAROTID SINUS PRESSURE

Fig. 3-25: Variations in mean arterial pressure and peripheral
resistance with changes in carotid sinus pressure in the dog.

Significant changes occur in the distribution of cardiac output to fulfill temporal variations in the requirements of the regional circulations in a variety of normal and abnormal states. As shown above, an increase in carotid sinus pressure produces a redistribution of cardiac output with blood flow decreasing in the renal and hepatosplanchnic areas, and increasing to the extremities or skeletal muscle. This pattern of blood flow changes is identical to those reported in pressor responses to carotid sinus nerve stimulation in the dog (40) to hypothalamic defense area stimulation (69), to acute emotional stress (70,71), to central sciatic nerve stimulation (72) and to intravenous norepinephrine infusion (73). Also, a similar pattern of blood flow redistribution occurs in moderate exercise in the dog which is associated with an elevation in arterial pressure (74). Finally, essential hypertension in man is also associated with the same change in blood flow distribution compared with normal man (75). In the case of acute, compensated stage of hemorrhagic shock in the dog, the exact opposite blood flow response has been reported (76).

Carotid Sinus and Blood Flow Distribution

Therefore, it appears that the distribution of cardiac output is strongly influenced by neural control mechanisms. These mechanisms can be viewed as representing the first line of control of the peripheral circulation. Obviously, other factors (such as hormonal, metabolic, etc.) interact with neural mechanisms to determine the overall response in a particular circumstance. However, the carotid sinus reflexes are more than simply blood pressure controllers.

HORMONAL CONTROL MECHANISMS

There are a large number of hormonal and chemical agents within the body which have significant effects upon the cardiovascular system. Since it is not possible to deal with all of these agents at this time, this discussion will concentrate on only two of them; angiotensin and vasopressin. These two hormonal agents have significant pressor effects on the vascular system. These effects are mediated in several ways and have a nonuniform effect on different elements of the cardiovascular system.

Angiotensin is formed in blood through the action of an
enzyme on a normally circulating plasma substrate. Through
a series of steps on octapeptide
Angiotensin   angiotensin II is formed in
plasma. The enzyme responsible
for the conversion of the inactive precursor to the active
angiotensin II is renin. Renin is released from the kidney
by a variety of mechanisms including a reduction in renal
perfusion pressure, increased renal sympathetic nerve activity,
circulating catecholamines, and reduced sodium delivery to
the distal nephron in the kidney (77).

Once angiotensin is formed by the action of renin, the
hormone circulates to all parts of the cardiovascular system
where it has profound effects both on the heart and on
vascular smooth muscle (78). The action of angiotensin on
the cardiovascular system is mediated in several ways.
Angiotensin has a direct action on the membrane of cardiac
and vascular smooth muscle. In addition, angiotensin potentiates
the action of circulating catecholamines on these two structures
as well. Angiotensin also has a stimulatory action on
sympathetic ganglia. The effects of angiotensin on the heart
are diverse with a net effect resulting from the direct
action of angiotensin on cardiac muscle and its indirect
effects mediated through changes in arterial pressure and
venous pressure. In the intact animal, low doses of angiotensin
generally have no effect on cardiac output. At high doses,
however, cardiac output is generally decreased in response
to angiotensin which is primarily the result of the increased
afterload, that is, arterial blood pressure.

On the peripheral circulation, angiotensin has a diverse
action. Blood flow in almost all vascular beds is decreased
in response to low and high doses of infused angiotensin
(79). As a fraction of cardiac output, however, blood flow
to skeletal muscle and bone are significantly increased
during angiotensin infusion. Renal, skin and splanchnic
blood flow response to angiotensin is qualitatively similar
to that produced by the carotid sinus baroreceptor mechanisms
described above. As a result, the total effect of circulating
angiotensin on blood flow distribution depends in part on
the action of the changes in cardiac output that accompany
changes in angiotensin concentration in plasma. In addition
to its effect on small blood vessels, angiotensin has a
direct vasoconstrictor action on large vessels such as the
femoral artery. Again, this action is the combined effect
of the direct action of angiotensin on the muscle as well as
a facilitation of the effects of norepinephrine.

Vasopressin is a peptide hormone released from the posterior pituitary gland. It is released in response to decreased extracellular fluid

Vasopressin   volume, reduced arterial blood

pressure, increased plasma osmotic pressure, and other stimuli such as pain, stress and exercise (80). Hemorrhage is a very potent stimulus for the release of pituitary vasopressin. In addition to its action on the kidney where it promotes water retention, vasopressin also has a significant action on the cardiovascular system. When infused intraarterially at physiological concentrations, vasopressin increases arterial blood pressure and peripheral resistance in a dose dependent manner. In addition, right atrial pressure is usually increased by vasopressin administration. Cardiac output generally decreases with the intravenous infusion of vasopressin primarily as a result of an increase in cardiac afterload (81). The action of vasopressin on the peripheral circulation is once again relatively nonhomogeneous. In general, the fraction of cardiac output delivered to the mesenteric and renal circulations increases whereas iliac artery blood flow decreases as a fraction of cardiac output. In absolute terms, all these regional blood flows decrease significantly in response to vasopressin.

Although both of these agents, angiotensin and vasopressin have significant actions on the cardiovascular system, their role in normal maintenance of blood pressure is not established. In the case of angiotensin there is no evidence that angiotensin contributes to the maintenance of arterial blood pressure in the normal person. Studies which have employed the use of angiotensin blocking agents or converting enzyme inhibitors have illustrated that no significant effect on arterial blood pressure occurs in normal man. While vasopressin certainly has an effect on circulating blood volume by virtue of its action on the handling of water by the kidney there is no evidence to suggest that it plays a significant role in the regulation of the distribution of cardiac output or of cardiac output, per se. Vasopressin is primarily involved in the regulation of blood volume.

PATHOGENIC SIGNIFICANCE OF CONTROL MECHANISM

From the above discussion, it should be apparent that neurohumoral factors exert a significant degree of control over arterial blood flow as well as the mechanical properties of large arteries. What is the significance of this control in the function of larger arteries as related to atherogenesis?

It is only possible to provide some speculation on possible
answers to this question. By virtue of their action on
contractile proteins, neurohumoral factors can and/or could
effect the following: a) arterial geometry, b) arterial wall
mechanics, c) vasa vasorum function, and d) endothelial
permeability.

Changes in arterial wall diameter in response to neurohumoral
signals can be substantial. The limited information available
in the literature suggests that
Effects on Wall   small changes in wall geometry can
Shear Stress   produce significant changes in wall
                         shear stress, by virtue of its
effects on blood velocity profile at the wall (82,83).
Changes in wall shear stress could occur as a result of
reflex adjustments in wall geometry, blood flow rate and
cardiac frequency. All of these factors can effect the
velocity gradient at the blood-wall interface, and therefore
wall shear stress. A direct link between wall shear stress
and atherogenesis has been suggested by several investigators
(84,85).

Neurohumoral control factors also modify the arterial
wall mechanical properties. The strain energy density
stored within the arterial wall depends upon its stress-
strain relations, i.e., its mechanical properties. Activation
of smooth muscle in large arteries produces an increase in
the strain energy density in the physiological pressure
range. Fry (86) has hypothesized that an increase in the
strain energy density of the arterial wall can facilitate
macromolecular transport across the endothelium. Again,
this provides a direct link with a proposed atherogenic
mechanism.

The outer layers of the media and the adventitia of
large to medium sized arteries have a vascular supply from
                         the vasa vasorum. This
Possible Role of   microcirculatory network has
Vasa Vasorum   been described as having
                         characteristics of small blood
vessels elsewhere, including its own "wall" containing
innervated smooth muscle. Do the vasa vasorum participate
in neurohumoral control? Specifically, is blood flow in the
vasa vasorum affected by neurohumoral agents? I am not
aware of any evidence in the literature on this subject.
Yet, the vasa vasorum has been suggested to play a role in
atherogenesis (87,88), especially in the relation between
hypertension and atherosclerosis (89).

The role of the vasa vasorum in the normal function of the arterial wall is not completely understood, nor is its relation to the arterial pathology. Much more work is needed in this area to clarify these relationships.

Recent studies have shown that the endothelial cells of large arteries contain the contractile proteins actin and myocin as well as the regulatory proteins, tropomyosin and troponin (90). It has been suggested that activation of these contractile proteins by angiotensin, epinephrine, cholesterol, prostaglandin E, and serum triglycerides produces an increase in endothelial permeability and the influx of macromolecules (91,92). Thus, another potential link exists between neurohumoral factors and atherogenesis in the contraction of endothelial cells. It should be pointed out that while this phenomenon is controversial, critical experiments remain to be performed. Thus, while endothelial cells contain contractile material, it has not been demonstrated to date that the myosin possesses ATPase activity. Furthermore, it has not been demonstrated that these agents have actions on endothelial cells per se, or on interendothelial cell junctions.

These speculations indicate that several important effects of neurohumoral agents exist on the arterial wall and various determinants of its function. Thus, neurohumoral factors may play an important modifying role in the response of the arterial wall to its environmental state and in particular to the events initiating atherosclerosis.

DR. DEWEY: One of the interesting questions that comes up with regard to the carotid sinus control is that the control arising from changes in configuration of the arterial wall could change as the properties of the carotid sinus itself change. For example during the course of disease. I could imagine that in a calcific artery the amount of stretch which would activate the nerves in the carotid sinus would change quite dramatically from the normal giving false signals to the regulatory functions of the body.

DR. COX: That is quite correct. There is very little information in the literature about this subject especially with regard to man. There are, however, at least three conditions which have been identified, associated with changes in baroreceptor function - one, of course, is hypertension and I am sure we are all very familiar with baroreceptor resetting in both experimental and natural forms of hypertension.

But recently Jennifer Angell-James has demonstrated that in
experimental atherosclerosis (64) and Vitamin D sclerosis
RABBIT (65) in the rabbit there are changes in aortic arch baroreceptor
afferent function. I stress afferent function because that
is as far as she went. She was able to show that there are
shifts in the relationship between nerve activity and pressure
within the aortic arch. Basically, the shift is in such a
fashion as to reduce the sensitivity of the aortic arch
baroreceptors. At a given level of transmural pressure
there is a smaller nerve activity so that one would expect
an increased arterial pressure. In the case of the experimental
atherosclerosis study, she did find an elevation of arterial
pressure in these animals over the controls, so there is at
least some evidence that altered baroreceptor function
exists in atherosclerosis. I don't really know of any
direct evidence of the effects of arterial wall pathology on
carotid sinus reflex in man other than that which can be
inferred from indirect information. I don't know any information
on the carotid sinus reflex in atherosclerosis, although
that may change next year.

     DR. CARO: I would like to comment that there is
strong evidence that the endothelial cells provide an important
resistance for the transport of macromolecules between the
blood and the artery wall, and suggest evidence that deformation
of them in some way enchances that transport. The important
point in the present context is that a decreased distensibility of the artery wall will diminish the deformation
suffered by the endothelial cells; their deformation will
largely become that due to shearing stress.

     DR. SCHWARTZ: I wonder if Dr. Cox would speculate on
the possible clinical implications of a non-deformable or
rigid carotid sinus. What intrigues me specifically is the
possible role that loss of the baroreceptor mechanism might
have in submitting the intercerebral circulation to a very
high peak of systolic ejection pressures. Could such peak
pressure be important in the development of cerebrovascular
disease, and, in particular, intercerebral hemorrhage?

     DR. COX: With regard to the control of blood pressure
there is no doubt that changes associated with atherosclerosis
will be of significance. There was a paper by Heath et al.,
(93) who showed some information on the morphology of
the human carotid sinus in atherosclerosis and there were
certainly some very impressive looking lesions in the carotid
sinus.

Winson et al., (94) studied force-length relations of
strips of carotid sinus from normal and from atherosclerotic
individuals. There is a very
What Sets Arterial Pressure   definite increase in stiffness in
the latter. There is no doubt
that it is going to effect carotid sinus reflex control of
blood pressure. Fortunately for us there is considerable
redundancy in neural control mechanisms. My feeling would
be that if the carotid sinus were the only site of disease,
the other arterial mechanoreceptor sites would have the
capacity to regulate arterial pressure. Probably the individuals
would lose their ability to minimize fluctuation in arterial
pressure so that a given degree of activity would produce
much larger arterial pressure responses. For example,
exercise, orthostatic changes or what have you. The other
interesting thing is this whole idea of baroreceptors resetting.
If baroreceptors can reset with chronic alterations either
in pressure or chronic alterations in mechanical properties
of the wall of the receptors, then what is it that determines
arterial blood pressure? Mechanoreceptors are really following
the lead of this controller which sets the level of arterial
pressure. Engineers like to think of control systems in
terms of a set point and if we translate this to man, we
think of something in the brain that determines blood pressure
and it is the dial on the temperature control in a room, or
it is the speedometer on the automobile. We don't know the
analogous function of the body that sets arterial pressure.

DR. CHIEN: How were the impedence measurements made?
What was the method?

DR. COX: Blood flow was measured with electromagnetic
flow meter and pulsatile pressures were recorded with strain-
gauge manometers. The pressure and flow data were subjected
to time series analysis, Fourier series. From Fourier
series analysis you get a series of harmonics at integral
multiples of the heart rate. For each of these multiples,
we take the ratio of pressure and flow and use that information
to compute impedance.

DR. CHIEN: The other question is, if there is any
separation of flow in the carotid sinus as Dr. Dewey showed
yesterday in the model, how would this affect the baroreceptor
reflex?

DR. COX: Our experiments were performed using a low
flow. It is creeping flow so that there is no separation.

As far as the physiological question is concerned in vivo
there is no information available on flow separation in the
carotid sinus. One of the things that I did not mention is
that the carotid sinus nerve activity is not only sensitive
to changes in diameter of the sinus wall, but also to longitudinal
deformation of the sinus as well. One could certainly
visualize the formation of an atherosclerotic plaque on the
free border of the sinus producing a very severe restraint
to the longitudinal motion of the wall.

This would certainly have an effect on the carotid sinus
reflex. Basically, it would reduce sensitivity because it
will not allow for longitudinal deformation to activate the
nerve endings, and there would be a smaller amount of afferent
nerve activity for a given arterial pressure pulse.

DR. KENYON: In terms of long term pressure regulation,
a stiff carotid sinus means the stretch activity of the cell
is diminished...What role do you see for kidney pressure
regulation in terms of it being able to overcome the deficiency
in the carotid sinus?

DR. COX: This is one of the arguments of the Guytonian
school. Alan Cowley in Arthur Guyton's group has demonstrated
that you can denervate the carotid sinuses, you can cut the
aortic arch afferent nerves, and you don't produce very
large changes in arterial blood pressure (95). If you
average pressure over 24 hours, you get essentially normal
values of arterial pressure. In other words, you do not get
neurogenic hypertension. What you do get is a very unstable
animal and any kind of perturbation produces very wide
fluctuations in arterial pressure, but the mean over 24
hours is pretty much unchanged. What basically they say,
therefore, is that there are other factors that regulate the
arterial pressure and I think, this group would say it is
the venous return. The latter is primarily determined by
extracellular fluid volume and that is in part one of the
functions of the kidney. I think I will shield my own prejudice
and not go any further on this question.

DR. MALLIANI: This first comment I would like to make
concerns the classic scheme of the neural control of the
circulation to which you referred. In an interdisciplinary
meeting like this one, I think that it should be clearly
pointed out that such a scheme, although useful for some
operational purposes, reflects a great deal of oversimplification.

This has been amply demonstrated in recent years. For
instance, in the case of the neural reflex mechanisms contributing
to the hypertensive state, the problem has been mainly
studied from the point of view of resetting of baroreceptive
reflexes. However, we know from very recent work of Mancia
et al., (96) that hypertensive patients do not necessarily
have a reduced efficiency of the baroreflexes with regard to
blood pressure control. Indeed, I believe that additional
spinal sympathetic reflexes, of which I shall speak may have
a relevant importance. Another point concerns in general
the variability of properties of cardiovascular receptors.

For example, the experiments of Recordati and co-workers
have recently confirmed that vagal atrial receptors of type
A and B can profoundly
Two Types of Atrial   modify their firing characteristics
Receptors   under difficult experimental
                                    states (changes in atrial loads,
in inotropic states, etc.). However, it seems that atrial
receptors of type B mainly signal static and dynamic changes
in atrial wall passive tension (97) while type A atrial
receptors appear to be mainly influenced by the active
tension developed by atrial muscle during contraction (98).
Thus, in conclusion, it is likely that any given receptor as
a sensor covers a wide spectrum of possibilities for detecting
the static and the dynamic components of mechanical stimuli.

DR. COX: I would agree with most of what you said. I
am not sure that I completely agree with the separation of
atrial receptors into types for the following reasons.
These receptors are mechanoreceptors and originally investigators
tried to relate their afferent activity to atrial pressure
changes. You have to remember that there are changes in the
deformation of the atrium other than those associated with
atrial pressure changes alone, for example, with movement of
the heart and of the great veins. So one has to be careful.
There is in fact a recent paper by Armour from Loyola (99)
in which he showed that even the receptors that appear to
possess higher afferent activity in diastole were responding
to deformation. He could probe around the atrium mechanically
until he found the receptor site and show by pushing on it
that it would respond. Again, this is a complex business
and that is not exactly a physiological demonstration of
control.

DR. STONE: The topic under discussion is the dynamics
of arterial flow which includes the fluid and mechanical
properties of the flowing medium and the vessel wall.

In the approach to this problem it is important to consider the dynamic properties of the vessels as influenced by the autonomic nervous system. In some physiological textbooks, (100) the pressure-volume characteristics of various vascular segments are shown to be influenced by the presence of catecholamines. The pressure at any volume has been found to be larger in both arteries and veins in the presence of the catecholamines. This would imply that the vessel has become stiffer by the action of the agent on either the smooth muscle cells or the matrix of the vessel. The catecholamine norepinephrine is felt to be the primary transmitter released by most of the sympathetic nervous system efferent terminals. Norepinephrine has also been shown to reduce the elastic modulus of blood vessel by Dobrin (101) and McDonald (102) and to influence the velocity of wave-propagation. The latter factors will impact on the fluid mechanics of the circulatory system. The effect of the autonomic nervous system on the dynamics of arterial flow must be considered. The cerebral and coronary circuits are of particular interest in this regard

Role of Autonomic
Nervous System

since only in recent years has information concerning the role of the autonomic nervous system in control of these circuits become available.

      Early studies by Penfield (103) and Chorobski and Penfield (104) demonstrated the presence of a dense nerve apparatus surrounding the large cerebral vessels. These authors found through nerve degeneration studies

Cerebral Circulation

that the nerves originated in the vicinity of the carotid artery as the artery enters the cranium. At this time the authors could not make a distinction between the nerves as to whether the nerves were part of the sympathetic or parasympathetic nervous system. Subsequently several authors (105,106,107) have shown that the sympathetic nervous system innervates the major cerebral vessels to at least the size of pial arteries (40-100 u dia.). These nerves form a rich ground plexus in the adventitia of the vessels and terminate in the tunica media of the vessel wall. In the monkey, a very consistent pattern of distribution of the postganglionic sympathetic fibers was apparent. The basilar, middle cerebral and anterior cerebial arteries were more densely innervated than the posterior cerebral and vertebral arteries. An example of the sympathetic postganglionic fiber can be seen in Fig. 3-26. The cerebral vessel was stretched on to a glass slide and exposed to paraformaldehyde vapor causing the catecholamine in the nerves and vesicles to produce a fluorescence when properly excited.

MONKEY

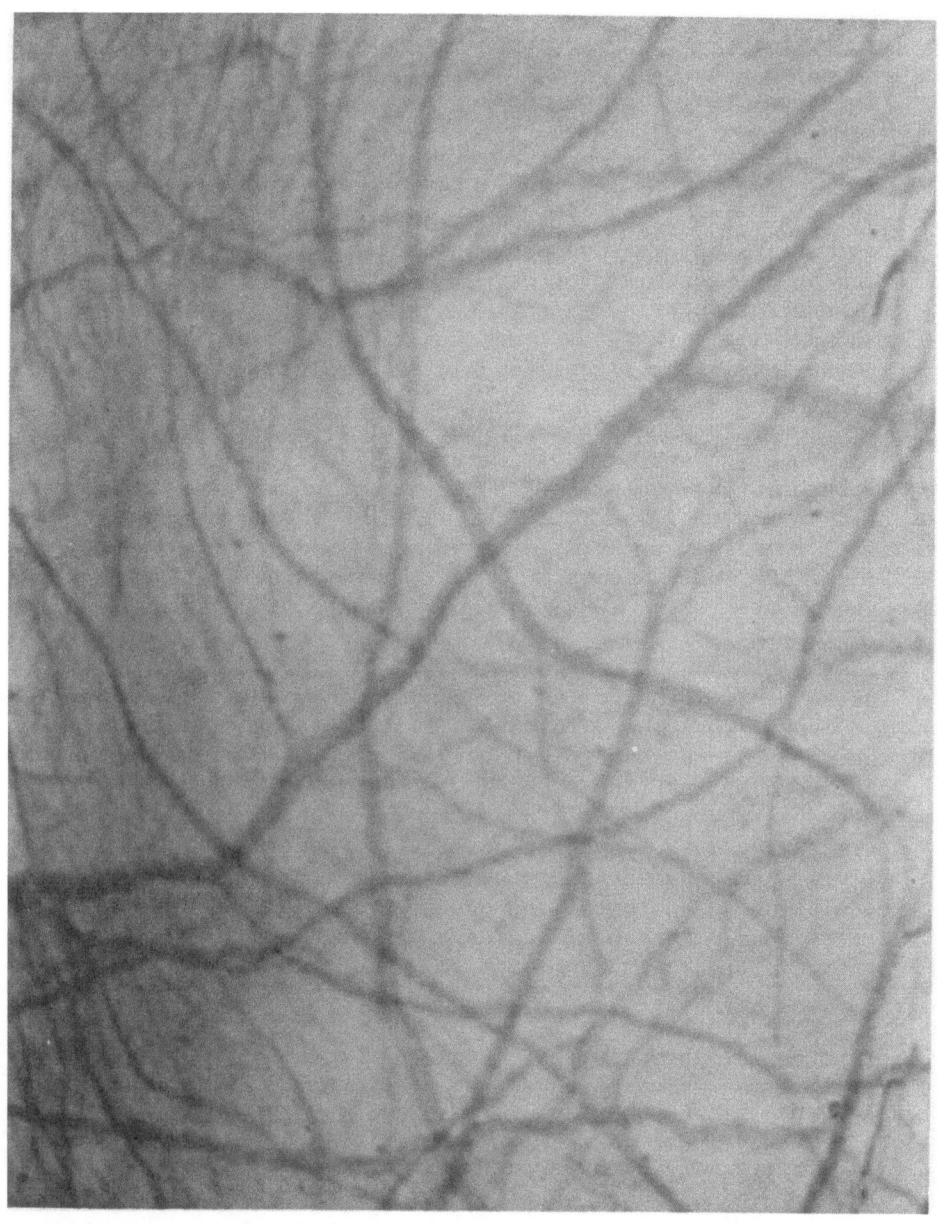

Fig. 3-26: Sympathetic Post Ganglionic Fibers.

The origin of many of the postganglionic sympathetic fibers
has been found to be the superior cervical ganglion (107).
Removal of the ganglion resulted in a loss of most of the
fibers on the larger cerebral vessels but in the small
vessels some fluorescence was still present. This could
indicate that there might be an intracranial source of
postganglionic sympathetic fibers. Hartman (108) and Itakura
(109) have shown that the small arterioles and possibly the
capillaries may receive a postganglionic sympathetic innervation
from an intracranial source. The intracranial source may be
the nucleus locus coerulius of the brain (108). These
findings imply that the sympathetic neural control extends
to the level of the capillary in the brain.

The parasympathetic nervous system has been shown to
innervate the arteries of the brain (110,111) also. A
representative example of the cholinergic innervation can be
seen in Fig. 3-27. The distribution of the parasympathetic
fibers is very similar to that
Source of Parasympathetic   of the sympathetic fibers. The
Fibers   parasympathetic nerves are found
in the adventitial layer of the
vessel wall and have been shown in cross section to enter the
tunica media. The posterior cerebral and vertebral arteries in
MONKEY the monkey were found to have a less dense innervation than
the other large vessels. Fibers that are apparently parasympathetic
have been shown to be present on the pial arteries. The origin
of the parasympathetic fibers found in associaiton with the
cerebral vessels has not been clearly identified. Suggestions
(110) have been made that the fibers arise from the seventh
cranial nerve and enter the cranium via the internal carotid
artery. An intracranial source of these fibers cannot be
ignored.

The intimate association of the parasympathetic and
sympathetic fibers in the adventitia of the blood vessels
may imply an interaction at the postganglionic terminal. A
schematic representation of this association can be seen in
Fig. 3-28. The transmitter released from either type of
postganglionic fiber must diffuse to the target cells, i.e.,
the vascular smooth muscle cells. Sympathetic postganglionic
fibers are felt to be vasoconstrictor while the postganglionic
parasympathetic fibers have been reported to cause vasodilation
of the vessels. Autonomic nerve fibers that transmit information
to the brain center (afferent fibers) have not been described
in relation to the cerebral vessels with the exception of
the extracranial carotid bifurcation region.

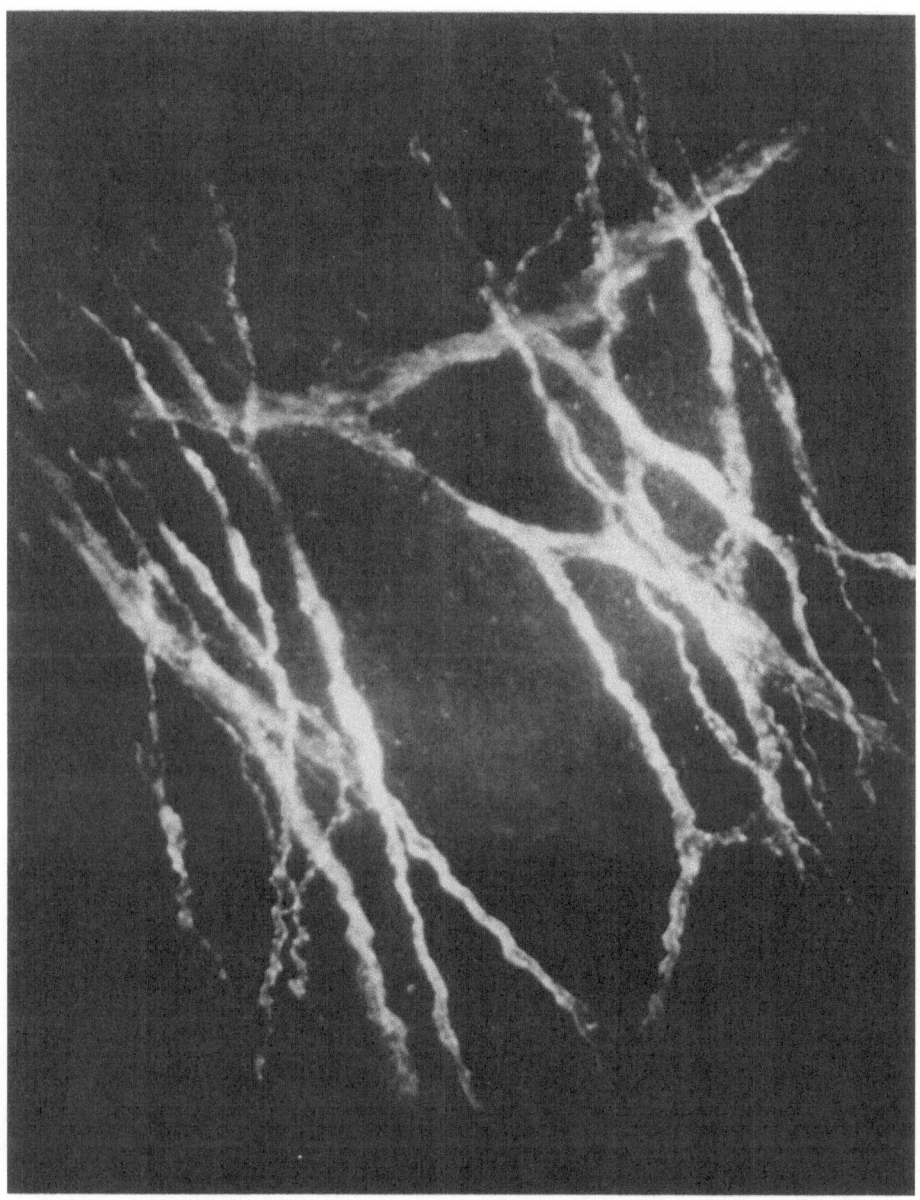

Fig. 3-27: Cholinergic Arterial Innervation.

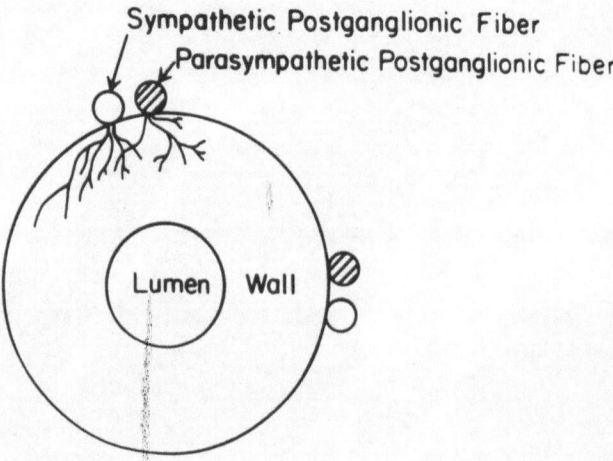

Fig. 3-28: Schematic representation of possible sympathetic –
parasympathetic wall interaction.

The real question to be asked in relation to the autonomic innervation of the cerebral vessels is the physiological role of the nerves in the dynamic response characteristic of the cerebral circulation. There are several ways to demonstrate the role of the sympathetic nervous system but the parasympathetic system has been much more difficult to characterize.

A method to determine the effect of the sympathetic nervous system in cerebral circulation would be to measure the change in resistance and flow during stimulation or removal of the superior cervical ganglion. Stimulation of the sympathetic nervous system to the cerebral vessels can cause an 80% reduction in cerebral flow and a tremendous increase in resistance (112). Removal of the superior cervical ganglion in the monkey resulted in a 25% increase in cerebral inflow (113). From these studies it was clear that the sympathetic nervous system when activated could cause cerebral vasoconstriction but more important the removal of the sympathetic innervation resulted in an increase in cerebral flow.

The latter point would indicate a tonic sympathetic activity to the major cerebral vessels. The finding of a tonic sympathetic activity to the vessels would indicate a possible role in the ability of the cerebral circulation to regulate cerebral flow when arterial driving pressure is changed. A comparison of the ability of the cerebral vascular bed to maintain flow over a pressure range was made in a group of animals with one superior cervical ganglion removed. A schematic representation of these results can be seen in Fig. 3-29. As arterial pressure was changed the cerebral flow in the intact side remained constant and began to decline as the arterial pressure approached 80 mm Hg. The sympathectomized side began with an increased cerebral flow and the relationship between flow and pressure was the same as the intact side. The unique characteristic of the cerebral vascular bed to maintain flow constant over a large pressure range was not affected except that cerebral flow was greater after sympathectomy. If the major site of pressure drop was in vessels larger than the pial arteries, this would indicate that the role of the sympathetic nervous system was predominantly on the larger cerebral vessels. A 50% reduction in pressure across vessels larger than 0.5 mm in diameter has been found by in situ pressure measurements (114).

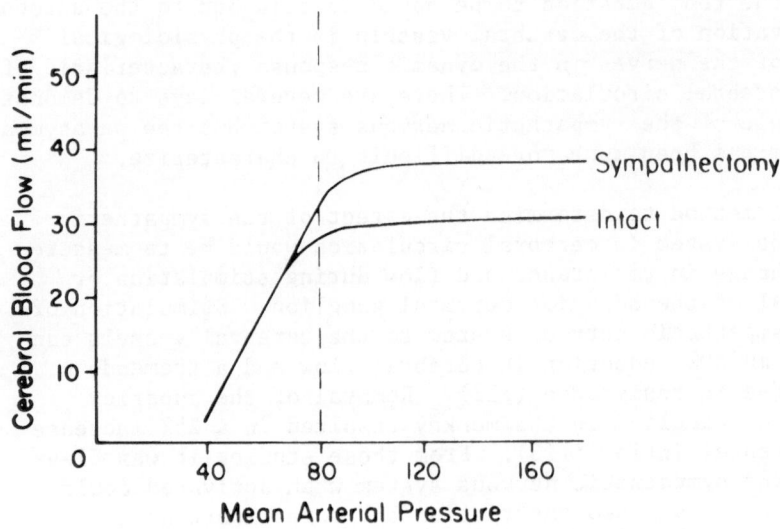

Fig. 3-29: Adaptation of cerebral blood flow to changes in arterial pressure.

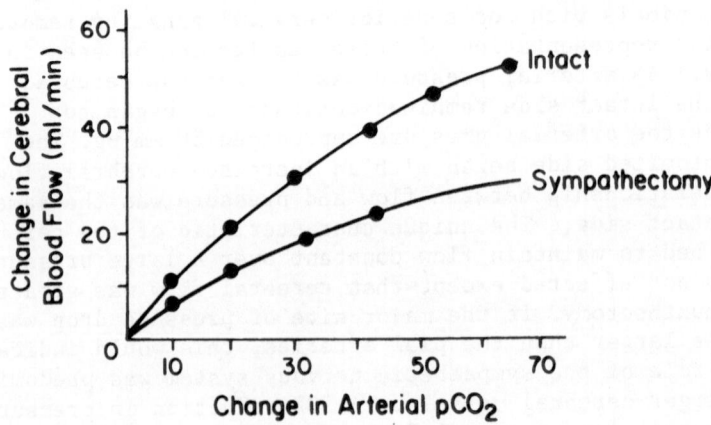

Fig. 3-30: Changes in cerebral blood flow related to arterial pCO_2.

The cerebral circulation is very sensitive to changes in the arterial carbon dioxide pressure. Is the sympathetic nervous system involved in

Arterial pCO_2 the response to carbon dioxide? Previous studies (115,116) have shown that when the arterial $pCO2$ was increased above normal, cerebral blood flow would increase and conversely if arterial $pCO2$ was decreased cerebral blood flow decreased also. This direct relationship can be seen schematically in Fig. 3-30 to increases in arterial pCO_2. In the intact animal, the slope of the relationship between the increases in cerebral blood flow and the increase in arterial pCO_2 was approximately 1 (117). Bilateral removal of the superior cervical ganglions resulting in near total sympathectomy reduced the sensitivity of the cerebral vessels to changes in arterial $pCO2$. Since there was a tonic sympathetic vasoconstrictor tone found in the cerebral vasculature, the change in pCO_2 through either a direct effect or by an increase in hydrogen ion concentration inhibited the release of sympathetic transmitter resulting in dilation. Removal of the sympathetic nervous system to the cerebral vessels reduced the effect of pCO_2. Recent evidence would indicate that the change in hydrogen ion concentration may be the mechanism of cerebral vasodilation instead of a direct action of pCO_2 on vascular smooth muscle (118). The role of the sympathetic nervous system in the dynamics of cerebral blood flow now seems very clear. This vascular bed certainly responds to the local needs of the tissue through local control, but the total inflow appears to be regulated by the autonomic nervous system. The mechanism outlined above would furnish the cerebral vascular bed with a central neural control and a fine local control mechanism.

The dynamic characteristics of the sympathetic innervation to the cerebral vessels was demonstrated in another study (119), by stimulation of the

Differential Effect of   cerebellum of the brain.
Sympathetic Nervous   Stimulation of the cerebellum
System on Circulation   result in a tremendous increase in mean arterial pressure in

the monkey. The increase in mean arterial pressure was found   MONKEY to be a result of a vasoconstriction of the splanchnic circulation indicating an increase in sympathetic nervous system activation. Cerebral blood flow was measured in intact monkeys and in monkeys with the sympathetic innervation of the cerebral vessels removed.

In the intact animals cerebral blood flow increased with
stimulation of the cerebellum and cerebral resistance decreased.
Removal of the sympathetic nerves to the cerebral vessels
reduced the flow response and the decrease in cerebral
vascular resistance. This study demonstrated a differential
effect of the sympathetic nervous system on the circulation.
A vasoconstriction in the peripheral vessels and a vasodilation
of the cerebral vessels was found. It was clear from this
data that the vasodilation found in the cerebral vascular
bed may also have been in part due to an increase in the
activity of cholinergic vasodilator nerves.

        In summary, the dynamic characteristics of the cerebral
vascular bed must encompass the autonomic nervous system and
its role in the minute to minute adjustment of flow to the
tissue. The sympathetic nervous system has clearly been
shown to influence cerebral flow and the presence of the
parasympathetic nervous system has been demonstrated while
its role at present in regulation is not known.

Coronary Circulation

        In the coronary circulation, the vessels have been
found to be innervated by efferent autonomic fibers as well
as afferent autonomic fibers particularly sympathetic efferent
fibers. The presence of both an afferent and efferent
innervation suggests very strongly the possibility of local
reflexes and feedback control that may influence flow in
large vessels as well as the distribution of flow across the
myocardial wall.

        Sympathetic afferent fibers arising from the coronary
arteries or near coronary arteries have been demonstrated
                                    (120). These fibers course
Activation of Afferent   with the sympathetic nerves to
Receptors   the heart only the afferent
                                    fibers do not synapse in the
paravertebral ganglion but have their cell bodies in the dorsal
root ganglion of the spinal cord. The afferent receptors
may be mechanoreceptors and activated by a decrease in
pressure in the vessel or the suggestion has been made that
some may be chemoreceptors and activated by a reduction in
oxygen supply to the myocardium. The exact nature of the
stimulus that activates these receptors is not known.
Efferent nerves from both the sympathetic and parasympathetic
nervous system have been identified in the adventitia of the
coronary vessels (121) as described for the cerebral vessels.

The efferent sympathetic nerves were found to be rather
dense in the adventitia of all major coronary vessels.
Removal of the stellate ganglion caused a loss of the sympathetic
nervous system innervation of the vessels. A gradient in
the degree of cholinergic innervation was found. The left
anterior descending coronary artery was more densely innervated
than either the left circumflex artery or the right coronary
artery. The cholinergic innervation was found to course at
two distinct levels in the vessel wall. One group of fibers
could be removed by stripping the adventitia of the vessel
while a second group adhered to the surface of the tunica
media. Section of the vagus nerve failed to eliminate the
cholinergic innervation as expected. The fibers running
along the coronary vessels must be postganglionic parasympathetic
fibers arising from the intrinsic cardiac ganglia.

The role of the autonomic innervation of the coronary
vessels has been much debated over the last few years.
Until recently the major
Debate over Role of determinant of coronary flow
Autonomic Innervation had been felt to be local factors
of Coronary Vessels liberated when oxygen need was
greater than supply (122). The
rich autonomic innervation and the possibility of reflexes were
not counted as being important in the coronary vascular bed.
Stimulation of the cardiac sympathetic nerves resulted in a
vasoconstriction (123) while activation of the parasympathetic
nerves to the heart caused a vasodilation (124). If the
local control of coronary flow were the dominant factor,
changes in coronary blood flow would not be expected to
occur until abnormal levels of oxygen supply had been achieved.
The question of sensitivity of the central system must be
answered. In studies in conscious dogs, the inspired oxygen   DOG
was lowered from a normal 20% to 5%. Fig. 3-31 shows the
transient response of arterial oxygen saturation, coronary
flow, and the maximum rate of rise of left ventricular
pressure to the exposure to 5% inspired oxygen. It should
be noticed that coronary flow has increased before there was
a significant decrease in arterial oxygen saturation. This
would clearly indicate that some neurogenic influence had
caused the coronary dilation and increase in coronary flow.
Blockage of beta-adrenergic receptors did not change the
transient response to hypoxia nor did drugs that blocked the
effect of adenosine. Thus neurogenic regulation of coronary
flow may be as important as local factors in the response of
coronary flow to decreases in oxygen supply.

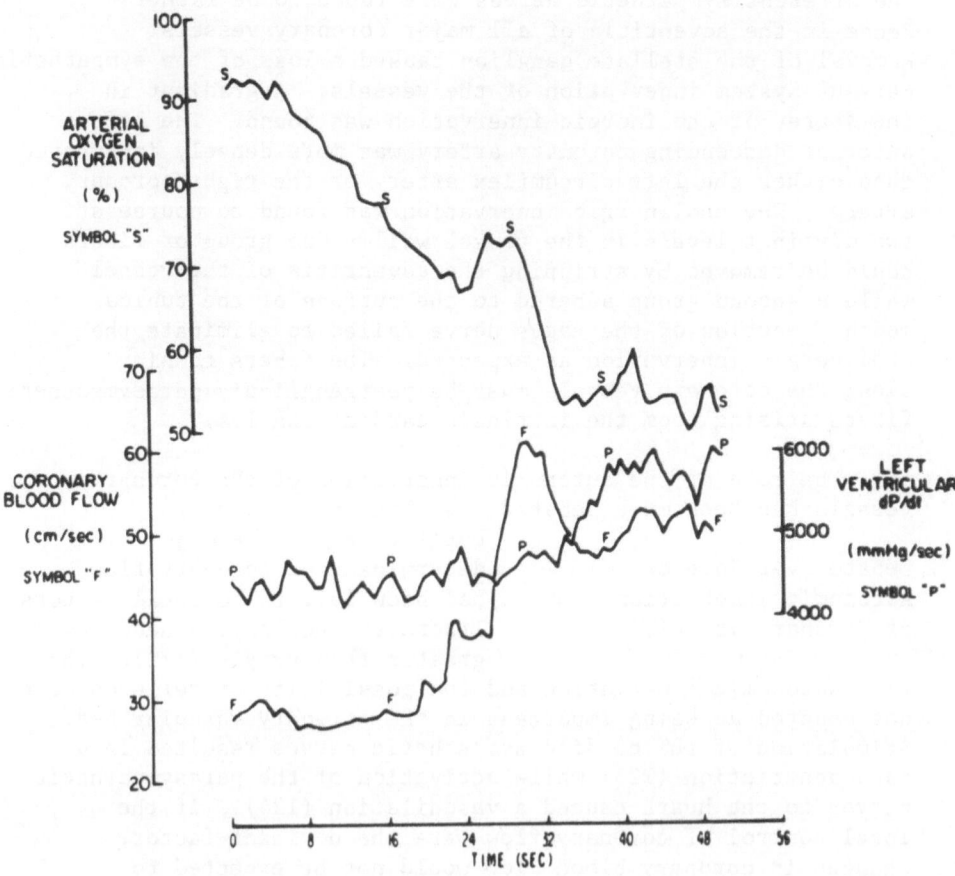

Fig. 3-31: Changes in left ventricular pressure and coronary blood flow during Hypoxia.

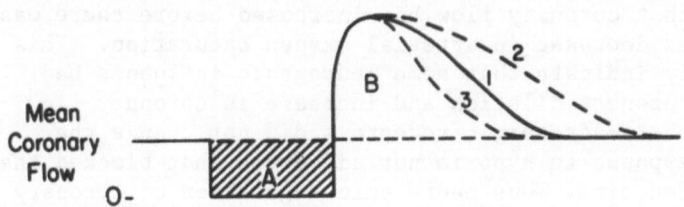

Fig. 3-32: Typical coronary reactive hyperemia response. The portion labeled A is the flow deficit and the portion labeled B is the payback following release of occlusion. See text for explanation of Figure.

Another approach to defining a possible role of the autonmic nervous system in the control of coronary flow is to challenge the system by very brief (10 sec.) occlusion of a coronary artery. Following the 10 second occlusion of a coronary artery, the flow rapidly increases above the control level and returns to control level over some time period. Fig. 3-32 Curve 1 shows a typical normal response of coronary flow to a brief occlusion. A comparison of the area B to area A provides an estimation of the overpayment of coronary flow to the occlusion. This response is termed reactive hyperemia and has been described previously (125,126). The normal reactive hyperemia was 476% in a group of dogs (127). In this same group of animals, the left stellate ganglion was removed and the experiment repeated. Curve 2 of Fig. 3-32 shows representative results of this experiment. The reactive hyperemia was increased to 622%. Beta-adrenergic blockage (Curve 3) reduced the hyperemic response to 390%. Alpha-adrenergic blockage mimicked the response of left stellate ganglionectomy. From these studies, we concluded that there was a tonic Alpha-adrenergic vasoconstrictive tone on the coronary vessels that did not permit a maximum vasodilation with brief (10 sec.) occlusions of the coronary artery. Beta-adrenergic blocade resulted in an opposite effect on the hyperemic response and may have been caused by a direct depression of myocardial metabolism by this blocking agent.

The distribution of coronary flow across the myocardial wall may also be influenced by the sympathetic nervous system. Various drugs have Dynamics of Coronary been shown to effect the Circulation must Include distribution of myocardial A Neurogenic Component flow (128). Removal of the left stellate ganglion was found to increase endocardial blood flow when all other conditions were the same as compared to the control conditions. These studies suggest that the control of coronary blood flow and distribution is influenced by the autonomic nervous system.

In the coronary vascular bed, the larger arteries course across the surface of the heart and give off branches which dive into the myocardial wall. The intramural vessels are subjected to the tension generated by the contracting myocardium and thus some degree of neural control of these vessels would be important.

It is entirely possible that the various vascular segments
in the myocardium have different adrenergic receptors on the
smooth muscle cells thus amplifying the control of flow. It
seems clear that sympathetic activation of the myocardial
cells and coronary circulation may be entirely separate thus
a high degree of coronary control can be achieved. As in
the case of the cerebral circulation, the dynamics of the
coronary circulation must include a neurogenic component.

      DR. WOLF: Dr. Stone's demonstration of increased
cerebral blood flow in association with increased blood
pressure raises an old story that was started by Cohnheim
and picked up by Heinbecker several years ago. They held
that the biological significance of essential hypertension
was to increase cerebral blood flow.

Aorta and Sympathetic Reflexes

      DR. MALLIANI: I shall try to analyze some of the
problems that may originate from the fact that the vessels
are richly innervated structures and, in particular, I shall
examine some new experimental data concerning the aorta.

      During recent years it has been amply demonstrated that
afferent sympathetic fibers with cardiovascular sensory
                              endings can mediate cardiovascular
Reflexes in Neural Control   reflexes. Moreover, as many of
of Cardiac Functions   these afferents have a spontaneous
                              impulse activity and, in addition,
are extremely sensitive to hemodynamic stimulii, we advanced
the hypothesis that they may participate in the tonic regulation
of the circulation (129). Thus, in the case of the neural
control of cardiac functions, as far as reflexes arising
from the heart are concerned, one should distinguish vago-
vagal, vago-sympathetic, sympatho-sympathetic and sympatho-
vagal reflexes (129).

      The same complexity holds true for reflexes arising
from the aorta. Afferent vagal fibers innervating the aorta
constitute one of the classic afferent pathways subserving
cardiovascular neural control. However, the aorta is also
possessed of a very abundant sympathetic sensory innervation.
Fig. 3-33 shows the activity of an afferent sympathetic
nerve fiber with its receptive field located in the proximal
third of the descending thoracic aorta. The calculated
conduction velocity was 5 m/sec (hence the fiber belonged to
the group A S (130). It is clear that the fiber was excited
by any increase in aortic pressure, however obtained.

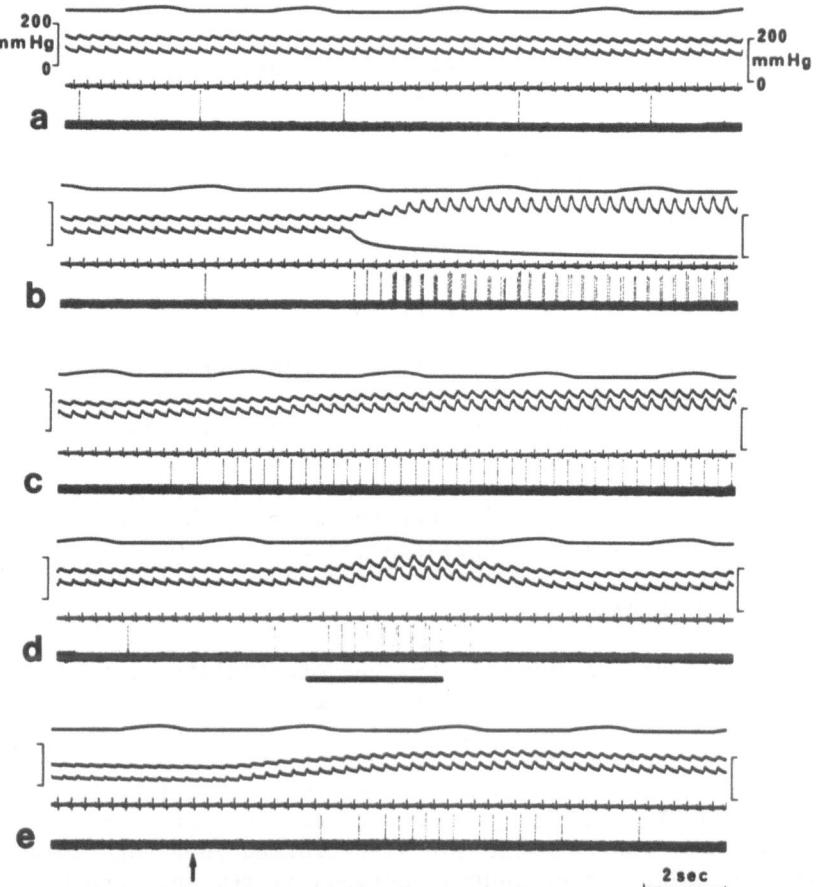

Fig. 3-33: Activity of an afferent sympathetic nerve fiber
Group A) with receptive field located in the proximal third of
the descending thoracic aorta. Calculated conduction velocity
5 m/sec. Tracings in a,b,c,d and e represent, from top to bottom,
the endotracheal pressure (inflations upwards) the aortic and
femoral arterial pressures, the e.c.g. and the nervous recording.
a, control. b, occlusion of the descending throacic aorta
(indicated by the diverging blood blood pressure traces). c,
effects of an I.V. injection of 2 ug angiotensin, performed just
before the beginning of the record. d, effects of a reflex blood
pressure rise produced by occluding the right carotid artery
(occlusion indicated by the bar). e, effect of an abrupt increase
in venous return produced by releasing, at the arrow, an occlusion
of the inferior vena cava. (from ref. 131, by courtesy of
J. Physiol.).

In Fig. 3-34 the impulse activity is displayed of an afferent sympathetic fiber belonging to the group C (130) (conduction velocity of 1 m/sec). That fiber was also studied post mortem by stretching the aortic wall with a balloon after the animal had been killed by bleeding. When the balloon was inflated (Fig. 3-34c and following parts of the figure) the highest impulse frequencies were attained during the rising phase of the pressure stimulus, followed thereafter by an adapted discharge (Fig. 3-34 e and h). A dynamic component of the stimulus was also proven by reaching the same level of absolute pressure at different speeds (Fig. 3-34 c and d) or from different initial pressures (Fig. 3-34 e and f). Finally a response which might be attributed to receptor fatigue and/or mechanical alterations of the vascular wall was observed: in Fig. 3-34 h, a pressure rise produced a much higher activation of the impulse activity than that that illustrated in Fig. 3-34 where the same step of pressure was applied after the stimulus had been sustained for 100 sec. and just released for a few seconds. These data were published recently and more details can be found in the original paper (131).

In order to investigate the potentiality of reflexes arising from sympathetic aortic receptors we stimulated them by means of a mechanical stretch (132). We used a special aortic cannula which made it possible to gradually stre+ch the aortic walls, without interfering with aortic blood flow. In Fig. 3-35a, the effects can be seen of such a stretch of the thoracic aorta, performed in a vagotomized CAT cat, with an intact central nervous system and with both common carotid arteries occluded. The reflex effects, mediated through an excitation of the sympathetic outflow, consist of an increase in arterial blood pressure, myocardial contractility and heart rate. The effects of propranolol administration are illustrated by Fig. 3-35b: aortic stretch, in these conditions, induced a smaller but clear increase in arterial and left ventricular dP/dtmax increased only very slightly and slowly during the period of stimulation.

On the basis of our understanding of blood pressure regulation (Fig. 3-36, upper diagram), the stretch of a reflexogenic area (R), simulating a rise in arterial blood pressure, Feedback Mechanisms produces a reflex decrease in systemic blood pressure through an inhibition of the sympathetic (S) discharge affecting vascular (V) resistances and thus blood pressure (BP).

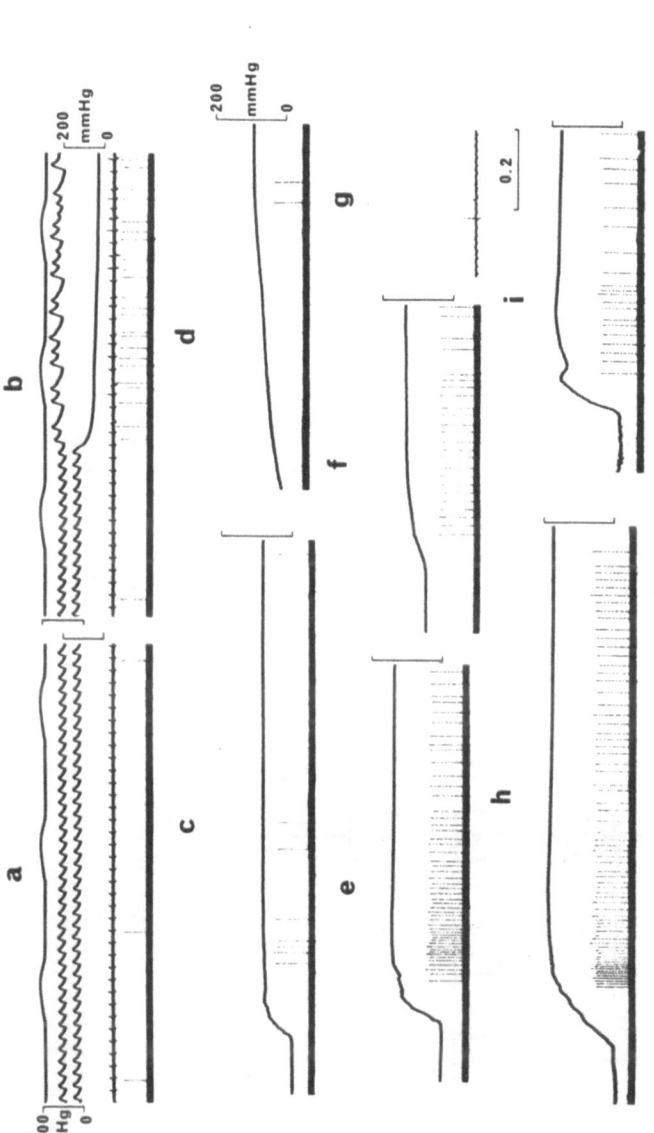

Fig. 3-34: Activity of an afferent sympathetic nerve fiber (Group C) with receptive field located in the distal third of the aortic arch. a, control. b, occlusion of the descending aorta. c,d,e,f,h and i, effects of stretching aortic wall by distending a latex balloon located in the distal part of the aortic arch (see text). g, electricl stimulation of the left inferior cardiac nerve activating the fiber. Approximate length of the fiber, 5 cm. Calculated conduction velocity 1 m/sec. Tracings in a and b as in Fig. 3-33; c,d,e,f,h, and i, top tracing; pressure applied to the distending balloon; bottom tracing: nervous activity (from ref. 131, by courtesy of J. Physiol.).

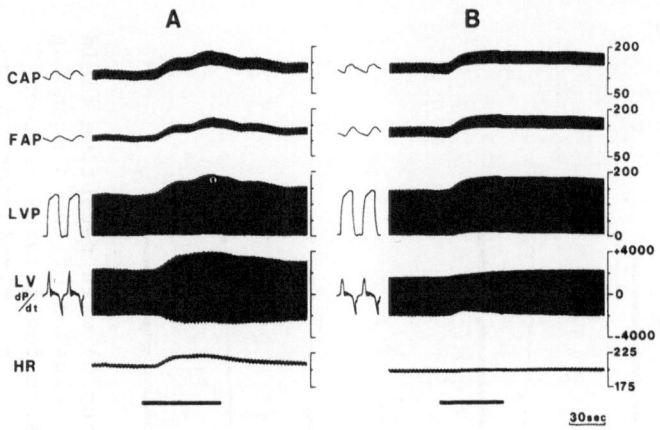

Fig. 3-35: Effects of stretching the thoracic aorta in a vagotomized cat with an intact central nervous system and both common
carotid arteries occluded. CAP = carotid artery pressure (recorded
proximal to the point of occlusion), FAP = femoral artery pressure,
LVP = left ventricular pressure (all in mmHg), LV dP/dt = rate of
change of left ventricular pressure (mmHg/sec), and HR = heart
rate (beats/min.). On the left of each section are fast-speed
records of each variable. The aortic stretch is indicated by a
bar. A: Control; B: After administration of propranolol (1 mg/kg,
iv). (from ref. 132 by courtesy of Circulation Res.).

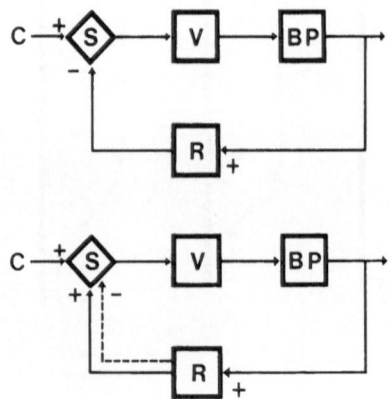

Fig. 3-36: Schema of suggested mechanisms underlying nervous
control of blood pressure regulation. For details see text.
(from ref. 133, by courtesy of Clin. Sci.).

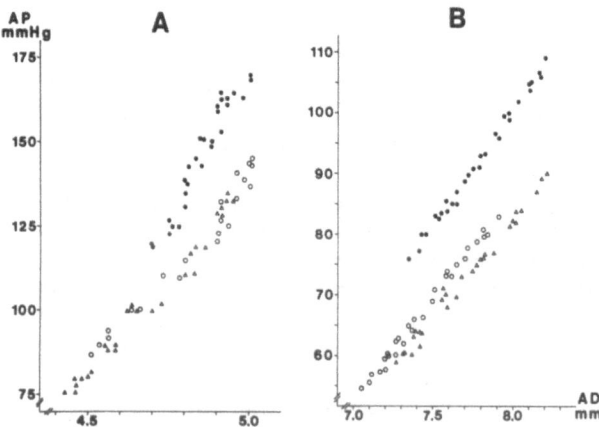

Fig. 3-37: Effect of stimulation of cut central end of ICN (A) and decentralized left thoracic sympathetic chain (B) on diastolic pressure (AP) and diameter (AD) relationship in 2 animals with both carotid arteries occluded. o Before stimulation; ● stimulation; and o after stimulation. (from ref. 135 by courtesy of Am. J. Physiol.).

In this closed loop a negative feedback assures a tonic
control of the system. Vice versa, our experiments, in
which supraspinal inhibitory mechanisms were not operative,
have revealed sympatho-sympathetic reflexes which seem to
exhibit positive feedback characteristics (Fig. 3-36, lower
diagram), as the stretch of aortic walls produced an excitation
of the sympathetic outflow. We have advanced the hypothesis
that these sympathetic reflexes may contribute to the tonic
maintenance of the effects of an increased central command
(c, in both diagrams in Fig. 3-36 and thus to the pathogenesis
of arterial hypertension (133).

However, it should be pointed out that electrophysiological
techniques have detected in the sympathetic efferent discharge
both excitations and inhibitions induced reflexly by a
similar aortic stretch (134):   the coexistence of these
inhibitory components in spinal sympathetic reflexes is
represented by the broken line in the lower diagram in Fig. 3-36.

Spinal sympathetic reflexes can also modify the mechanical
properties of the thoracic aorta (135).   In Fig. 3-37a the
effect is shown of the electrical stimulation of the cut
central end of the inferior cardiac nerve (CN) on the aortic
diastolic pressure (AP) and diameter (AD) relationship.   It
can be seen that during a sympathetic reflex the diastolic
aortic diameter is reduced for any given pressure.   Such a
reflex response is similar to that obtained with direct
electrical stimulation of sympathetic efferents (Fig. 3-37b).

It is important to realize that sympathetic reflexes
can therefore arise from the aorta and can be distributed
back to the aorta. Moreover, reflexes that modify the
aortic pressure-diameter relationship are also likely to
modulate the sensitivity of aortic mechano-receptors and the
characteristics of the reflexes initiated by them.

In the hypothesis that these concepts may provide some
understanding for the interpretation of some pathophysiological
sites, one should consider, however, that pathophysiological
alterations often represent the result of mechanisms progressing
for years and that it is impossible to ask an acute experiment
for more than a trace in the world of possibilities. On the
other hand, a phenomenon which may appear of a non-relevant
magnitude during the short span of an experiment, may indeed
constitute the core of a fundamental dynamic process.

To end up, I would like to say that most of this complexity, in my opinion, will never be solved unless multidisciplinary approaches are devised. In other words, we should be ready not only for multidisciplinary meetings, but for a real multidisciplinary strategy of research.

DR. COX: Where did you measure carotid blood flow?

DR. STONE: Internal carotid.

DR. COX: Do you feel all those changes represent intracranial blood flow?

DR. STONE: Yes. Many years ago we compared three things. Xenon 133 washout, internal or middle cerebral flow directly with internal carotid. We found that directionally all of these things changed in the same direction with interventions. The magnitude of changes ... was certainly different in the three places but directionally they were always constant.

DR. COX: In your cerebellar stimulation, you had a decreased carotid resistance that is internal carotid again?

DR. STONE: Yes.

DR. COX: What about peripheral resistance?

DR. STONE: Peripheral resistance has gone up.

DR. COX: Did you measure that?

DR. STONE: We have not measured it, but other people have.

DR. COX: This is not a cardiac output?

DR. STONE: No, cardiac output goes up a little bit, but, we have not measured that either. The reports in the literature say that cardiac output goes up slightly. Although there is a tremendous vasoconstriction in the limbs, the increased arterial pressure seems to be from an increase in splanchnic resistance. One of the questions that obviously comes out of that is what is the carotid sinus doing?

DR. COX: Was it not a chronic output response primarily?

DR. STONE: Not entirely.

DR. COX: If it were entirely a cardiac output response it might explain why you were getting more blood flow.

DR. STONE: I don't think so.

DR. CAREW: I want to address my question to Dr. Stone. I thought the information about the stellate ganglion was a fascinating observation and I wondered if you would expand on that a little bit, by telling us to what extent you think the regional distribution of flow in the heart is determined by neurogenic factors. Could you also give us more details as to how this was measured, I presume by microspheres, and whether that increase in endocardial flow is a relative increase and epicardial flow an absolute increase and whether, for example, heart rate and blood pressure were controlled during the experiments.

DR. STONE: Yes, we did measure the distribution of flow with microspheres, they were 15 microns in diameter and measure distribution fairly well. We actually directly measured a circumflex flow in these studies. These were anesthetized dog studies where we did the distribution. We held heart rate constant and measured MVO2 across the heart during the experiment both control and after removal of the left stellate ganglion. We also measured contractility. So all these parameters were controlled or were constant and what we had in those conditions was that a greater increase in the endo-epi ratio with a constant inflow, and no change in flow through the circumflex which would indicate a reduction in epicardial flow and an increase in endocardial flow.

DR. BJORKERUD: I am not too familiar with mechanics and this may be a very silly question. If you increase the pressure in the aorta, could there be two alternative effects on the coronary circulation --either a constriction or a dilatation with either an increased flow or a decreased flow? Is that right? -- Of course what I am getting at is the possible balance between the cholinergic and the sympathetic effects.

DR. STONE: On the coronary vessels?

DR. BJORKERUD: Yes, and if there is, that will then explain why trained people behave differently from untrained people, in a number of cardiovascular aspects, for instance, the increase of heart rate in response to physical exercise.

DR. STONE: As far as the interaction on the coronary vessels, I cannot answer that because no one really looked at a situation where you get large changes in flow and what that vasculature is going to do in the absence of cholinergic fibers. So, unfortunately, I cannot answer that. My feeling is that it may be a balance between the two but that is just a feeling.

DR. BJORKERUD: Because there is a significantly lower mortality in patients with heart infarction treated with B-receptor blocking agents in comparison to untreated patients. That is thought to be due to reduced incidence of arrhythmias but it could, of course, be due to other factors which are more related to what you have been talking about.

DR. STONE: Well, yes and also the reduced overall energy requirements in the myocardium. We have shown that many arrhythmias are directly coupled to the sympathetic nervous system and part of it is probably due to some of the electrical properties as well as possible flow properties. You can't separate the two.

DR. CHIEN: If I understand you correctly, the sympathetic innervation to the brain can cause both vasoconstriction and vasodilatation because if we look at the control data comparing the denervated and innervated sides, the sympathetic nerves seem to be causing vasoconstriction; but when you look at the PO_2 experiments, or the cerebellar stimulation experiments, the innervation seems to be causing vasodilation. Do you think there are two separate receptors such as alpha and beta receptors that are mediating these different changes in the cerebral circulation?

DR. STONE: Owman and Edwidsson (136) have shown very well that there are both receptors present in the vasculature of the brain. We are seeing a tonic constriction in the brain that if removed, there occurs a dilation on that side. Certainly there is also a cholinergic innervation, as the Russians have shown. It may well produce vasodilation as well, as Penfield showed back in the 30's. So how that enters I don't know but with PO_2 there is also a direct effect on the vasculature. I don't know what the relationship at this point between the sympathetic and cholinergic innervation would happen to be but, yes, I would make the assumption that a withdrawal of a tonic activity would cause vasodilation or a decrease in resistance.

DR. NEREM: Were you saying that the primary innervation of the coronary system is the extramural vessels and thus that primary neurogenic control is in these extramural vessels?

DR. STONE: No. We have looked at vessels as small as
we could visibly dissect them and found that the distribution
of the innervation decreases with vessel size. So that I
will not say where the major site of resistance is in the
coronaries. The brain studies have shown that the major
site of pressure drop is in vessels larger than .5 millimeter
which excludes the pial circuit. So here we are talking
about relatively large small arteries, let us say. In the
coronaries the picture is not quite clear.

BIBLIOGRAPHY

1.   Gow, B.S.: The influence of vascular smooth muscle on
      the viscoelastic properties of blood vessels.
      Cardiovascular Fluid Dynamics. D.H. Berge (Ed.)
      Vol. II. London and New York Academic Press,
      pp. 65-110, 1972.

2.   Furchgott, R.F.: The pharmacology of vascular smooth
      muscle. Pharmacol. Rev. 7:183-265, 1955.

3.   Wissler, R.W.: The arterial medial cell, smooth muscle or
      multifunctional mesenchyme? J. Atheroscler. Res.
      8:201-213, 1968.

4.   Aars, H.: Effects of altered smooth muscle tone on
      aortic diameter and aortic baroreceptor activity in
      anesthetized rabbits. Circ. Res. 28:254-262, 1971.

5.   Cox, R.H.: Determinants of systemic hydraulic power in
      unanesthetized dogs. Am. J. Physiol. 226:579-587,
      1974.

6.   Pagani, M., Schwartz, P.J., Bishop, V.S. and Malliani, A.:
      Reflex sympathetic changes in aortic diastolic
      pressure-diameter relationship. Am. J. Physiol.
      229:286-290, 1975.

7.   Roach, M.R. and Burton, A.C.: The reason for the shape
      of the distensibility curves of arteries. Can. J.
      Biochem. Physiol. 35:681-690, 1957.

8.   Wolinsky, H. and Glagov, S.: Structural basis for the
      static mechanical properties of the aortic media.
      Circ. Res. 14:400-413, 1964.

9.   Apter, J.T.: Correlation of viscoelastic properties with
      microscopic structure of large arteries. Circ. Res.
      21:901-918, 1967.

10. Fischer, G.M. and Llaurado, J.G.: Collagen and elastin
    content in canine arteries selected from functionally
    different vascular beds. Circ. Res. 19:394-399, 1966.

11. Harkness, M.L.R., Harkness, R.D. and McDonald, D.A.: The
    collagen and elastin content of the arterial wall in
    the dog. Proc. Roy. Soc. London, Series B. 146:
    541-551, 1957.

12. Benninghoff, A.: Blutgefasse und Herz. In: Handbuch der
    mikroskopischen Anatome. Berlin, Springer-Verlag.
    Vol. VI., pp. 1-225, 1930.

13. Cox, R.H.: Anisotropic properties of the canine carotid
    artery in vitro. J. Biomechanics 8:293-300, 1975.

14. Bergel, D.H.: The dynamic elastic properties of the
    arterial wall. J. Physiol. 156:458-469, 1961.

15. Siegman, M.J., Butler, T.M., Mooers, S.U. and Davies, R.E.:
    Crossbridge attachment, resistance to stretch, and
    viscoelasticity in resting mammalian smooth muscle.
    Science 191:383-385, 1976.

16. Dobrin, P.B. and Rovick, A.A.: Influence of vascular
    smooth muscle on contractile mechanics and elasticity
    of arteries. Am. J. Physiol. 217:1644-1651, 1969.

17. Gore, R.W.: Wall stress: a determinant of regional
    differences in response of frog microvessels to
    norepinephrine. Am. J. Physiol. 222:82-91, 1972.

18. Speden, R.N.: Muscle load and constriction of the rabbit
    ear artery. Am. J. Physiol. 248:531-533

19. Dobrin, P.B.: Isometric and isobaric contraction of
    carotid arterial smooth muscle. Am. J. Physiol.
    214:561-565, 1968.

20. Cox, R.H.: Mechanics of canine iliac artery smooth
    muscle in vitro. Am. J. Physiol. 230:462-470, 1976.

21. Herlihy, J.T. and Murphy, R.A.: Length-tension relation-
    ship of smooth muscle of the hog carotid artery.
    Circ. Res. 33:275-283, 1973.

22. Furness, J.B. and Marshall, J.M.: Correlation of the
     directly observed responses of mesenteric vessels of
     the rat to nerve stimulation and noradrenaline with
     the distribtuion of adrenergic nerves. J. Physiol.
     239:75-88, 1974.

23. Davis, D.L. and Dow, P.: Intraluminal pressures and
     rate and magnitude of arterial constrictor responses.
     Am. J. Physiol. 227:1149-1157, 1974.

24. Davis, D.L. and Baker, C.H.: Arterial segment constriction
     under constant-pressure and constant in-flow perfusion.
     Am. J. Physiol. 227:1149-1157, 1974.

25. Abboud, F.M.: Control of the various components of the
     peripheral vasculature. Fed. Proc. 31:1126-1239, 1972.

26. Gow, B.S.: Viscoelastic properties of conduit arteries.
     Circ. Res. 26 and 27, Suppl. II:II-113-II-122, 1970.

27. Cox, R.H.: Pressure dependence of the mechanical properties
     of arteries in vivo. Am. J. Physiol. 229:1371-1375,
     1975.

28. Shepard, J.T.: Intrathoracic baroreflexes. Mayo Clin.
     Proc. 48:426-437, 1973.

29. Koushanpour, E. and Kelso, D.M.: Partition of the carotid
     sinus baroreceptor response in dogs between the
     mechanical properties of the wall and the receptor
     elements. Circ. Res. 31:831-845, 1972.

30. Pelletier, C.L., Clement, D.L. and Shepard, J.T.: Comparison
     of afferent activity of canine aortic and sinus nerves.
     Circ. Res. 31:557-568, 1972.

31. Koushanpour, E. and Kelso, D.M.: Partition of the carotid
     sinus baroreceptor response in dogs between the
     mechanical properties of the wall and the receptor
     elements. Circ. Res. 31:831-845, 1972.

32. Koushanpour, E.: Quantitative analysis of whole nerve
     action potentials recorded from the carotid sinus
     baroreceptors. J. Electrophy. Tech. 3:39-45, 1975.

33. Angell-James, J.E. and Daly, M. de B.: Comparison of the
     reflex vasomotor responses to separate and combined
     stimulation of the carotid sinus and aortic arch
     baroreceptors by pulsatile and non-pulsatile pressures
     in the dog. J. Physiol. 209:257-293, 1970.

34. Ninomiya, I. and Irisawa, H.: Aortic nervous activities in
    response to pulsatile and nonpulsatile pressure.
    Am. J. Physiol. 213:1504-1511, 1967.

35. Bagshaw, R.J.: Pressure dependence of the carotid sinus
    elastic modulus in the dog. M.I.T. J. Life Sci.
    5:43-48, 1975.

36. Bagshaw, R.J. and Peterson, L.H.: Sympathetic control of
    the mechanical properties of the canine carotid sinus.
    Am. J. Physiol. 222:1462-1468, 1972.

37. Alarcon, J.E., Campbell, K.B. and Peterson, L.H.: Effect
    of norepinephrine on the carotid sinus. The Physiologist
    17:171, 1974.

38. Wurster, R.D. and Trobiani, S.: Effects of cervical
    sympathetic stimulation on carotid occlusion reflexes
    in cats. Am. J. Physiol. 225:978-981, 1973.

39. Cox, R.H., Bagshaw, R.J., Detweiler, D.K and Peterson, L.H.:
    Effects of aging on the carotid sinus control of
    canine arterial hemodynamcis. IRCS Med. Sci.
    3:293, 1975.

40. Vatner, S.F., Franklin D., Van Citters, R.L. and
    Braunwald, E.: Effects of carotid sinus nerve
    stimulation on blood-flow distribution in conscious
    dogs at rest and during exercise. Circ. Res.
    27:495-503, 1970.

41. Bjurstedt, H., Rosenhamer, G. and Tyden, G.: Cardiovascular
    responses to changes in carotid sinus transmural
    pressure in man. Acta Physiol. Scand. 9:497-505, 1975.

42. Moissejeff, E.: Zur Kenntnis des Carotissinus-reflexus.
    Z. Ges. Exptl. Med. 53:696-704, 1926.

43. Angell-James, J.E. and Daly, M. de B.: Effects of graded
    pulsatile pressure on the reflex vasomotor responses
    elicited by changes of mean pressure in the perfused
    carotid sinus-aortic arch regions of the dog.
    J. Physiol. 214:51-64, 1971.

44. Schmidt, R.M., Kumada, M. and Sagawa, K.: Cardiac output
    and total peripheral resistance in carotid sinus
    reflex. Am. J. Physiol. 221:480-487, 1971.

45. Cox, R.H. and Bagshaw, R.J.: Baroreceptor reflex control
        of arterial hemodynamcis in the dog. Circ. Res.
        37:772-786, 1975.

46. Bond, R.F. and Green, H.D.: Cardiac output redistribution
        during bilateral common carotid occlusion. Am. J.
        Physiol. 216:393-403

47. O'Rourke, M.F. and Taylor, M.G.: Vascular impedance of
        the femoral bed. Circ. Res. 18:126-139, 1966.

48. Taylor, M.G.: The input impedance of an assembly of
        randomly branching elastic tubes. Biophysical J.
        6:29-51, 1966.

49. Levy, M.N., NG, M.L. and Zieske, H.: Cardiac and
        respiratory effects of aortic arch baroreceptor
        stimulation. Circ. Res. 19:930-939, 1966.

50. Hainsworth, R., Ledsome, J.R. and Carswell, F.: Reflex
        responses from aortic baroreceptors. Am. J. Physiol.
        218:423-429, 1970.

51. Pelletier, C.L., Edis, A.J. and Shepard, J.T.: Circulatory
        reflex from vagal afferents in response to hemorrhage
        in the dog. Circ. Res. 29:626-634, 1971.

52. Ott, N.T. and Shepherd, J.T.: Modifications of the aortic
        and vagal depressor reflexes by hypercapnia in the
        rabbit. Circ. Res. 33:160-165, 1973.

53. Pelletier, C.L. and Shepherd, J.T.: Effect of hypoxia
        on vascular responses to the carotid baroreflex.
        Am. J. Physiol. 228:331-336, 1975.

54. Mancia, G.: Influence of carotid baroreceptors on vascular
        responses to carotid chemoreceptor stimulation in the
        dog. Circ. Res. 36:270-276, 1975.

55. Mancia, G., Shepherd, J.T. and Donald, D.E.: Role of
        cardiac, pulmonary, and carotid mechanoreceptors in
        the control of hind-limb and renal circulation in
        dogs. Circ. Res. 37:200-208, 1975.

56. Bagshaw, R.J., Lizuka, M. and Peterson, L.H.: Effect of
        interaction of the hypothalamus and the carotid sinus
        mechanoreceptor system on renal hemodynamics in the
        anesthetized dog. Circ. Res. 25:569-585, 1972.

57. Kumada, M., Schramm, L.P., Altmansberger, R.A. and
     Sagawa, K.: Modulation of carotid sinus baroreceptor
     reflex by hypothalamic defense response. Am. J. Physiol.
     228:34-45, 1975.

58. Symth, H.S., Sleight, P. and Pickering, G.W.: Reflex
     regulation of arterial pressure during sleep in man:
     A quantitative method of assessing baroreflex
     sensitivity. Circ. Res. 24:109-121, 1969.

59. Bristow, J.D., Brown, E.B., Cunningham, D.J.C.,
     Howson, M.G., Peterson, E.S., Pickering, T.G. and
     Sleight, P.: The effect of bicycling on the
     baroreflex regulation of pulse interval. Circ. Res.
     28:582-592, 1971.

60. Higgins, C.B., Vatner, S.F., Eckberg, D.L. and Braunwald, E.:
     Alterations in the baroreceptor reflex in conscious
     dogs with heart failure. J. Clin. Invest. 51:715-724,
     1972.

61. Epstein, S.E., Beiser, G.D., Goldstein, R.E., Stampfer, M.,
     Wechsler, A.S., Glick, G. and Braunwald, E.:
     Circulatory effects of electrical stimulation of the
     carotid sinus nerves in man. Circ. 40:269-276, 1969.

62. McCubbin, J.W., Green, J.H. and Page, I.H.: Baroreceptor
     function in chronic renal hypertension. Circ. Res.
     4:205-210, 1956.

63. Angell-James, J.E.: Characteristics of single aortic and
     right subclavian baroreceptor fiber activity in
     rabbits with chronic renal hypertension. Circ. Res.
     32:149-161, 1974.

64. Angell-James, J.E.: Arterial baroreceptor activity in
     rabbits with experimental atherosclerosis. Circ. Res.
     34:27-39, 1974.

65. Angell-James, J.E.: Pathophysiology of aortic baroreceptors
     in rabbits with vitamin D sclerosis and hypertension.
     Circ. Res. 34:327-338, 1974.

66. Pickering, T.G., Gribbin, B.and Sleight, P.: Comparison of
     the reflex heart rate response to rising and falling
     arterial pressure in man, Cardiovascular Res.
     6:277-283, 1972.

Rothbaum, D.A., Shaw, D.J., Angell, C.S. and Shock, N.W.:
Age differences in the baroreceptor response of rats.
J. Gerontology 29:488-492, 1974.

68.   Cox, R.H., Fronek, A. and Peterson, L.H.: Effects of
carotid hypotension on aortic hemodynamics in the
unanesthetized dog. Am. J. Physiol. 229:1376-1380,
1975.

69.   Forsyth, R.P., Hoffbrand, B.K. and Melmon, K.L.: Hemodynamic
effects of angiotensin in normal and environmentally
stressed monkeys. Circ. 44:119-129, 1971.

70.   Forsyth, R.P. and Harris, R.E.: Circulatory changes during
stressful stimuli in rhesus monkeys. Circ. Res.
26 and 27 Suppl. I:I-13-I-20, 1970.

71.   Caraffa-Braga, E., Granata, L. and Pinotti, O.: Changes
in blood-flow distribution during acute emotional
stress in dogs. Pflugers Arch. 339:187-205, 1973.

72.   Fell, C.: Changes in blood flow distribution produced by
central sciatic nerve stimulation. Am. J. Physiol.
214:561-565, 1968.

73.   Hoffband, B.I. and Forsyth, R.P.: Regional blood flow
changes during norepinephrine, tyramine and methoxamine
infusions in the unanesthetized rhesus monkey.
J. Pharmacol. and Exp. Ther. 184:656-661, 1973.

74.   Vatner, S.F., Higgins, C.B., White, S., Patrick, T.
and Franklin, D.: The peripheral vascular response
to severe exercise in untethered dogs before and
after complete heart block. J. Clin. Invest.
50:1950-1960, 1971.

75.   Brod, J.: Essential hypertension haemodynamic observations
with a bearing on its pathogenesis. The Lancet
2:773-778, 1960.

76.   Kaihara, S., Rutherford, R.B., Schwentker, E.P. and
Wagner, H.N., Jr.: Distribution of cardiac output
in experimental hemorrhagic shock in dogs. J. Appl.
Physiol. 27:218-222, 1969.

77.   Davis, J.O.: Viscoelastic properties of conduit arteries.
Am. J. Med. 55:333-350, 1973.

78.   Oparil, S. and Haber, E.: The renin-angiotensin system.
New Eng. J. Med. 291:389-401, 446-457, 1974.

79. Forsythe, R.P., Hoffbrand, B.I. and Melmon, K.L:
    Hemodynamic effects of angiotensin in normal and
    environmentally stressed monkeys. Circ. 44:119-129,
    1971.

80. Ganong, W.F.: Medical Physiology, 5th Ed., Lange Med.
    Publications, Los Altos, California

81. Schmid, P.G., Abboud, F.M., Wendling, M.G., Ramberg, E.S.,
    Mark, A.L., Heistad, D.D. and Eckstein, J.W.:
    Regional vascular effects of vasopressin: plasma
    levels and circulatory responses. Am. J. Physiol.
    227:998-1004, 1974.

82. Lutz, R.J., Cannon, J.N. and Monroe, R.E.: Shear stress
    measurements in model arteries during steady and
    pulsatile flow. Fluid Dynamic Aspects of Arterial
    Disease. Columbus, Ohio, State University Press,
    pp. 5-8, 1974.

83. Nerem, R.N., Rumberger, J.A., Jr., Gross, D.R., Hamlin, R.L.
    and Geiger, G.L.: Hot-film measurements of coronary
    blood flow in horses. Fluid Dynamic Aspects of Arterial
    Disease. Columbus, Ohio, State University Press,
    pp. 28-31, 1974.

84. Fry, D.L.: Responses of the arterial wall to certain
    physical factors. Atherogenesis: Initiating Factors.
    Ciba Foundation Symposium, Amsterdam, Associated
    Scientific Publishers. pp. 93-125, 1973.

85. Caro, C.G. and Nerem, R.M.: Transport of ^{14}C-4-Cholesterol
    between serum and wall in the perfused dog common
    carotid artery. Circ. Res. 32:187-205, 1973.

86. Fry, D.L.: Certain chemorheologic considerations regarding
    the blood vascular interface with particular reference
    to coronary artery disease. Circ. 39 and 40, Suppl.
    4:IV-38-IV-59, 1969.

87. Nakata, Y., Shionoya, S., Matsubara, J. and Shinjo, K.:
    An experimental study on the vascular lesions caused
    by disturbance of the vasa vasorum and the periaortic
    vein. Jap. Circ. J. 36:945-951, 1972.

88. Glagov, S.: Mechanical stresses on vessels and the non-
    uniform distribution of atherosclerosis. Medical
    Clinics of North America. 57:63-77, 1973.

89. Sacks, A.H.: The vasa vasorum as a link between hypertension
     and arteriosclerosis. Angiology 26:385-390, 1975.

90. Blose, S.H.: Contractile proteins and cytoplasmic filaments
     in cloned venous endothelial cells. Fed. Proc.
     35:234, 1976.

91. Shimamoto, T.: New concept of atherogenesis and treatment
     of atherosclerotic diseases with endothelial cell
     relaxant. Jap. Heart J. 13:537-562, 1972.

92. Robertson, A.L. and Khairallah, P.A.: Effects of angiotensin
     II and some analogues on vascular permeability in the
     rabbit. Circ. Res. 31:923-931, 1972.

93. Heath, D., Smith, P., Harris, P., and Winson, M.: The
     atherosclerotic human carotid sinus. J. Path.
     110:49-58, 1973.

94. Winson, M., Heath, D. and Smith, P.: Extensibility of the
     human carotid sinus. Cardiovasc. Res. 8:58-64, 1974.

95. Cowley, A.W., Jr., Laird, J.F. and Guyton, A.C.: Role of
     the baroreceptors in daily control of arterial blood
     pressure and other variables in dogs. Circ. Res.
     32:564-576, 1973.

96. Mancia, G., Ludbrook, J., Ferrari, A., Gregorini, L.,
     Zahchetti, A.: Baroreceptor Reflexes in Human
     Hypertension. Circulation Res. 43:170-177, 1978.

97. Recordati, G., Lombardi, F., Bishop, V.S., Malliani A.:
     Response of type B atrial vagal receptors to changes
     in wall tension during atrial filling. Circulation Res.
     36:682-691, 1975.

98. Recordati, G., Lombardi, F., Bishop, V.S., Malliani, A.:
     Mechanical stimuli exciting type A atrial receptors in
     the cat. Circulation Res. 38:397-403, 1976.

99. Armour, J.A.: Physiological behavior of thoracic
     cardiovascular receptors. Am. J. Physiol. 225:
     177-185, 1973.

100. Guyton, A.C.: Textbook of Medical Physiology. W.B.
     Saunders, Philadelphia, PA, 5th Ed., 1976.

101. Dobrin, P.D. and Rovick, A.A.: Influence of vascular
     smooth muscle on contractile mechanics and elasticity
     of arteries. Am. J. Physiol. 217:1644-1651, 1969.

102. McDonald, D.A.: <u>Blood Flow in Arteries</u>. William &
      Wilkins, Co., Baltimore Md., 2nd Ed., 1969.

103. Penfield, W.: Intracerebral vascular nerves. <u>Arch.
      Neurol. Psychiat.</u> (Chic). 27:30-44, 1932.

104. Chorobski, J. and Penfield, W.: Cerebral vasodilator
      nerves and their pathway from the medulla oblongata.
      With observations on the pial and intracerebral
      vascular plexus. <u>Arch. Neural. Psychiat.</u> 28:
      1257-1289, 1932.

105. Falck, B., Nielsen, K.C. and Owman, C.: Adrenergic
      innervation of the circulation. <u>Scand. J. Clin.
      Lab. Invest.</u> Suppl. 102, VI:B, 1968.

106. Nielsen, K.C., and Owman, C.: Adrenergic innervation
      of pial arteries related to the circle of Willis in
      the cat. Brain <u>Research</u> 6:773-776, 1967.

107. Hernandez-Perez, M.J. and Stone, H.L.: Sympathetic
      innervation of the circle of Willis in the macaque
      monkey. <u>Brain Research</u> 80:507-511, 1974.

108. Hartman, B.K.: Immunofluorescence of dopamine-beta-
      hydroxylase. Application of improved methodology to
      the localization of the peripheral and central nora-
      drenergic nervous system. <u>J. Histochem. Cytochem.</u>
      21:312-332, 1973.

109. Iwayama, T., Furness, J.B and Burnstock, G.: Dual
      adrenergic and cholinergic innervation of cerebral
      arteries of the rat. An ultrastructural study.
      <u>Circ. Res.</u> 26:635-646, 1970.

110. Forbes, H.S., Schmidt, C.F. and Nason, G.I.: Evidence of
      vasodilator innervation in the parietal cortex of
      the cat. <u>Am. J. Physiol.</u> 125:216-219, 1939.

111. Denn, M.J. and Stone, H.L.: Cholinergic innervation of
      monkey cerebral vessels. <u>Brain Research</u> 113:394-399,
      1976.

112. D'Alecy, L.G., and Feigl, E.O.: Sympathetic control of
      cerebral blood flow in dogs. <u>Circ. Res.</u> 31: 267-283,
      1972.

113. Hernandez-Perez, M.J., Raichle, M.J., Stone, H.L.:
      The role of the sympathetic nervous system in cerebral
      blood flow autoregulation. Stroke 6:284-292, 1975.

114. Stromberg, D.D. and Fox, J.R.: Pressures in the pial
      arterial microcirculation of the cat during changes in
      systemic arterial blood pressure. Circ. Res. 31:
      229-239, 1972.

115. Raichle, M.E. and Stone, H.L.: Cerebral blood flow
      autoregulation and graded hypercapnia. Proceedings
      of the 5th International Symposium on Cerebral Blood
      Flow Regulation (S. Karger) pp. 1-5, 1972.

116. Reivich, M.: Arterial pCO_2 and cerebral hemodynamics.
      Am. J. Physiol. 206: 25-35, 1964.

117. Betz, E.: Cerebral blood flow: Its measurements and
      regulation. Physiol. Rev. 52: 595-630, 1972.

118. Stone, H.L., Raichle, M.E., Hernandez-Perez, M.J.: The
      effect of sympathetic denervation and cerebral CO_2
      sensitivity. Stroke 5: 13-18, 1974.

119. McKee, J.C., Denn, M.J. and Stone, H.L.: Neurogenic
      cerebral vasodilation from electrical stimulation of
      the cerebellum in the monkey. Stroke 7: 179-186,
      1976.

120. Malliani, A., Parks, M., Tuckett, R.P., Brown, A.M.: Reflex
      increases in heart rate elicited by stimulation of
      afferent cardiac sympathetic nerve fibers in the cat.
      Circ. Res. 32:9-14, 1973.

121. Denn, M.J. and Stone, H.L.: Autonomic innervation of dog
      coronary arteries. J. Appl. Physiol. 41:30-35, 1976.

122. Berne, R.M.: Regulation of coronary blood flow. Phsyiol.
      Rev. 44:1-29, 1964.

123. Feigl, E.O.: Sympathetic control of coronary circulation.
      Circ. Res. 20:262-271, 1967.

124. Feigl, E.O.: Parasympathetic control of coronary blood
      flow in dogs. Circ. Res. 25:509-519, 1969.

125. Olsson, R.A., Gregg, D.E.: Metabolic responses during
      myocardial reactive hyperemia in the unanesthetized
      dog. Am. J. Physiol. 208:231-236, 1965.

126. Eikens, E., Wilcken, D.E.L.: Myocardial reactive
      hyperemia and coronary vascular reactivity in the
      dog. Circ. Res. 33:267-274, 1973.

127. Schwartz, P.J. and Stone, H.L.: Tonic influence of the
      sympathetic nervous system on myocardial reactive
      hyperemia and on coronary blood flow distribution
      in dogs. Circ. Res. 41:51-58, 1977.

128. Fortnun, N.J., Kaihara, S., Becker, L.C., Pitt, B.:
      Regional myocardial blood flow in the dog studied
      with radioactive microspheres. Cardio. Res. 5:
      331-336, 1971.

129. Malliani, A., Lombardi, F., Pagani, M., Recordati, G.,
      and Schwartz, P.J.: Spinal cardiovascular reflexes.
      Brain Res. 87:239-246, 1975.

130. Burgess, P.R., and Perl, E.R.: Cutaneous mechanoreceptors
      and nociceptors. In: A. Iggo (Ed.), Handbook of
      Sensory Physiology, Vol. 2, Somatosenory System,
      Berlin, Springer-Verlag, pp. 851, 1973.

131. Malliani, A. and Pagani, M.: Afferent sympathetic nerve
      fibers with aortic endings. J. Physiol. 263:157-169,
      1976.

132. Lioy, F., Malliani, A., Pagani, M., Recordati, G., and
      Schwartz, P.J.: Reflex hemodynamic responses
      initiated from the thoracic aorta. Circ. Res.
      34:78-84, 1974.

133. Malliani, A., Lombardi, F., Pagani, M., Recordati, G.,
      and Schwartz, P.J.: Spinal sypathetic reflexes in
      the cat and the pathogenesis of arterial hypertension.
      Clin. Sci. Mol. Med. 48:259s-260s, 1975.

134. Pagani, M., Schwartz, P.J., Banks, R., Lombardi, F. and
      Malliani, A.: Reflex responses of sympathetic
      preganglionic neurones initiated by different
      cardiovascular receptors in spinal animals. Brain
      Res. 68:215-225, 1974.

135. Pagani, M., Schwartz, P.J., Bishop, V.S., and Malliani, A.:
      Reflex sympathetic changes in aortic diastolic
      pressure-diameter relationship. Am. J. Physiol.
      229: 286-290, 1975.

Chapter 4   HYDRODYNAMIC EFFECTS ON ENDOTHELIAL CELLS

DR. WEINBAUM: I would like to discuss how fluid
mechanics may be changing the transport of macromolecules
                              and augmenting vesicle transport
Models for Vesicle   and also how endothelial cells
Transport   establish intracellular channels
                              with typical 100 to 200 angstrom
spacing. I think it would be useful to show what models for
vesicle transport have been developed and to show how these
models tie in with the experimental information which is
just now being gathered. Let us look at the first three
figures.

I should mention that all these figures were made when
I was at Imperial College working with Dr. Colin Caro. Dr.
Clifford Lewis of the Zoology Department at Imperial prepared
the EMs I will now show.

Figure 4-1. The interesting feature observed in the
first figure is that when an artery is in a relaxed state,
with no transmural pressure, but stretched back to in vivo
length, numerous blebs are noticed all around the periphery
of the endothelial cell. You are able to easily remove
these blebs by applying transmural pressure. Another feature
which I think will be critical in understanding how vesicle
motion can be enhanced, is what is happening to the nucleus
when mechanical stresses are applied. The nucleus obviously
occupies a large fraction of the volume of an endothelial
cell.   It is not known whether a tethering exists between
the nucleus and the plasmalemma membrane of the endothelial
cell. I think it is reasonable to assume that this tethering,
if it exists, is not rigid, but rather flexible. In other
words, if you can produce a slushing motion of the cytoplasm
the nucleus will also move. To turn the nucleus around, one
can hypothesize that you may need very long exposure to
stress, as in Dr. Fry's experiment. To change the orientation
of the endothelial cell, one must change the flow direction.
The time scale for this type of realignment of the nucleus
is several weeks. These long time scale changes should have
little effect on vesicle transport rate.

Figure 4-2. In Fig. 4-2 notice that the blebs are
gone. There is no flow here and the artery is at 100 mmHg
transmural pressure.

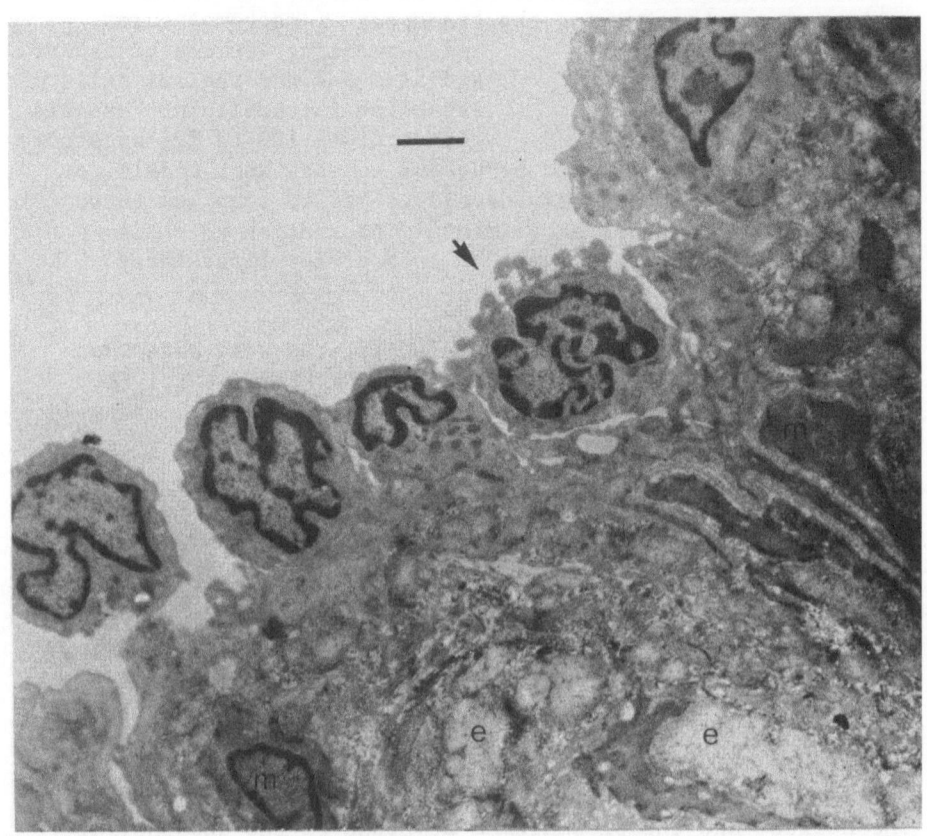

Fig. 4-1: Low magnification (13,000 X) electron micrograph of
canine carotid endothelium in relaxed state. Note numerous blebs
in plasmalemma when there is no transmural pressure. (Courtesy
of C. Lewis). (Reduced 30% for purposes of reproduction.)

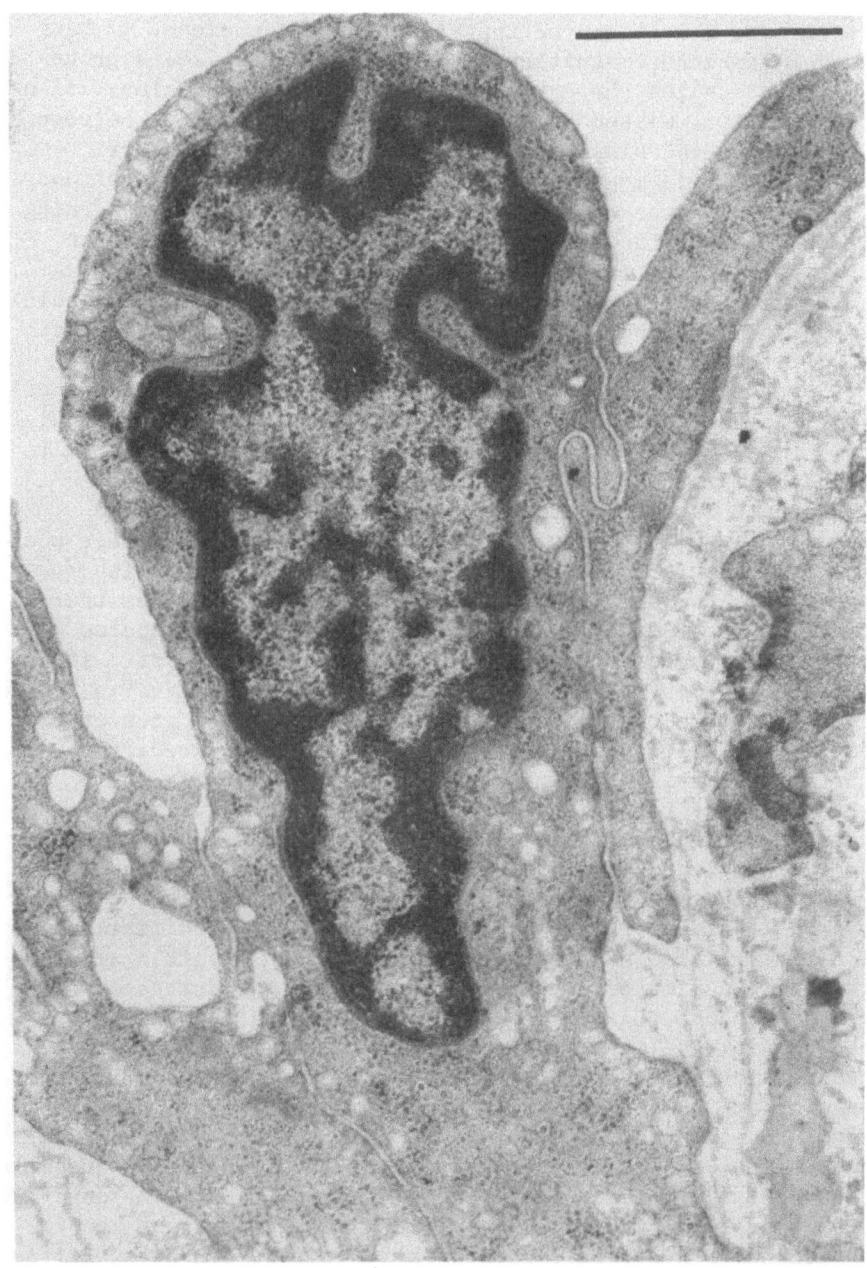

Fig. 4-2: High magnification (45,000 X) electron micrograph of canine carotid endothelial cell with 100 mmHg transmural pressure. Note involuted appearance of nucleus and long tortuous extracellular channel. Blebs have disappeared. (Courtesy of C. Lewis). (Reduced 20% for purposes of reproduction.)

Transmural pressure removed all the blebs. The other interesting
feature is the involuted appearance of the nucleus. I have
looked at higher magnification Ems from Dr. Palade's group
and have studied the cytoplasm surrounding the nucleus.   In
particular, I wished to see if there is a tethering between
the nucleus and plasmalemma in that region. The other
feature that is beautifully shown here are the long tortuous
intracellular channels. The question I raised this morning
was how the extracellular channels form? The information
that is of great interest to us is the magnitude of the
force required to spread the channel apart. It is difficult
to perform an experiment where one could quantify this, but
I will tell you my current thoughts. In many endothelial
cells, the ciliary body, the gall bladder, arterial endothelium,
you find out that the extracellular channel has a strikingly
uniform spacing that runs between 100 and 200 angstrom units
when there is no flow and which widens to perhaps 1000 A
when there is active transport with a large water flow
accompanying it. There are also localized regions where the
spacing diminishes to 20A or less. This latter spacing
determines the cutoff between the size macromolecules that
traverse the intracellular clefts and the size molecules
that cross the endothelium through vesicle transport. It is
reasonable to hypothesize that there are attractive Van der Waals
forces between the two lateral membranes on each side of the
extracellular channel. We also know that the exterior
surfaces of cell membranes have small negative charges
which provide repulsive forces. Those two forces in balance
establish the equilibrium spacing. The surface charge can
be redistributed, that is, there are localized regions where
you can have more or less surface charge. This is the
reason I believe the equilibrium spacing can be diminished
locally. I also have seen experiments with lecithin and
related experiments with low molecular weight dextrans where
you can change the polarization of molecules comprising the
phospholipid bilayer or the intervening medium. This also
causes a change in the equilibrium spacing. The equilibrium
spacing by itself does not tell you anything about the
absolute magnitude of the forces. All you know is that the
two forces are equal because they are in balance. To determine
the magnitude of each force, one is interested in the departure
from the equilibrium spacing. One wishes to measure the
additional separation caused by a force that can be quantified.
The extracellular channel water flux creates a pressure
force which can be calculated from hydrodynamic theory if
the flow rate is known. These two measurements, the flow
rate in a channel, and the change in channel spacing should
provide a reasonable estimate of the magnitude of the forces
that hold the channel together.

Ems showing this change in spacing are available --unforuntately, the people who are most active in this research: Dave Tormey and Jared Diamond, are in California and hard for me to visit. The Ems these investigators have taken of the gall bladder beautifully show the changes in channel spacing as a function of the flow rate.

Figure 4-3. The next figure shows a flattened endothelial cell at 100 mmHg pressure. The flow direction is from top to bottom. It is evident from this figure that the endothelial cell can deform very easily due to hydrodynamic forces at its surface. The nucleus here looks symmetric; it really isn't if you look carefully. The principal transport of vesicles does not occur in the nuclear or perinuclear region because of the large resistance offered by the endoplasmic reticulum which is concentrated in these areas. I believe that the important vesicular transport occurs in the periphery of the cell which has relatively little volume. Small movements of the nucleus could easily generate sizeable velocities in the cell periphery.   The fluid response time for these changes is almost instantaneous. Thus, if one can establish a cytoplasmic circulation to augment the Brownian diffusion of vesicles, in the periphery of the cell, one could have a nice mechanism for increasing or changing the macromolecule transport rate. Another thing which is very nicely illustrated in this figure is the two phase structure of the underlying tissue which is comprised of smooth muscle cells and interstitial space. The endothelium and the underlying tissue are ultrastructural opposites from the standpoint of macromolecule transport. The macromolecules cross the endothelium through vesicles, since the extracellular channels are too narrow. The macromolecules, once they are released by the vesicles at the tissue front, can easily pass through the large gaps between adjacent smooth muscle cells since these gaps are 1000 A or more.

Vesicular Transport

Macromolecule Transport

Figure 4-4. I wish I could show you some of Dr. Palade's electron micrographs of vesicles interacting with the plasmalemma membranes. The electron micrographs show the various stages during the attachment and with rupture processes. Fig. 4-4 is a schematic showing the various steps in the vesicle attachment process.

Vesicles Interacting with Plasmalemma Membranes

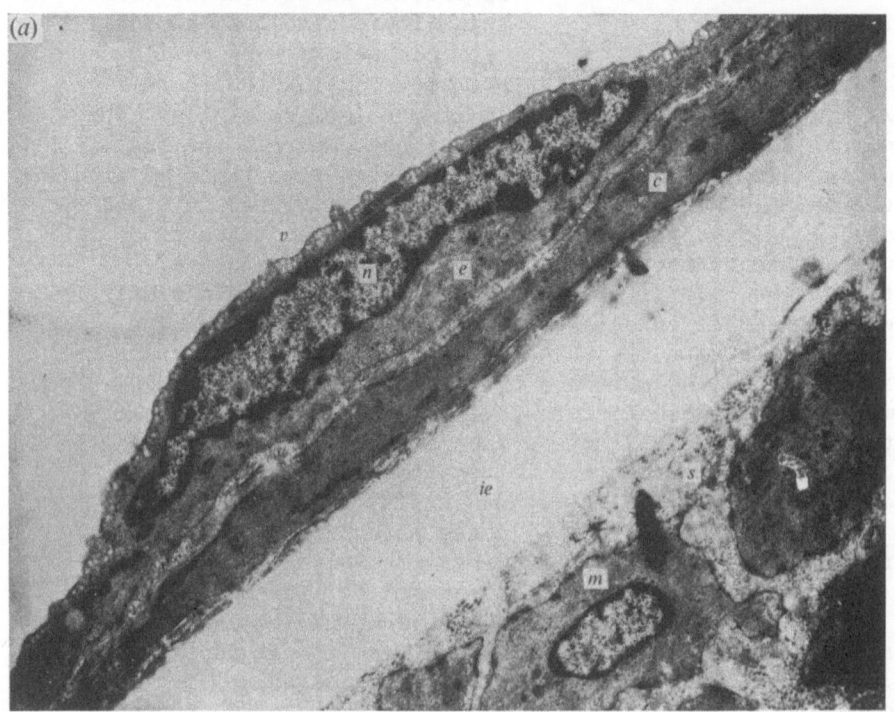

Fig. 4-3: Electron micrograph of flattened endothelial cell
in canine carotid artery with flow in lumen. Transmural
pressure 100 mmHg. 17,000 X (Courtesy of C. Lewis). From
Weinbaum and Caro (1).

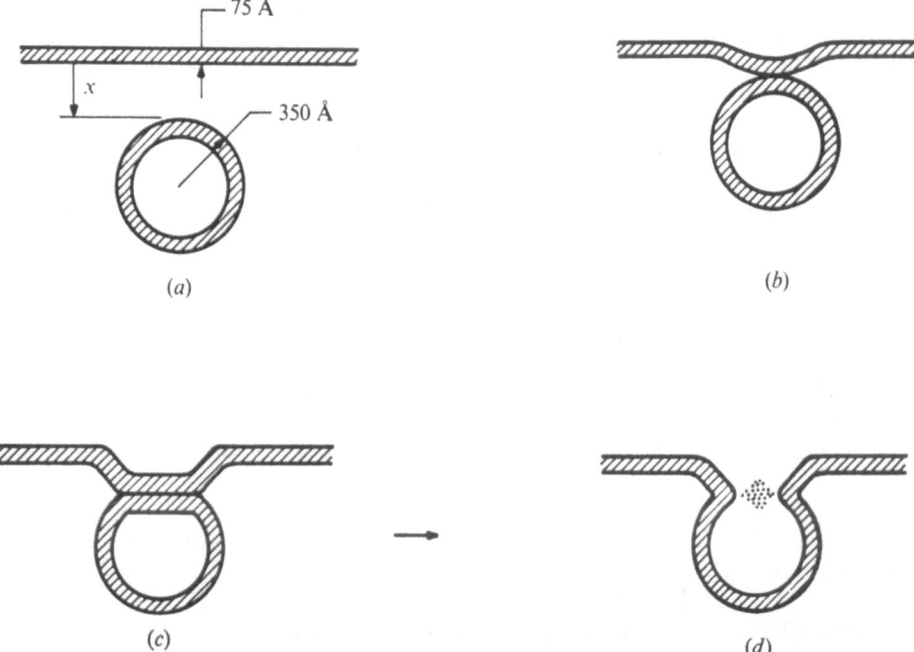

Fig. 4-4: Sketch of proposed sequence of events leading to the attachment of free vesicle to plasmalemma. (a) X 200 Å region of strong hydrodynamic interaction, (b) indentation of plasmalemma due to Van der Waals force interaction, (c) configuration before formation of vesicle neck and (d) attached vesicle. From Weinbaum and Caro (1).

When a vesicle approaches to within roughly one radius of
the plasmalemma it starts to experience a very strong hydrodynamic
interaction. At even closer spacings one encounters the
Van de Waals force interaction that we talked about earlier.
While exterior surfaces of membranes have a small negative
surface charge, it appears that the interior surface is
devoid of charge. You have to look at many pictures to
catch a vesicle in the transitory step before attachment.
If the plasmalemma had a negative surface charge on its
interior surface, you would expect an equilibrium spacing
like one observes in the intracellular channel. It does not
exist. There is no fluid gap between the vesicle and the
plasmalemma prior to reattachment. The configuration where
the vesicle and the plasmalemma abut against one another
forming a double membrane is unstable.

    What appears to happen is that the protein heads of the
bilayer membrane flow radically outward leaving the lipids
behind in the middle of the newly formed vesicle attachment
stalk. It is difficult to estimate the time scale of this
process or how long the lipid diaphragm remains in the
vesicle neck. The next question is how an attached vesicle
ruptures? The most likely hypothesis is that this is due to
Brownian motion. We are currently trying to develop a theory
to predict how far an attached vesicle will zig-zag in its
attached state.

    DR. NEREM: I am confused on one point. What were you
implying what the long channel was?

    DR. WEINBAUM: The long intracellular channel.

    DR. NEREM: The other question is: Do you want to say
anything about the relative importance of pressure versus
shear stress in enhancing some type of vesicular transport?

    DR. WEINBAUM: I don't know the answer to this. We are
going to have to perform more sophisticated EM studies to
show how a nucleus moves inside a cell. We need to find out
what kind of internal circulation is established in the
periphery of the endothelial cell due to hydrodynamic forces
at its surface.

    DR. BJORKERUD: I think one should also then try to
account for some other factors when trying to make a hypothesis
of how vesicles fuse with the plasma membrane.

I mean, if this were so, the cells would have difficulty in discerning between mitochondria, vesicles of other types, etc. The membrane would pick up things rather unselectively. People have discussed the matter and it has been shown that concommitantly with fusion or before fusion of vesicles with the plasma membrane, there is a rearrangement of the protein part of the membrane, i.e., of the intramembranous particles. These are rearranged when a vesicle will form. This is thought to reflect some selective mechanism by which the plasma membrane can identify structures. As a consequence, something which should not leave the cell does not fuse with the membrane. I think you must also incorporate these features into your theory before we would be able to accept it.

DR. WEINBAUM: The vesicle's membrane is undoubtedly the same phospholipid bilayer as the plasmalemma membrane. The two membranes are indistinguishable. The vesicles are passive bodies. There are many other bodies in the interior of the cell which have the specialization you are talking about, but the vesicle membrane is just extra membranous material which is identical in structure as far as I know to plasmalemma.

DR. BJORKERUD: It is very probable that the outer leaf of the membrane has different phospholipid distribution as compared to the inner one which would be difficult to reconcile with your theory.

DR. WEINBAUM: No, the vesicle membrane is inside out compared to the plasmalemma.

DR. COLTON: When the vesicle fuses to the surface, the inside is like the outside of the plasma membrane.

DR. WEINBAUM: That is the reason I think there is a difference in surface charge, between the exterior surface of the vesicle and the exterior surface of the plasmalemma.

DR. COLTON: But then you need a separate mechanism which is not charge dependent which prevents all the other organelles in the cell from going through and fusing with the plasmalemma.

DR. KENYON: I would like to ask you about your hypothesis on the junction characteristics during pressurization and how you are going to calibrate, essentially, this hydraulic resistance because if you don't calibrate you still don't get, I believe, the pressure difference across the endothelial surface.

DR. WEINBAUM: In a gall bladder epithelium you have a
tight junction at the luminal surface. The gall bladder
water flux can be arrested by poisoning the active transport.
Jared Diamond (1) has shown that the active transport--in
the gall bladder is electrically neutral. The chloride ions
are pumped and the Na ions follow to satisfy electroneutrality.
The water movment is passive and follows the local osomotic
gradient produced by the ion pumps. By collecting exuded
fluid and estimating the geometry of the cell layer, you can
make an estimate of the flow rate in the extracellular
channel. With this information, I can calculate the pressure
distribution in the channel.

DR: KENYON: Which are you considering known--the
dimension of the channel or the flux?

DR. WEINBAUM: I only know the dimension at the base of
the channel. I would like to determine the distorted geometry
of the channel during flow using a lubrication theory approach.

DR. COLTON: Are you suggesting that you are going to
do this with endothelial cells?

DR. WEINBAUM: No, not with endothelial cells, with gall
bladder epithelium. While it is not the same endothelium
cell layer, I expect the membrane molecular force to be
similar.

DR. CAREW: I would again like to bring up the point
that not all vesicles are equal with regard to this model.
                              I would also point out that
Not All Vesicles Are Equal   the total picture may not be
                              as simple as all vesicles
having the same sort of Van der Waals interaction in attaching.
There is some experimental evidence for there being differences
in attachment as a function of what is inside the vesicle.
Some work done by the Steins in Jerusalem, (2) when they
were on sabbatical in La Jolla, with regard to the binding
of endocytic vesicles, primarily lysosomes, in cultured
fibroblasts, showed that they could block the fusion of the
primary lysosome with the endocytic vesicle by pre-incubating
the cells with Concanavalin A and that suggests that what
may be found on the inner membrane of the vesicle could
sufficiently alter the outer membrane leaflet so that you
may have different fates for different sorts of vesicles and
it raises a question of what is responsible for the attachment
of vesicles to one body or the other, to what extent, are
the phospholipids important, to what extent are the lipolipids
important, and membrane fluidity?

How do things change with what is carried in the vesicle?

DR. WEINBAUM: I agree with all the things that you have just said. There are many intracellular bodies which are membrane-bound. The very striking feature about plasmalemma vesicles is their homogeneity in size. If you look at the statistical distribution of plasmalemma vesicles sizes you will find that they are seven hundred angstroms with a standard deviation of less than fifty angstroms.

DR. SCHWARTZ: Be careful, because they have looked largely at capillary vesicles and there are very real differences between arterial and capillary endothelium.

DR. WEINBAUM: I agree. The internal structures of capillary and arterial endothelial cells are quite different. The vesicles themselves appear to be quite similar.

DR. FRY: Hemodynamic forces interact with the arterial wall in two ways: 1, to convey blood borne substances and cellular elements to and from the wall, and 2, to exert a mechanical force directly on the endothelial surface and its subjacent tissues. This presentation concerns only the latter, the effects of hemodynamic forces on the endothelial surface. For simplicity these forces may be resolved into two components, a perpendicular force field, "pressure stress," and a field of force acting parallel to the surface, a "shear stress." Pressure stresses are related mostly to the arterial blood pressure whereas shear stresses are related mostly to the drag of the adjacent blood flow.

The response of the endothelial surface to shear stress appears to depend on the magnitude of the stress and also upon the stability of the stress field. At relatively physiologic levels of stress exposure the endothelial cells are seen to be elongated with elliptically shaped nuclei having major semiaxes that are oriented in the direction of the adjacent streamlines of the blood flow (3). If the adjacent streamlines are changed by certain experimental surgical techniques, the patterns of endothelial cell orientation are seen to realign to the new pattern of streamlines within a matter of weeks (4). Thus many of the structural features of the normal endothelial surface appear to be determined, at least in part, by the adjacent hemodynamic forces.

The permeability of the endothelial surface to macromolecules in the blood also appears to be sensitive to the adjacent hemodynamic stress fields.

Permeability of Endothelial Surfaces

Permeability increases monotonically with actuely increased levels of stress exposure (5,6,7). Surface permeability is also increased in regions of turbulence (5).

Under conditions of exposure to chronically elevated shear stress, such as in an artery supplying a surgically induced arteriovenous fistula, the permeability is seen gradually to decrease over a matter of weeks. Thus it appears that under chronic conditions compensatory mechanisms are apparently invoked which tend to return the endothelial permeability to normal values (8).

The levels of shearing stress considered up to this point, although increased, are unassociated with any significant structural evidence of endothelial damage. However, if shearing stress is elevated to levels ranging from 200 to 700 dynes/cm ^{2}, endothelial structural changes become evident even by light microscopy. These consist of cellular swelling, deformation, and vacuolization

Acute Critical Yield Stress

of the cytoplasm followed by progressive endothelial cell disintegration and erosion. The level of stress in an individual that is associated with the occurence of these changes has been defined as the acute critical yield stress of the endothelial surface for that individual at that site (5,9). Erosion of the endothelial surface is associated with a massive influx of plasma substances into the intimal surface as well as the deposition of platelets, leucocytes, and fibrin on the exposed intimal surface. It is of interest to note that small areas of endothelial erosion can be found in the arterial trees of normal animals (8) suggesting that this process may be a recurring event throughout the lifetime of an individual. Whether these sites represent regions that have been exposed momentarily to an intense hemodynamic force or whether the acute yield stress of the endothelial surface at these sites has been lowered by certain metabolic or hemodynamic events (8) remains to be explored.

Pressure stress can also be shown to alter endothelial surface permeability. Pressure can increase the permeability of the arterial wall by stretching the endothelial surface (3) and also by increasing the driving pressure across the wall to increase the flux of plasma substances (10).

In principle, an increased pressure stress may also influence the endothelial surface permeability indirectly by producing a deformation of the normally streamlined conduit geometry thereby predisposing the normally stable streamlined flow patterns to unstable patterns at various points along the arterial trees. To the extent that shear stress patterns that are changing in magnitude and directions are associated with chronically endothelial surface permeability, this indirect effect of increased pressure on flow stability may be important (3,8).

Altered Endothelial Permeability in Experimental Atherogenesis

Thus a variety of hemodynamic events can be shown either directly or by inference to alter endothelial structure and permeability. Data presented elsewhere (3,8,11) suggest that altered endothelial permeability plays one of the central roles in experimental atherogenesis and by inference perhaps also in human atherosclerosis.

DR. MANSFIELD: Our interest in the endothelial cell, its growth in tissue culture, and its function as an in vivo lining for artificial vascular prosthesis is an outgrowth of our work with a left ventricular assist device and the problems of thrombus generation associated with the use of that device. (12-17).

During our evaluation of several anticoagulation techniques designed to reduce thrombus in these devices, we have used a model for thrombus generation which is shown in Fig. 4-5.

Anticoagulation Studies

With this technique, we remove a segment of the descending aorta in the calf and replace it with a non-porous, prosthetic graft containing an inside lining which we wish to study. The graft is attached to the ends of the aorta using continuous suture (2-0 Ticron) techniques currently used in clinical vascular surgery. One of the most promising materials we have used has been polypropylene microfiber. With this lining surrounded by a non-porous polyurethane back and a dacron sleeve to permit suturing to the ends of the individual aorta, we have studied thrombus generation with and without anticoagulants.

When anticoagulants were not utilized in this model with the polypropylene microfiber surface, thrombus, rapidly deposited on the surface up to depths of 1 to 3 millimeters was found after 7 days implantation.

Thrombus Generation

See Fig. 4-6. Frequently, thrombus hung downstream into the lumen of the aorta, but where the aortic endothelium was intact there was no thrombus attachment.

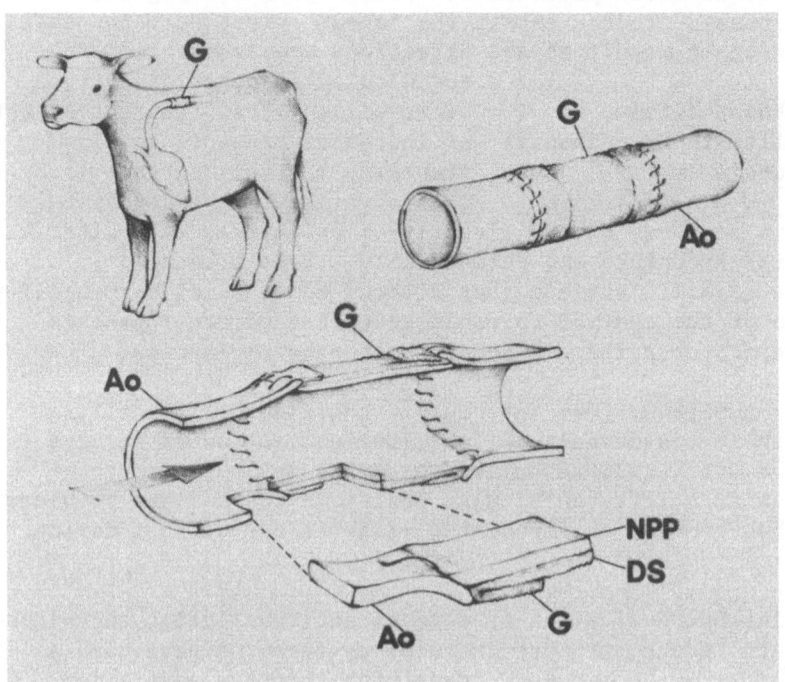

Fig. 4-5: Thrombus generation model used in these studies. A
segment of the descending aorta in the calf is removed and
replaced with a vascular prosthesis (G). Commonly used clinical
vascular surgical techniques are used to anastomose the graft
and the aorta (AO). The graft, shown in cut-out, is composed
of an external dacron sleeve (DS) used for sutering, a non-
porous polypropylene backing tube (NPP), and an inner lining
surface which is varied according to the study in progress.
Flow in the aorta is shown by the arrow. Because of its
location in the descending aorta, emboli which may originate
from the graft can be evaluated by inspection of the kidneys for
infarcts. This serves as a sensitive indicator of distal emboli.

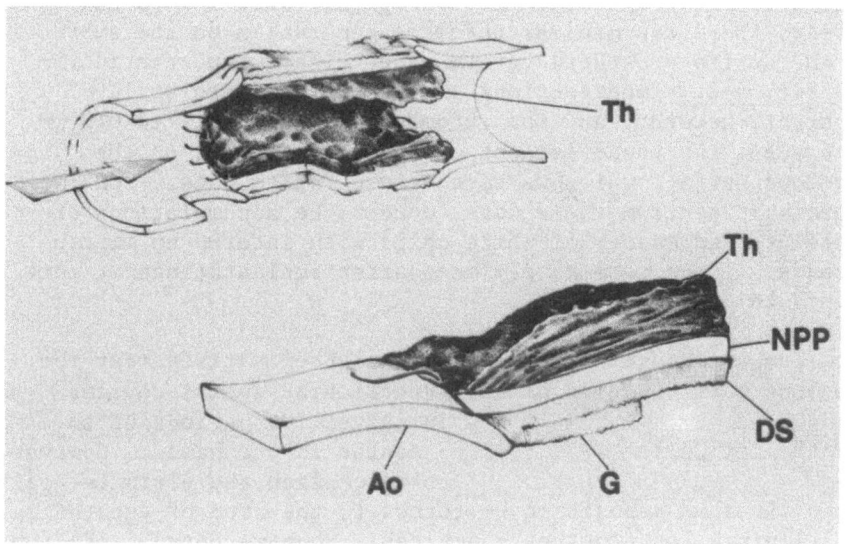

Fig. 4-6: Drawing of thrombus generation on aortic tubular
graft, 7 days after implantation. No anticoagulants used.
Thrombus (TH) originates only from the bare surface of the
graft (polypropylene microfiber) and hangs downstream into
the lumen of the aorta. Embolic infarcts found in the kidneys.
NPP: non-porous polyurethane backing, DS: dacron sleeve,
AO: aorta, G: graft.

Placing the graft in the descending aorta permitted us to
evaluate the incidence of peripheral emboli which could be
seen as multiple infarcts within the kidney. Multiple
infarcts were found when no anticoagulation was used.

After evaluating 11 different anticoagulation protocols
in nearly 100 calves, we found the most effective protocol
was a combination of coumadin, persantine, and aspirin (18).
With this anticoagulation protocol, initiated 5 days before
surgey, there was minimal thrombus generation on the surface
of the aortic prosthetic graft after 7 days implantation.
See Fig. 4-7. Imperfections in the surface were still
apparent, however, and the thrombus depths of 0.1 to 0.3 mm
were seen. We found islands of whitish material on the
thrombus surface which we have termed "white caps." On
histologic section these were found to be accumulations of
platelets and masses of white cells with interwoven fibrin
strands. These were rarely seen after implantations of more
than 3 to 4 weeks.

The anticoagulation protocol has been satisfactory for
the long-term function of left ventricular assist devices
in calves for periods up to
3 months in our hands. However,
to accomplish the ultimate goal
of no thrombus deposition we turned to the area of endothelial
cell linings for prosthetic devices. When we began, (17) the
techniques for serial passage of viable endothelial cells in
tissue culture had not been developed.

Endothelial Cells

We initially utilized cells from the inferior vena cava of
calves and more recently have used endothelial cells from
the carotid artery of the
calf. The technique we developed
for obtaining these cells is
shown in Fig. 4-8a & b. The
blood vessel is washed with Hanks Salt Solution (calcium and
magnesium free) cut longitudinally and exposed to 0.02%
versene-trypsin (0.25% solution) (pH 8.0). After 25 minutes
the incubating solution is gently pipetted over the endothelial
surface and the dislodged cells collected. Complete tissue
culture medium was added to the cell suspensions as a source
of calcium and serum protein to inhibit the action of versene
and tryspin. Following centrifugation the cell pellet was
resuspended in complete tissue culture medium and seeded
into plastic flasks. Using this technique we have now had
multiple cell lines which have had over 25 serial passages
in tissue culture.

**Technique for Endothelial
Tissue Culture**

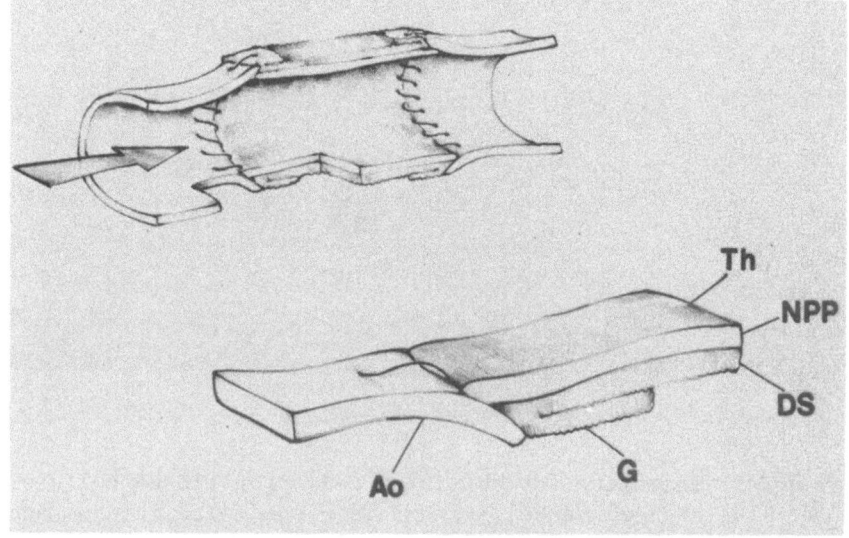

Fig. 4-7: Drawing of thrombus generation found on aortic tubular graft using coumadin, persantin and aspirin anti-coagulation protocol. Graft implantation for 7 days. Maximum thrombus depth 0.3 milimeters. No renal embolic infarcts found. TH: thrombus layer, NPP: non-porous polyurethane backing layer, DS: dacron sleeve, AO: aorta, G: tubular graft.

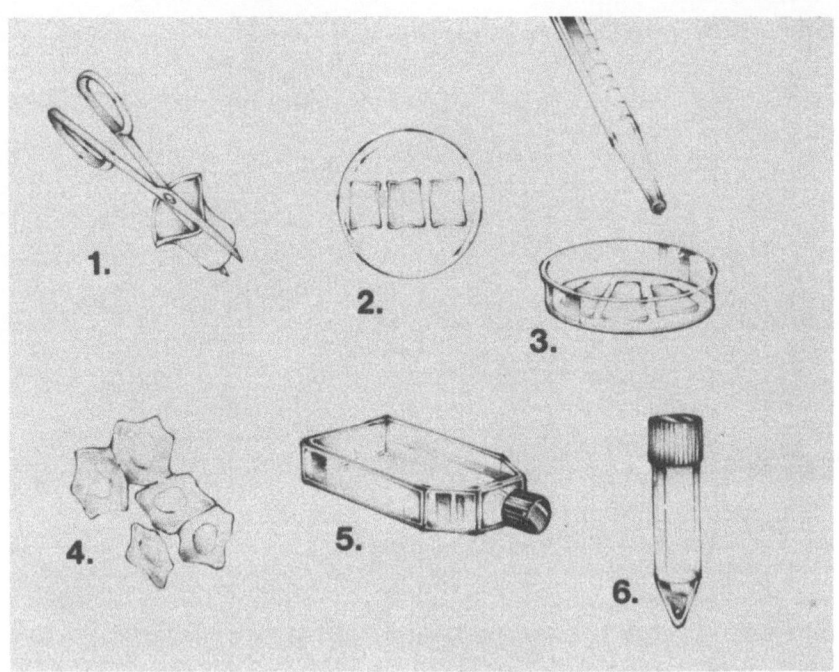

Fig. 4-8A: Technique for obtaining cells for tissue culture.
A: 1. The excised vessel segment is washed with calcium and
magnesium-free Hanks Balanced Salt Solution to remove residual
blood. Carotid artery cut into three sections after the
surrounding adventitial tissue had been dissected away.
2. The segments are placed endothelial surface up in a petri
dish containing 0.02% versene solution in calcium and magnesium-
free phosphate buffered saline (pH 7.0). After 5 minutes at
room temperature, the specimens are transferred to a second
petri dish containing 0.02% versene tryps in (0.25%) solution
(pH 8.0). After 25 minutes at 37° C in a humidified atmosphere
of 5% CO_2 and 95% air, the incubating solution is gently
pipetted (3) over the endothelial surface, and the dislodged
cells collected (4).

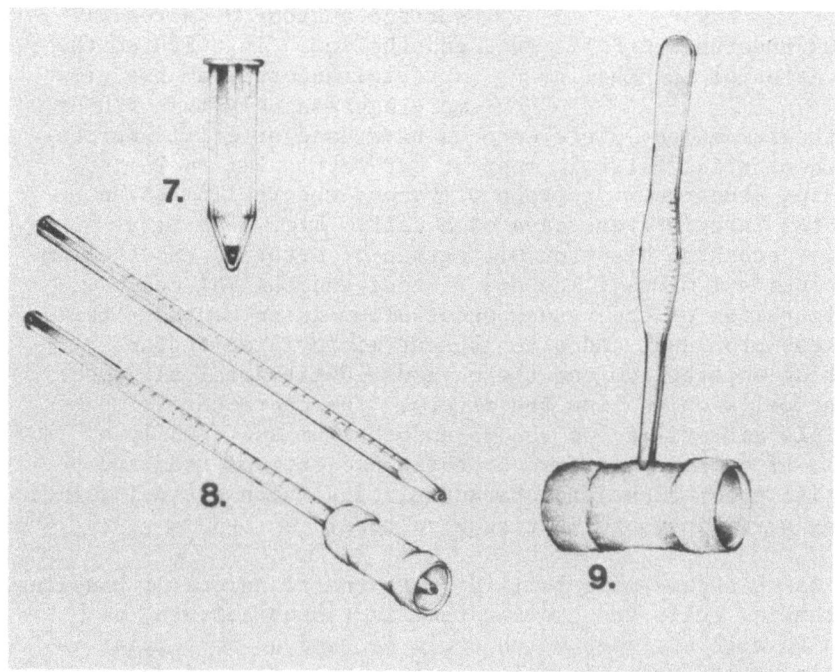

Fig. 4-8B: These cells were then transferred to flasks for
further growth. When a satisfactory number of cells had been
grown, they were centrifuged into a pellet (6). When approximately 35 X 10^6 cells were available they were resuspended and
gently distributed evenly over the inside lining of the aortic
tubular graft (8). The cells were cultured for 7 days before
implantation in animals (9).

The endothelial cells grow well in plastic as well as on glass surfaces.

We feel it is significant that the surface anatomy of venous endothelium is significantly different from the surface anatomy of arterial endothelium. In culture, the arterial endothelium has grown more aggressively than venous endothelium and by preference we have used arterial sources for endothelial cells in most of our work. Fig. 4-9a is a scanning electron micrograph of venous endothelium taken from the inferior vena cava of a calf. Fig. 4-9b is a similar scanning electron micrograph of arterial endothelium. The prominent microvillae and rounded endothelial cell configuration of the venous endothelium is in contrast to the less prominent and often absent microvillae in the arterial endothelium and the obvious longitudinal alignment of the cells which line the artery. The characteristics of multiple microvillae on venous endothelium and usually a single or occasionally two or three projections from the arterial endothelium are characteristics which are maintained during serial passage in tissue culture.

Venous Endothelium Different from Arterial Endothelium

As we became more familiar with the technique of handling endothelial cells and growing them in tissue culture, we began to seek surfaces which could be used as artificial vessels or linings for assist devices on which the cells would grow. Our experience has shown that polypropylene microfiber, parylene c-coated (Type B) from Union Carbide Corporation has been an excellent substrate for endothelial cell growth. Figure 4-10 is a scanning electron micrograph of the microfiber surface. We have found the endothelial cell to be rather fastidious as to the substrate to which it likes to adhere. It prefers a relatively regular surface and has difficulty in covering areas where there are large gaps between supporting structures. Polypropylene microfiber of identical chemical composition and surface characteristics if physically teased apart during manufacture often leads to poor endothelial cell coverage.

To test the adherence characteristics of the endothelial cells to the underlying prosthetic substrate we devised a technique of applying a jet of fluid onto the surface of the cells. The fluid passes through a tapered glass nozzle and is directed vertically toward the cells.

Adherence of Endothelial Cells to Prosthetic Materials

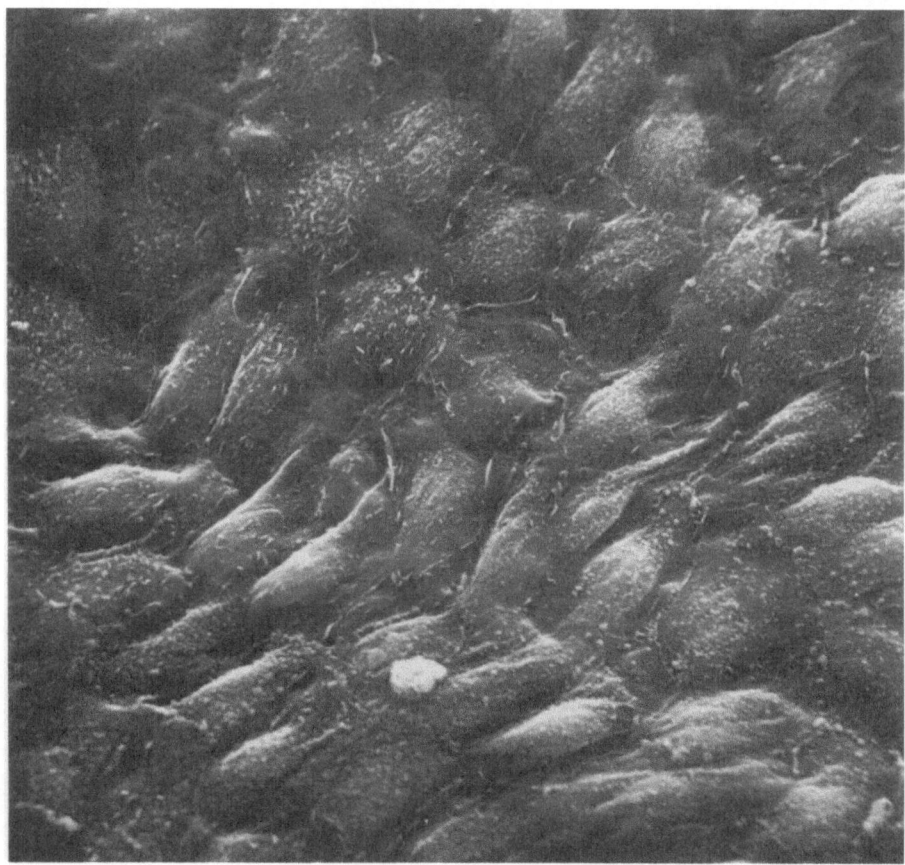

Fig. 4-9A: In vivo venous and arterial endothelium. A.
Scanning electron micrograph of Bovine venous endothelium.
Surface microvillae are numerous and cellular arrangement is
cobblestone in appearance (X 1180).

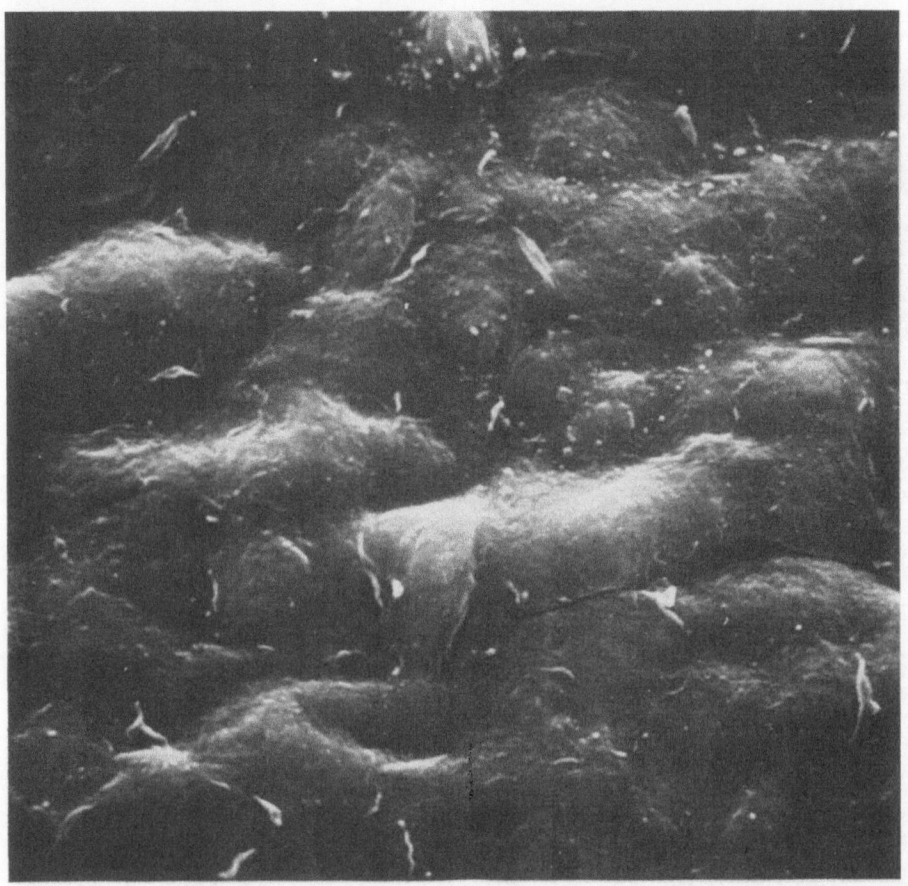

Fig. 4-9B: Scanning electron micrograph of Bovine arterial
endothelium showing single or double projections from the
surface of each cell. These projections have a different
configuration than the microvillae as seen on venous endothelium
in Fig. 4-5A. (X 1599).

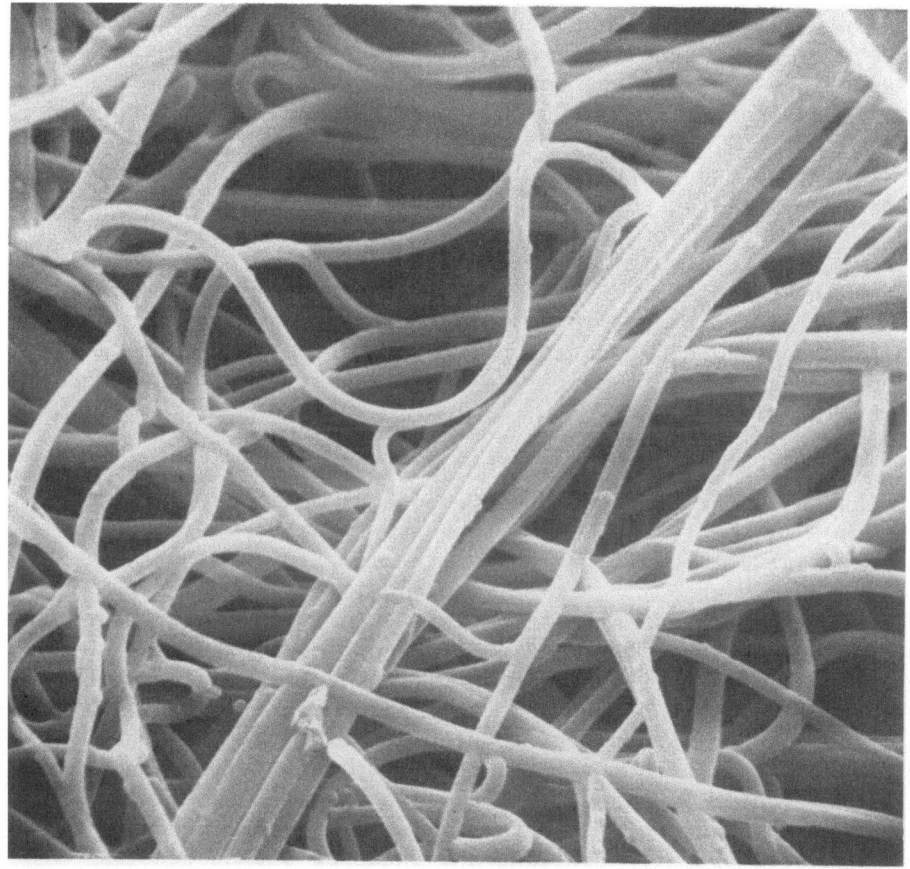

Fig. 4-10: Scanning electron micrograph of polypropylene microfiber, parylene C coated (Type B). Microfiber distribution is random, the fibers are fairly uniform in diameter. (Approximately 1 micron). (X 2210).

By maintaining a constant pressure and velocity and therefore
force of the fluid hitting the cell surface from sample to
sample, it is possible to compare qualitatively the adherence
characteristics of each of the substrates on which the cells
have been grown. See Figure 4-11. Vital staining of the
cells after shear testing demonstrates which cells have
survived and over how great a surface area the cells have
disrupted from the substrate below. Our calculations, which
can only be considered approximate, would suggest that we
have used shear stresses (which vary over the surface in a
predictable way from the center of the fluid jet) between no
stress to approximately 600-800 dynes per centimeter squared.

Once we had learned to line discs for study in the shear
apparatus, we proceeded to line tubular grafts which had the
polypropylene microfiber surface. This was done in tissue
culture prior to surgical implantation into the thrombus model
shown in Figure 4-5. Figure 4-12 is a histologic section of
endothelial cells pre-lining the polypropylene microfiber
surface prior to implantation into the aorta. Note the
monolayer and ability of the cells to conform to the surface
irregularities.

When the endothelial cell lined tubular grafts were
implanted in the aorta without the use of anticoagulants, we
                                 found no thrombus where the
Endothelial Cell Grafts   endothelium remained intact.
                                 Figure 4-13 is a drawing of
the findings of such a graft implanted for 4 weeks in the
descending aorta of the calf. We found a monolayer of viable
endothelial cells (these were autologous cells obtained from
the carotid artery of the same calf into which the graft was
later implanted) lining the tubular graft at the time the
animal was sacrificed. Minute bits of thrombus were found at
the anastomotic junctions, but nowhere else in these animals.
(Compare to Figure 4-6). Obviously, the endothelial cell
linings were able to withstand the shear of the descending
aorta, remain viable, and were as effective in preventing
thrombus as the normal aortic endothelium above and below
the graft. Figure 4-14 is a scanning electron micrograph of
the endothelial surface of a 4 week tubular implant. One
can see that the endothelial cells have aligned in the
direction of flow and have remained as a confluent monolayer.
No such flow alignment was present at the time of implantation.

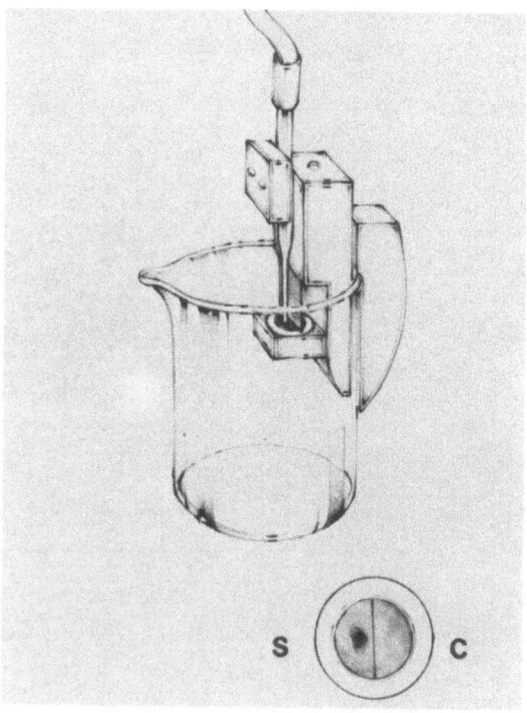

Fig. 4-11: Shear testing apparatus. A disc supporting the substrate and a covering of endothelial cells (S: shear tested side, C: control side) is placed on a support stand within the beaker. A glass nozzle is mounted immediately above the surface, and fluid at a known pressure and velocity impinges on the endothelial cell surface at right angles for 30 seconds. The disc is then removed, vital staining done to determine cell distribution and cell death. As can be seen, an area of significant staining has occurred on the shear tested side of the disc in comparison to the control side.

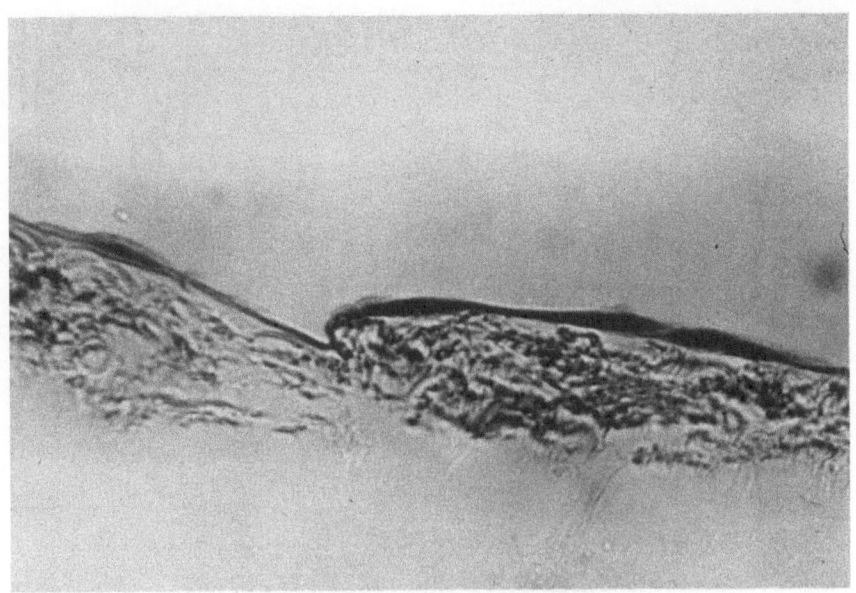

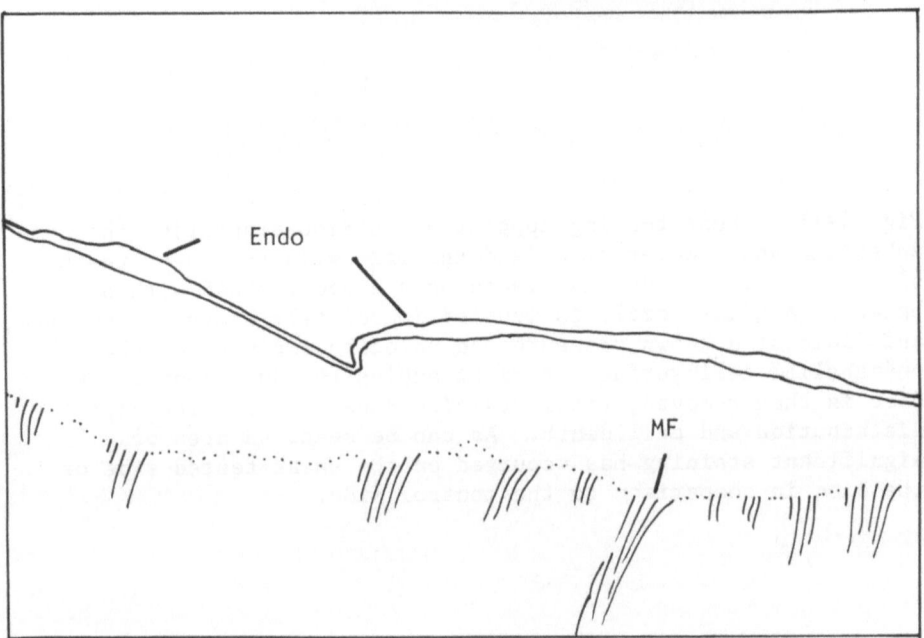

Fig. 4-12: Histologic section of endothelial lined polypropylene microfiber. Note the monolayer of endothelial
cells and ability to conform to surface irregularities.
Line drawing defines the microfiber (M) and the endothelial
cell (N) (X 670). (Reduced 30% for purposes of reproduction.)

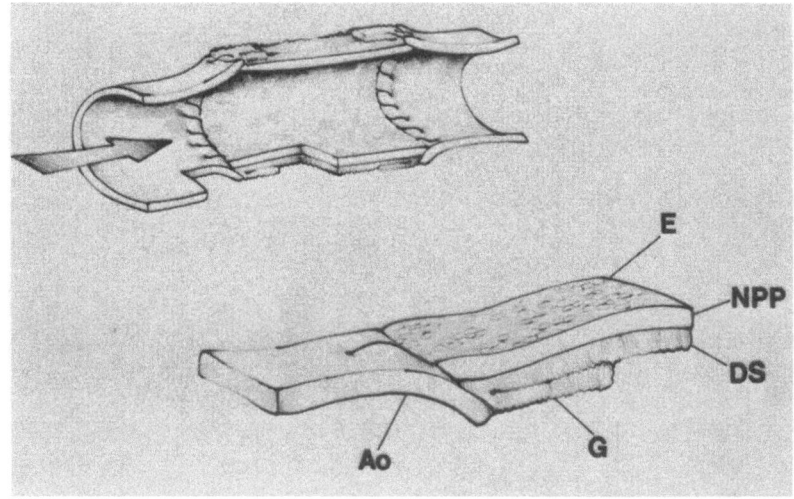

Fig. 4-13: Aortic tubular graft prelined with autologous
arterial endothelium in tissue culture. No significant
thrombus was found on the surface of this graft. No anticoagulants were used. Minute amounts of thrombus were seen
at the anastomotic junctions. An endothelial monolayer
covered the polypropylene microfiber lining of this graft, and
cell orientation was parallel to that of blood flow through
the vessel. E: endothelial monolayer, NPP: non-porous
polyurethane backing, DS: dacron sleeve, G: aortic tubular
graft, AO: aorta.

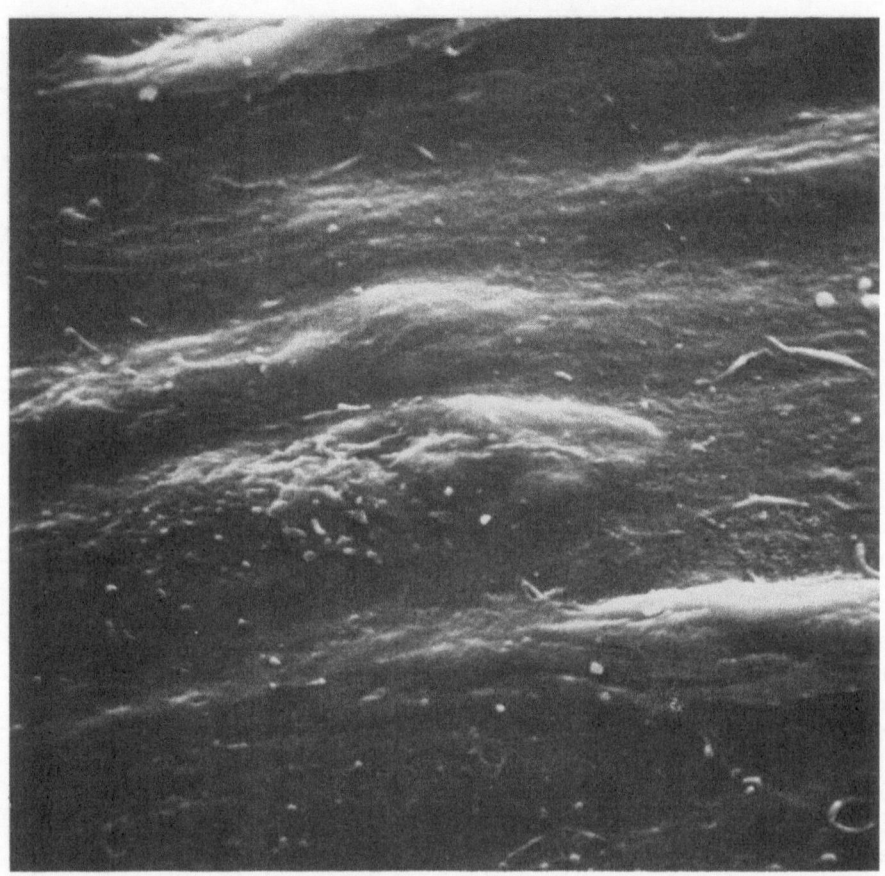

Fig. 4-14: Scanning electron micrograph of autologous
endothelial cell-lined tubular aortic graft after 4 weeks
implantation. The cells have aligned in the direction of flow
and no thrombus is evident. The surface remains a monolayer
of endothelial cells. (X 4609).

In addition to preventing thrombus generation, we found that viable endothelial cells lining the prosthetic graft have a significant influence on the tissue reaction at the anastomotic junctions between the graft and the normal aorta. Figure 4-15 is a drawing of the findings at 4 weeks of a control graft surface (no cell lining, no anticoagulants). There has been a continuous in-growth of pannus (19) which has begun to digest and organize the thrombus present on the surface of the polypropylene microfiber. We have found this pannus continues to progress for at least 2 centimeters from the anastomotic margins in experiments lasting up to 4 months. Macrophage activity within the thrombus itself precedes the in-growth of pannus over the surface of the thrombus and leads to actual thinning of the thrombus. In contrast, the endothelial cell lined grafts had no such pannus in-growth and aortic endothelium to graft attachment occurred with minimal underlying tissue reaction. No macrophage involvement beyond the anastomosis was seen. It appears that viable endothelium has the ability (even after multiple serial passages in culture) of communicating a message to normal arterial endothelium inhibiting a hyperactive healing response to an implanted prosthetic material. This may be a form of in vivo contact inhibition.

We have been interested in the method by which endothelial cells attach to their underlying substrate, be it sub-endothelial tissues in the wall of a vessel, or the glass or plastic vessels in tissue culture.

Role of Microfilaments in Endothelial Cell Attachment

In tissue culture there are no sub-endothelial tissues present and all cellular components must therefore be of endothelial cell origin. Dr. Schwartz showed slides which suggested there were filaments, very fine microfilaments, if you will, under the endothelial cell and suggested that these might play a role in endothelial cellular attachment to underlying tissues. We have found similar structures under endothelial cells in tissue culture. Figure 4-16 demonstrates these very fine filaments, far finer than retraction fibrils in dimension. These transmission electron micrographs suggest that there may be physical connections between these filaments and structures within these bovine endothelial cells, possibly the endoplasmic reticulum. Certainly our results demonstrate that whatever the mechanism, endothelial cell attachment to suitable substrates is more than adequate to withstand the shear stresses within the descending aorta of the calf. In addition to the bovine endothelial cell we have been able to grow and serially passage human endothelial cells in tissue culture also.

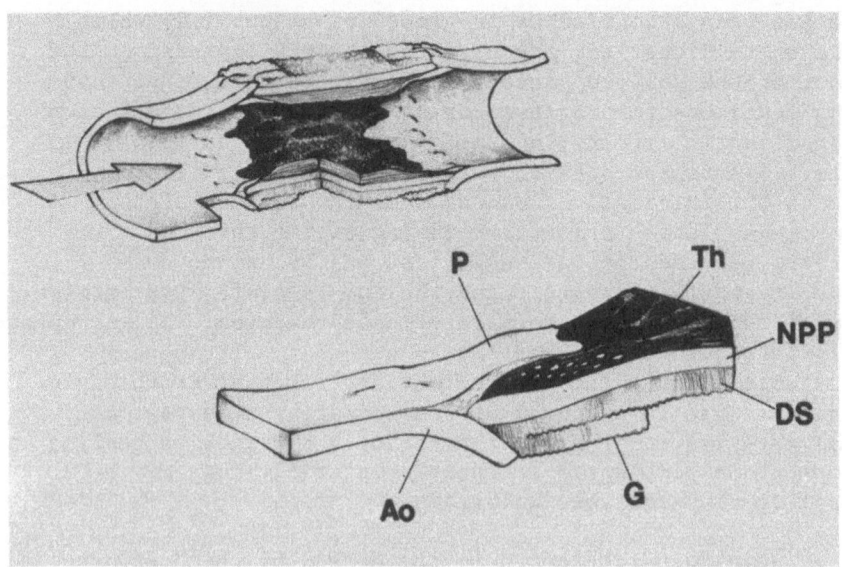

Fig. 4-15: Drawing of findings of aortic tubular graft after
4 week implantation. No pre-implant cellular linings and no
anticoagulants were used in this study. The cutaway section
demonstrates pannus (P) ingrowth over the previously deposited
thrombus (TH) on the microfiber surface lining this control
graft. Diagrammatic representation of macrophage activity
leading the pannus ingrowth is seen as white dots in the
thrombus. No such pannus activity was seen when grafts were
prelined with autologous endothelium. See Fig. 4-13. NNP:
non-porous polyurethane backing, DS: dacron sleeve, G: graft,
AO: aorta.

This is technically much more difficult and it is only rarely possible to obtain a true endothelial cell of human origin to serially passage in culture. It is interesting to note that when fibroblasts of either human or bovine origin are studied in a similar manner, no such microfilamentous structures between the cell and the underlying substrate have been seen in our studies. Figure 4-17 shows typical Weibel-Palade bodies seen after serial passage of human endothelial cells in tissue culture. We have found that the Weibel-Palade bodies are not as frequently encountered within endothelial cells of animals as compared to humans. Structures within the cell shown may be similar to microfilaments seen in bovine endothelial cells. Fig. 4-16.

The ability to provide a monolayer of true vascular endothelial cells on the surface of a porous microfiber substrate has suggested to us the possibility of using this approach to study transport mechanisms across endothelial cell linings. The polypropylene microfiber aortic tubular grafts have polyurethane backing to support them. However, it seems conceivable to us as is shown in Fig. 4-18, that it may be possible to line such a fabric with endothelial cells support-mounted between two rings. The ring becomes the connection between two fluid media-containing chambers. Ionic and molecular movement between the chambers which was passed through the endothelial cell lined disc could provide valuable information with regard to endothelial cell transport mechanisms. While our laboratory does not have the biochemical capability to perform such studies, we hope this suggestion will encourage others more capable in that area to consider this possible approach. Difficulties, of course, will be in proving that there is 100% coverage of the microfiber with endothelial cells at the time the experiments are performed.

Transport Mechanisms across Endothelial Cell Linings

Although there are similarities in the endothelial cells of human and of bovine origin, there are also differences. Endothelial cells of human origin can be separated out to individual cells and can survive alone. We have been unable to get bovine arterial endothelial cells to survive as single cells. They require other endothelial cells in contact with them to survive.

Human vs. Bovine Endothelial Cells

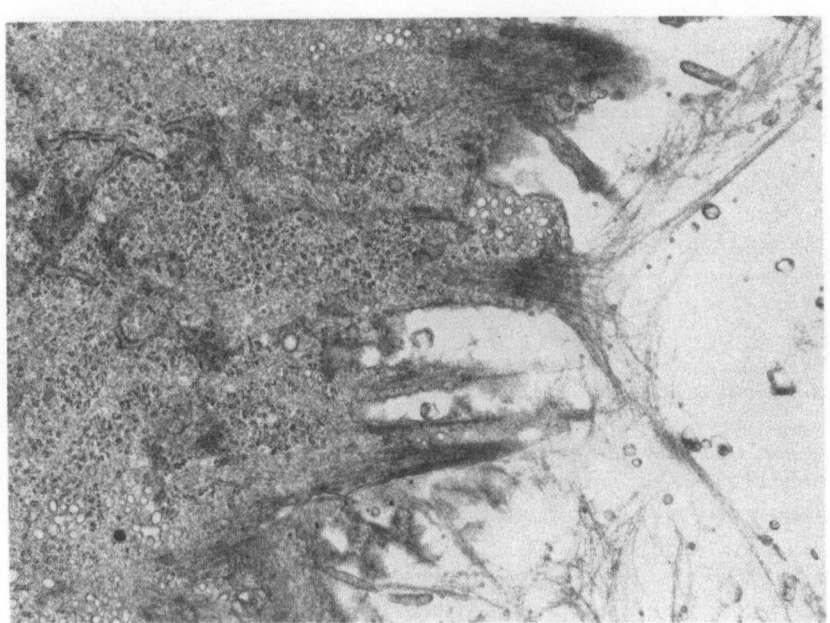

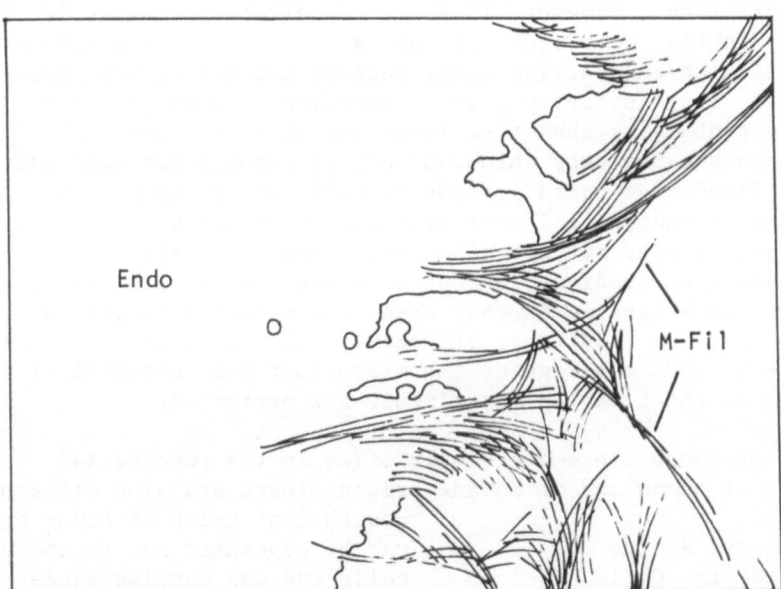

Endo

M-Fil

Fig. 4-16: Transmission electron micrograph of Bovine endothelium grown in tissue culture on plastic. A section is taken
at the junction between the cell and the plastic and demonstrates
the microfilaments discussed in the text. (X 7600). (Reduced
30% for purposes of reproduction.)

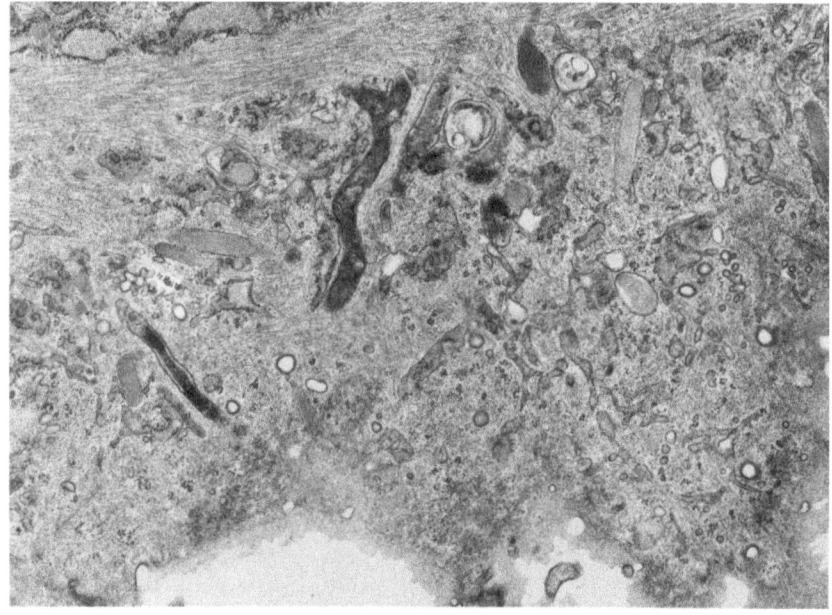

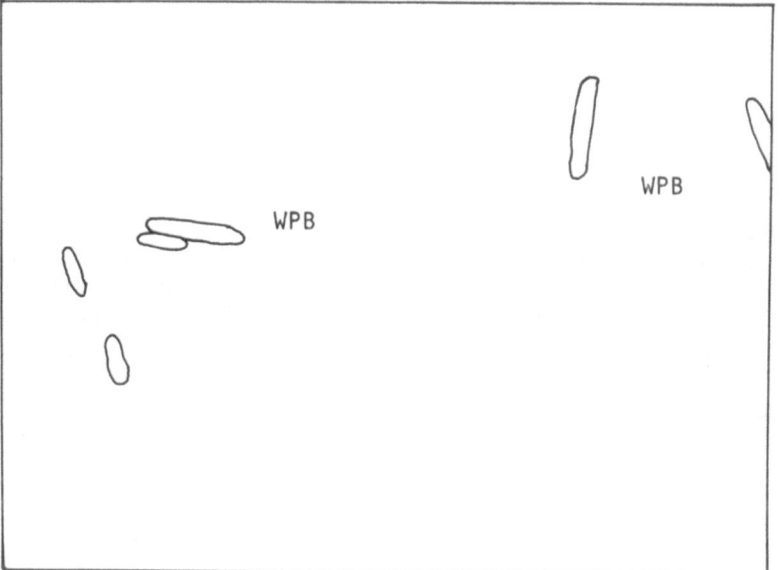

WPB

WPB

Fig. 4-17: Transmission electron micrograph of human endothelial cells after serial passage and culture demonstrating Weibel-Palade bodies characteristic of endothelial cells.

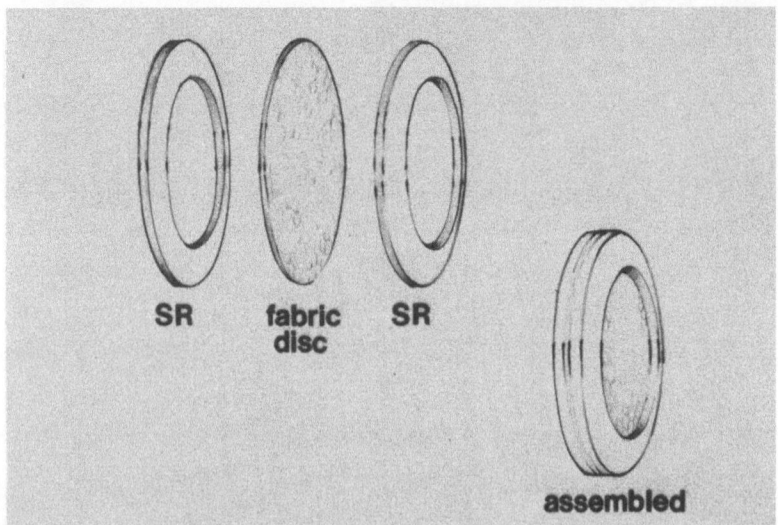

Fig. 4-18: Design concept for the study of endothelial cell
transport mechanisms. Now that endothelial cells can be grown
as monolayers covering a porous microfiber, we suggest the
use of this technique to study endothelial cell transport
mechanisms. By supporting the microfiber between discs
connecting two chambers, it should be possible to study the
ionic and molecular movement between the chambers and across
the cells.

In addition, the bovine arterial cells are very dominant in cell culture. They will overgrow fibroblast cultures and replace them, an exceedingly unusual occurrence in tissue culture work. We have also seen in bovine cultures that endothelial linings may pile up to 2 or 3 cells deep. Once they have been implanted in the aorta of the autologous calf, upon removal they are found to be monolayered. The fate of the other cells which were previously present is unknown. We have not seen this pile up of endothelial cells in human culture. If the antithrombogenic capability of the endothelial cell is not dependent on cell viability but rather on a surface structure or a bio-chemical matrix, it is exciting to think of the possibilities should that matrix or surface be generated on the inside of a vascular prosthesis. If indeed monocellular linings which are 100% confluent can be grown on porous backing, studies of transport across endothelial cell linings may give us new insight into the development of arteriosclerotic vascular disease.

DR. DEWEY: Referring to the differences in the shear resistance that you measured between bovine and human endothelial cells, did you actually obtain quantitative values for the shear stresses which would remove endothelial cells from the surface?

DR. MANSFIELD: It is extremely difficult to get a precise number. You can get a ball park figure and I might say you would be plus or minus a factor or two. We are talking in general; they did seem to shear in the range of four to six hundred dynes per centimeter squared, as we would calculate it.

DR. DEWEY: Do these values refer to human or bovine cells?

DR. MANSFIELD: No, the humans would be the upper limit of that and the bovine at the lower limit. There is a distinct separation between the two.

DR. SCHWARTZ: I would like to make a comment. I thought that was an excellent presentation, Dr. Mansfield. There are a lot of questions I would like to ask but I guess I will have to ask some of them later. I was very intrigued first of all with the polypropylene Type V. This presumably does not permit any cell growth from the adventitial surface into the luminal surface?

    DR. MANSFIELD: No, none at all. It is completely
separated from the adventitia by a one millimeter backing of
polyurethane which is absolutely solid.

    DR. SCHWARTZ: So then it is completely solid. The
influence of the combination of coumarin, persantin, and
aspirin on thrombosis in the graft is particularly interesting.
I wonder if you might tell us why you chose persantin as
part of the package, and how much you gave?

    DR. MANSFIELD: Surely. We have studied heparin,
coumarin, persantin, coumadin, persantin, aspirin and dextran
and several other anticoagulants. The best results were
obtained from a combination of coumadin, persantin and
aspirin, a combination found useful by Harker and Schlichter
in prosthetic valve surgery. (20). The population doubling
time for the human from saphenous vein origin is approximately
from 2 to 96 hours. The doubling time for the bovine calf
arterial endothelial cell is approximately 32 hours. See
Table 1.

    We have further studied the interaction of platelet-
rich plasma and the surface of tissue cultured fibroblasts
                                and endothelial cells of
Effects of Platelet-rich   bovine origin. When platelet-rich
Plasma on Cultured Cells   plasma is added to tissue cultured
                                fibroblasts of bovine origin,
clumping, pseudopod formation, and evidence of a release
reaction can be seen. See Figures 4-19 and 20. If under the
influence of versene fibroblasts contract and separate on a
plastic surface in culture, and platelet-rich plasma is
added, the platelets adhere to the fibroblast cell margins
and surface, but do not adhere to the exposed area of the
plastic.

    When an endothelial cell culture is exposed to platelet-
rich plasma of similar platelet concentration we have not
seen any attachment to the endothelial cell surfaces but
merely a pooling of non-creative platelets in the valleys
between the nuclei of the endothelial cells. If versene is
added to the culture and endothelial cells retract (leaving
fibrils between cells) the platelets adhere to these retractile
processes. Attachment and some pseudopod formation is seen
but the release reaction has not been identified in our
studies. (21). See Figures 4-21 & 4-22. We have not seen
platelets adhere to areas between endothelial cells under
the influence of versene, except where there are retraction
fibrils.

TABLE 1

Cell Characteristics	Human	Bovine
Source	Adult Vein	Yearly Artery
Attachment	Individual	Clump
Single-Cell Viability	High (90%)	Low (30-40%)
Density Dependent	Yes	No
Dominance	Non-Dominant	Dominant
Population Doubling Time	96 Hours	32 Hours
Maximum Passages	7	25
Weibel-Palade Bodies	Present	Present
Extra Cellular Microfilaments	Present	Present

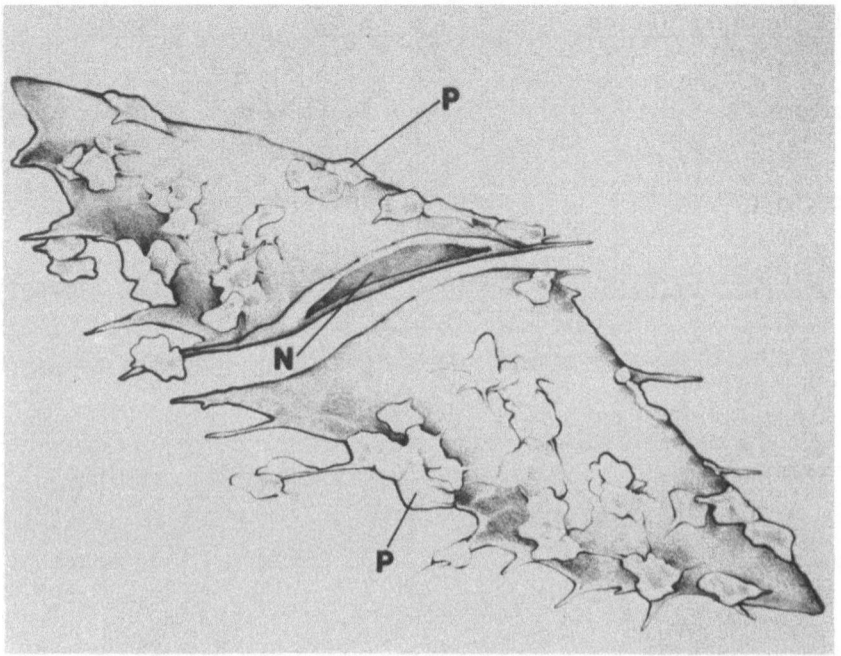

Fig. 4-19: Artist's concept of reaction between platelet-rich plasma and Bovine fibroblasts in culture. Note clumping, pseudopod formation and evidence of release reaction on the surface of the fibroblast.

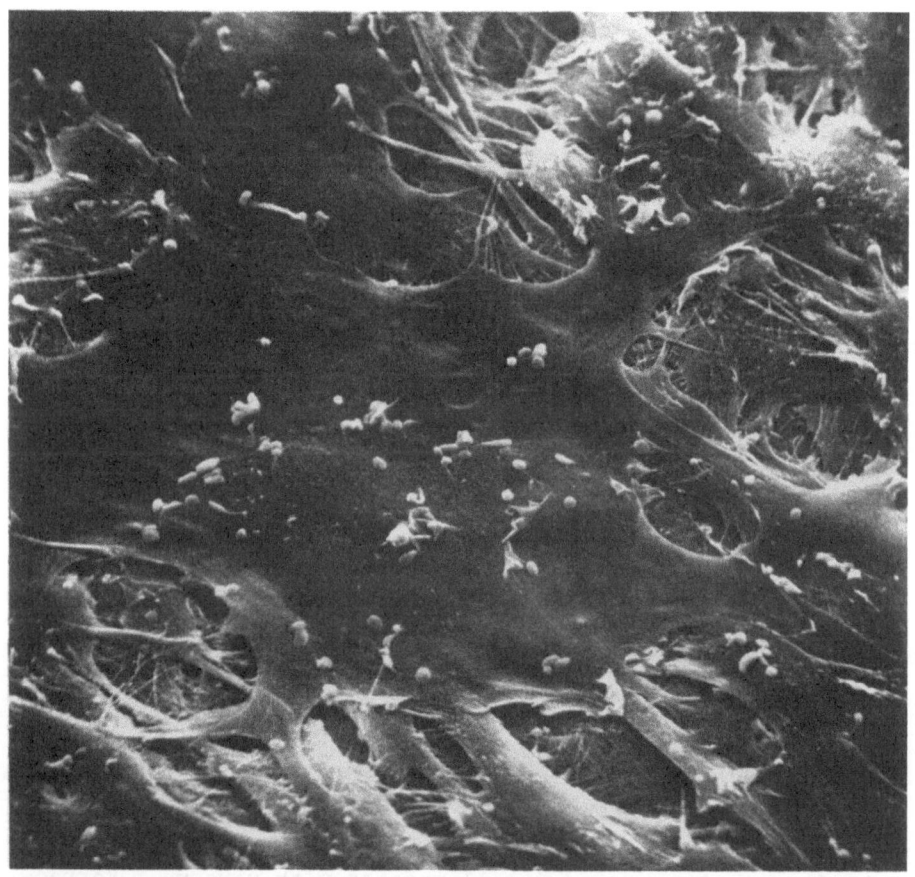

Fig. 4-20: Scanning electron micrograph of reaction between
platelet-rich plasma and Bovine fibroblasts in culture. Note
clumping, pseudopod formation and evidence of release reaction
on the surface of the fibroblast.

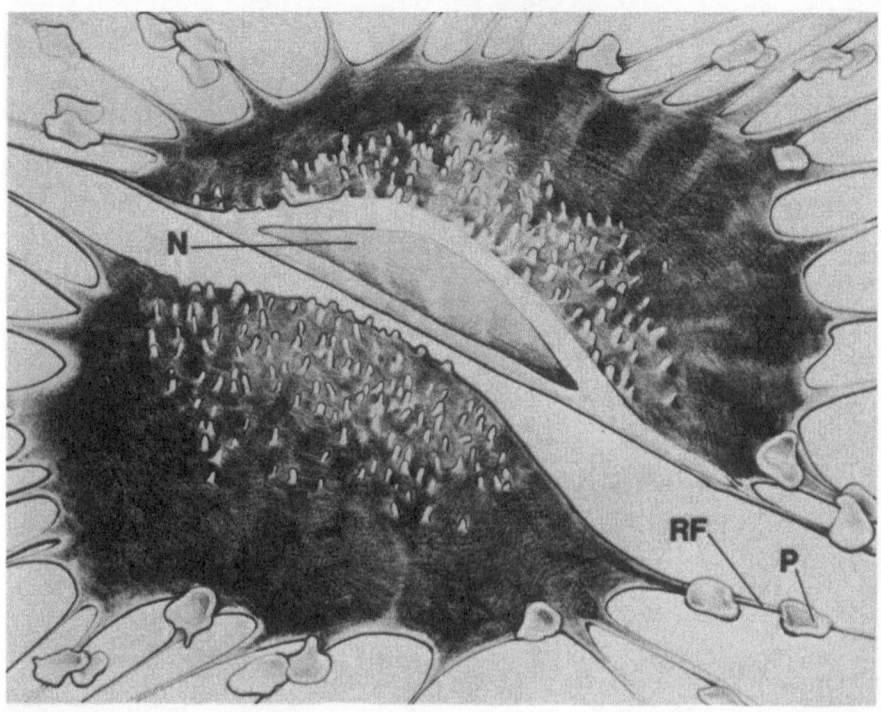

Fig. 4-21: Artist's concept of reaction seen between platelet-rich plasma and endothelial cell treated with versene. Retraction fibrils are prominent, platelet attachment is only to these retraction fibrils (RF). Attachment and pseudopod formation has been seen, but no release reaction has been identified in these studies. P: platelet.

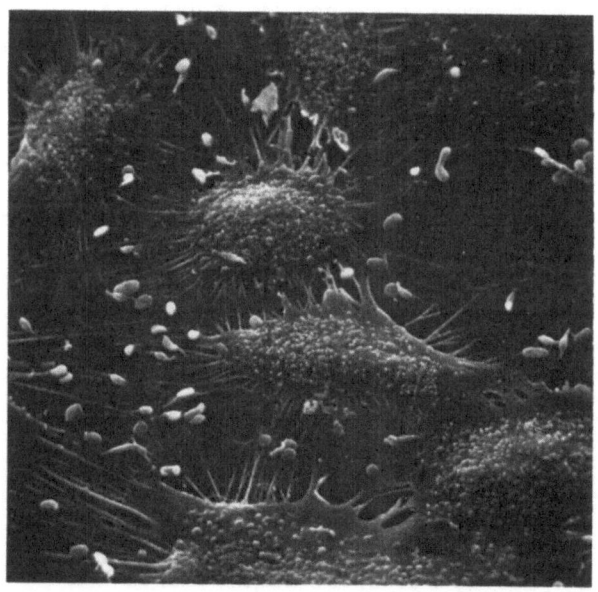

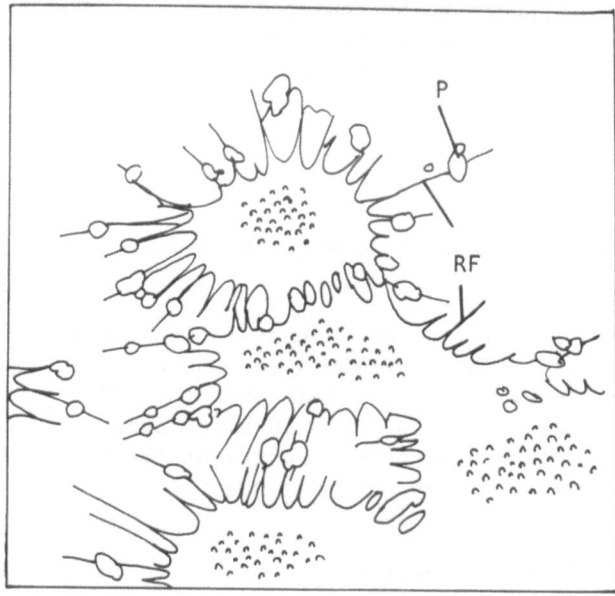

Fig. 4-22: Scanning electron micrograph of platelet-rich plasma and endothelial cells on plastic treated with versene to create retraction. Note platelets are attached only to the retraction fibrils and not to the body of the endothelial cells. Pseudopod formation is seen, but no evidence of release is apparent. RF: retraction fibrils, P: platelets (X 1465). (Reduced 30% for purposes of reproduction.)

See Figure 4-23. Thus, we have not been able to determine
whether the microfilament processes seen on transmission
electron microscopy have an affinity for platelet attachment
or not. Occasionally, with transmission microscopy there
has been the suggestion that attachment has occurred in the
area of microfibril distribution, but we have not been able
to consistently document this finding. We have some evidence
to suggest in early experiments that the ability of the
endothelial cell to avoid triggering platelet release reactions
is not dependent on metabolic integrity. Endothelial cells
fixed with glutaraldehyde did not appear to activate platelets
in studies similar to those described above. This work and
the other tissue culture work which I have described has
been the work of Ms. Arlene Wechezak, who is the tissue
culture supervisor at our laboratory.

Thus the ability to obtain and serially passage true
endothelial cells in tissue culture opens a vast area for
future research in blood vessel disease. We can now utilize
these cells totally separate from their subendothelial structures
for studies of their specific metabolic requirements and
capabilities. There appears to be some potential for the
use of these cells as antithrombogenic linings for vascular
prosthetic devices in the future. In the calves when we
were using 400 mgs of persantin a day orally and 1.2 grams
of aspirin a day with coumadin we maintained their prothrombin
time at 1.7 and two times their control. This was done for
four days prior to surgery and also after surgery. (18).

DR. STONE: What is the half life of the normal arterial
endothelial cell?

DR. MANSFIELD: I believe that depends on its location
within the arterial tree, most certainly. Turnover seems
greatest at bifurcations. (22,23). Tritiated thymidine
studies have shown very active turnover in bifurcations
whereas, for example, in the descending aorta at the mid
points it is much longer. I can't give you a specific time
in that regard.

DR. WEINBAUM: I have a question as to when you will
get the re-endothelialization. I look at it as a dual
problem. The one which we
have dealt with, as you have so
beautifully shown today, is the
development of the fibrous
attachments underneath. The
other aspect which is what I have been interested in, is the
ability of two endothelial cells to form intercellular

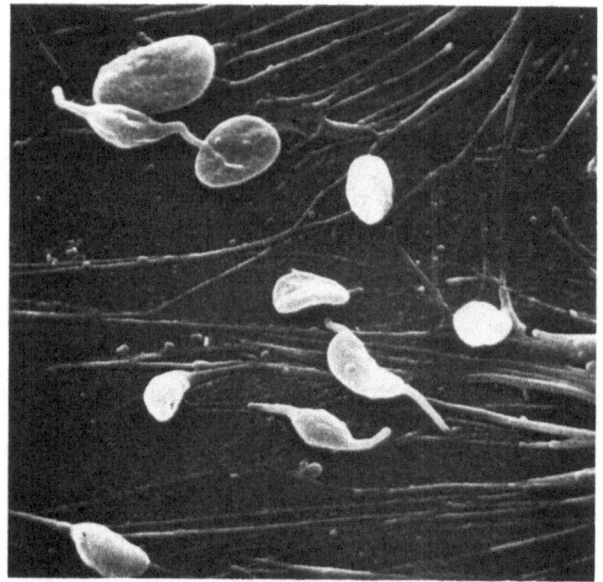

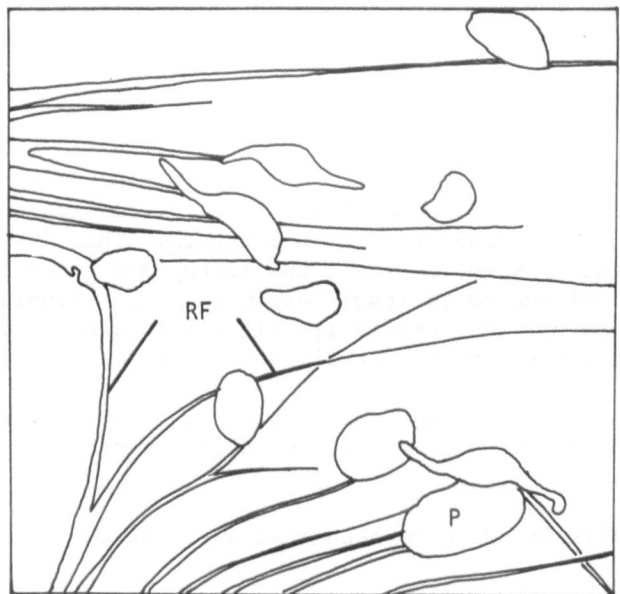

Fig. 4-23: High power scanning micrograph of portion of
Fig. 4-22. Note the attachment of platelets to retraction
fibrils with pseudopod formation, but no evidence of release
reaction. We have been unable to identify microfilaments with
scanning electron microscopy. RF: retraction fibrils. P:
platelets. (X 7540). (Reduced 30% for purposes of reproduction.)

channels with a typical spacing of 100-200A. The force
balance between two adjacent endothelial cell membranes
appears to be a balance between Van der Waals attractive
forces and a repulsive force due to a small surface charge
on the exterior surface of the endothelial cell. The repulsive
force is the same elastic bilayer effect that Dr. Shu Chien
has been studying in rouleaux formation between red cells.
Although I don't know the magnitude of the forces that
determine the equilibrium spacing, I do see a way of getting
an approximate answer to this problem.   In epithelial cell
layers where you have active transport with lots of water
movement, electron micrographs show that there is a change
in spacing in the extracellular channel due to this water
movement.   One can get some estimate of the pressure build
up at the closed end of the channel, thus some idea of the
magnitude of the forces that develop between two adjacent
endothelial cells across the intercellular channel.   I
wonder whether you know or have some idea of the magnitude
of the forces present in your endothelial grafts and if
surface electric effects might be present.   Unless the
endothelial cell is able to develop this small negative
surface charge, you can't establish an extracellular channel.

DR. MANSFIELD: Well, we certainly don't have any
answers as to why it goes on but it certainly does. We have
seen areas within an endothelial lined graft where the cells
are gone and thrombus has formed. When this occurs, the
endothelial cells from the tissue culture origin will grow
up over the thrombus and cover it. It is interesting that
they do not organize the thrombus underneath. This is in
contrast to the anastomosis where the macrophage comes in
from the wall of the aorta itself organizing and thinning
the thrombus layer. The endothelium itself apparently does
not have that capability but merely covers it over.

DR. BJORKERUD: For how long a time did you study that
phenomenon? How long did you follow the re-endothelialized
thrombus?

DR. MANSFIELD: We have seen that at eight weeks and at
twelve weeks.

DR. COLTON: On the plastic dishes did you in fact get
tight junctions?

DR. MANSFIELD: Yes.

DR. COLTON: Have you seen filamentous material bridging
to endothelial cells?

DR. MANSFIELD: We have not seen it in bridging. We are now trying to find various types of junctions between the endothelial cells in a tissue culture as compared to what is seen for example, on a Hautchen preparation. We have had no meaningful results so far, but it is an area that needs and deserves a tremendous amount of work and effort. Microfilaments have been described I believe, at least once before, in smooth muscle cells near the basement membrane area.

DR. COLTON: Have you tried growing endothelial cells on a substrate which is microporous?

DR. MANSFIELD: The discs that you saw in the slides do not have the polyurethane backing and yet the cells grow very well on them. The problem that you get into is that if you have something that is too porous the cells can't bridge the gap and you get an incomplete endothelial covering.

DR. COLTON: That may make a very interesting substrate for transport studies.

DR. MANSFIELD: Exactly. That is what I was suggesting.

DR. CARO: One question to Dr. Mansfield and one question to Dr. Fry. Continuing the present line of discussion, does versine cause the cells to retract?

DR. MANSFIELD: Yes.

DR. CARO: What does it do? Do the junctions between the cells open?

DR. MANSFIELD: It may tend to do that. The cells pull away from the substrate leaving fibrils that are attached to the plastic where the entire cell body was attached before.

DR. CARO: Do you have any explanation of how this comes about?

DR. MANSFIELD: The versine binds the calcium but we can't give you any further reason than that. One of the key techniques in obtaining endothelial cells that survive, rather than to strip them physically from the lining of a carotid artery, is to use versine first instead of trypsin and we used modifications of the two. Trypsin tends to damage the cells except at very low concentration. Since versine worked, we used it.

DR. SCHWARTZ: Concerning Dr. Mansfield's use of versine,
I suspect that this effect reflects the removal of calcium
                                and the need for a calcium
Role of Calcium   dependent ATPase for cell
                                adhesion to a surface.

DR. CARO: You are implying that the cell is becoming
spherical and it is the attachment that is weakened by the
versine.

DR. SCHWARTZ: No, I am simply suggesting that the
attachment ultimately is an energy dependent process, and
that a calcium dependent ATPase is involved in the energy
system.

DR. MANSFIELD: I think there is no question that it is
an energy dependent system because by any means that you
kill or damage cells, they do separate from the plastic or
whatever their connection is. The difference is that when
the fibroblast separates it leaves nothing. The endothelial
cell separates and leaves these microfilaments which are
incredibly reactive with platelets, far more so than any
other surface we have studied.

DR. WERTHESSEN: I am recalling the work we did with
Florey and Poole a number of years ago. (24). We used the
DeBakey prosthesis in a baboon's aorta. It provides a blood
clot. It was very disappointing work as far as I was concerned
because what I wanted out of that experiment was the ingrowth
of individual cell populations. With that I could have
disentangled which one synthesized the lipids. But the
conclusion of the study was that all of the cells were
pluripotential. I won't go through all of the data. I
should like to ask Dr. Mansfield whether in the experiments
he described earlier he tried to raise the transplanted
endothelium on a clot or put a clot into his fibers?

DR. MANSFIELD: No, we did not.

DR. WERTHESSEN: I regret that, since you could have settled
an issue. In one of our experiments a capillary grew into
the lumen of the aorta from the outside of the clot and then
spread out. All the cells were in the sheet of tissue over
the prosthesis lumen. This was true also of the ingrowth
tissue from the edge. Your findings surprised me.

DR. MANSFIELD: We actually have seen that now in
humans. We have designed filamentous dacron prostheses which
do accelerate transmural healing. We have now seen almost

total endothelialization in an actual femoral graft, after
three years in a human, which does not occur otherwise. It
would appear that this was not fall-out seeding, but rather
transprosthetic ingrowth with what turned out to be true
endothelial cells.

DR. WERTHESSEN: Then did you see smooth muscle
underneath?

DR. MANSFIELD: What looks like smooth muscle underneath,
yes.

DR. DEWEY: Could you expand that statement about the
sub-endothelial material?

DR. MANSFIELD: We are talking about a very porous
prostheses which when inserted has to be pre-potted in a very
specific way. We end up with a very high concentration of
heparin, trying to remove the thromboplastin on the surface.
We have found that there is ingrowth with the endothelial
cells lying on top of what appears to be compacted fibrin and
on occasion what appear to be smooth muscle cells, again which
have to have come from either the clot itself or outside. As
compared to the type of graft we are using here which is,
of course, not graft at all, it is totally impervious. This
makes a very major difference. We have done this also in the
baboon, but the baboon will heal a non-porous graft with
endothelium completely in six weeks. So it doesn't help us
a bit.

DR. CARO: I would like to ask Dr. Fry a question,
naemely, why he thinks that fluctuating shearing stresses
affect the permeability of
Regional Variation of   the wall differently from steady
Macromolecular Permeability   ones. I am not sure of the
significance of his results. He
has shown that wall permeability is initially increased and
then falls with time in his arterio-venous shunt but I am
not convinced that this is a normal situation or how to relate
it to the normal situation. Thus there are normally fluctuating
shearing stresses in arteries and blood flow can normally be
turbulent in the aorta. Nevertheless, it is generally agreed
that there are, in the steady state, regions where arterial
macromolecule permeability is relatively high and others
where it is relatively low.

DR. FRY: I doubt that I can convince you since I don't
have the necessary hard data. Rigorously designed experiments
to evaluate endothelial surface permeability directly as a
function of acute changes in magnitude as opposed to changes

in direction of the shear stress are extremely difficult to do and as yet have been technically unsuccessful. Similar studies to evaluate these responses in the chronic situation are even more difficult. The A/V shunt preparation seems at present to be the best approach to evaluation of the chronic response to changes in magnitude of the stress. As was noted, it appears that with chronically elevated exposure, compensatory processes are occurring in the endothelial cell surface that end to return the permeability toward normal values.

DR. CARO: What is the evidence that the wall was normal, especially during the early stage when permeability in the arterio-venous shunt was increased?

DR. FRY: The chronically exposed endothelial surface when viewed by scanning electron microscopy is not "typically normal" in the sense that endothelial cellular hyperplasia and cellular elongation in the direction of flow have occurred. Surprisingly, however the ultra structure by transmission electron microscopy is completely normal.

DR. STONE: I would like to ask Dr. Fry a question. You intimated that there is a tremendous difference with elevated pressures. What about the effect of sustained elevated flow rates on critical shear stress?

DR. FRY: You mean the tissue response to the increased shear stresses in the A/V shunt preparations?

DR. STONE: Yes.

DR. FRY: The flow rates are increased many fold in the arteries supplying the shunt. We have never seen endothelial erosion in either the carotid or iliac preparations suggesting that these elevated flows are associated with stresses less than the acute critical shear stress at these sites. Acutely one sees an occasional endothelial surface bleb by scanning electron microscopy and questionable subendothelial edema by transmission electron microscopy. Both disappear chronically and except for the aforementioned endothelial cell hyperplasia and elongation in the direction of flow, the wall appears essentially normal by ultrastructural criteria.

DR. STONE: Is there intimal thickening in that A/V shunt?

DR. FRY: In normolipemic animals one sees surprisingly little intimal fibromuscular hyperplasia in response to this chronically increased stress exposure. In hyperlipemic animals, however, intimal thickening is much more prominent.

BIBLIOGRAPHY

1. Diamond, J.M.: The mechanism of isotonic water transport. J. Gen. Physiol., 48:15, 1964.

2. Stein, O., Weinstein, D.B., Stein, Y., Steinberg, D.: Binding, internalization and degradation of low density lipoprotein by normal human fibroblasts and by fibroblasts from a case of homozygous familial hypercholesterolemia. Proc. Nat'l Acad. of Sciences, 73:14-18, 1976.

3. Fry, D.L.: Responses of the arterial wall to certain physical factors. In: Atherogenesis: Initiating Factors., pp. 93-125, Assoc. Sci. Pub., Amsterdam, 1972.

4. Flaherty, J.T., Pierce, J.E., Ferrans, V.J., Patel, D.J., Tucker, W.K., and Fry, D.L.: Endothelial nuclear patterns in the canine arterial tree with particular reference to hemodynamic events. Circ. Res. 30: 23-33, 1972.

5. Fry, D.L.: Certain histological and chemical responses of the vascular interface to acutely induced mechanical stress in the aorta of the dog. Circ. Res. 24:93-108, 1969.

6. Carew, T.E.: Mechano-chemical Response of Canine Aortic Endothelium to Elevated Stress In Vitro. Ph.D. Thesis, The Catholic University of America, Wash., D.C., 1971

7. Caro, C.G. and Nerem, R.M.: Transport of ^{14}C-4 cholesterol between serum and wall in the perfused dog common carotid artery. Circ. Res. 32:187-205, 1973.

8. Fry, D.L.: Hemodynamic forces in atherogenesis. Cerebro. Dis. 77-95, 1976.

9. Fry, D.L.: Acute vascular endothelial changes associated with increased blood velocity gradients. Circ. Res. 22:165-197, 1968.

10. Fry, D.L.: In preparation.

11. Fry, D.L.: Aortic Evans Blue dye accumulation: Its measurement and interpretation. Am. J. Physiol.: Heart and Circ. Physiol., Vol. 1, No. 2, pp. H204-H222, 1977.

12. Mansfield, P.B.: Tissue cultured endothelium for
     vascular prosthetic devices report to medical
     devices applications program. NIH-NHL-71-2060-1
     National Heart, Blood, and Lung Institute of
     HEW. Public Health Service, Bethesda, MD., 1971.

13. Mansfield, P.B.: Tissue cultured endothelium for
     vascular prosthetic devices report to medical
     devices application program. NIH-NHL-71-2060-1
     National Heart, Blood, and Lung Institute of
     HEW. Public Health Service, Bethesda, MD., 1972.

14. Mansfield, P.B.: Tissue cultured endothelium for
     vascular prosthetic devices report to medical
     devices applications program. NIH-NHL-71-2060-1
     National Heart, Blood, and Lung Institute of
     HEW. Public Health Service, Bethesda, MD., 1973.

15. Mansfield, P.B.: Tissue cultured endothelium for
     vascular prosthetic devices report to medical
     devices applications program. NIH-NHL-71-2060-1
     National Heart, Blood, and Lung Institute of
     HEW. Public Health Service, Bethesda, MD., 1973-1975.

16. Mansfield, P.B., Wechezak, A.R. and Sauvage, L.R.:
     Preventing thrombus on artificial vascular surfaces:
     True endothelial cell linings. Trans. Amer. Soc.
     Artif. Int. Organs. 21:264-272, 1975.

17. Wechezak, A.R.: and Mansfield, P.B.: Isolated and growth
     characteristics of cell lines from bovine venous
     endothelium in vitro. 9:39-45, 1973.

18. Mansfield, P.B., Sauvage, L.R. and Smith, J.C.: Factors
     influencing thrombus generation in artifical hearts.
     Symposium on Coronary Artery Medicine and Surgery
     (February, Surgery: Concepts & Controversies. N.Y.)
     Appleton-Century-Crofts, pp. 968-985, 1975.

19. Sauvage, L.R., Berger, K., Wood, S., Yates, S., Smith, J.C.,
     Mansfield, P.B.: Interspecies healing of porous
     arterial prostheses: Observations 1960-1974
     Arch. Surg. 109:698-705, 1975.

20. Harker, L.A. and Schlichter, S.J.: Studies of platelet
     and fibrinogen kinetics in patients with prosthetic
     heart valves. N. Eng. J. Med. 283:1302-1305, 1970.

21. Wechezak, A.R., Mansfield, P.B., and Way, S.A.: Platelet interation with cultured endothelial cells following in vitro injury. Artery 1:507-517, 1975.

22. Poole, J.C.F.: Regeneration of aortic tissues in fabric grafts of the aorta. Symp. Zool. Soc. London 11:131-140, 1964.

23. Wright, H.P.: Endothelial Turnover. Thromb. Diath. Haemorr. Suppl. 40:79-84, 1970.

24. Poole, J.C., Sanders, A.G. and Florey, H.W.: The regeneration of aortic endothelium. J. Path. Bact. 75: 133, 1958.

Chapter 5 METABOLIC ACTIVITIES IN THE ARTERIAL WALL

DR. SMITH: The review has been prepared in collaboration with my husband, Dr. R. H. Smith.

A fundamental requirement for all cells is energy production. In most cells in the presence of a normal oxygen supply the energy pathway is through the metabolism of glucose to pyruvate, which goes into the Krebs cycle and through the cytochrome system (Fig. 5-1, left side): this is the pathway of oxidative phosphorylation and produces a large amount of energy - 32 molecules ATP and 417 kilo calories. In the absence of molecular oxygen glucose is again converted to pyruvate but then the cell has to regenerate NAD by reduction of pyruvate to lactate, which cannot be metabolised further (Fig. 5-1, right side). This anaerobic glycolysis produces less energy - only 2 molecules of ATP and 32 kilo calories and lactate accumulates in the tissue (1).

Energy Production in Arterial Wall

As soon as oxygen is readmitted lactate production ceases and the system switches over to the aerobic pathway again, and this is known as the Pasteur Effect (1). It was first described by Pasteur in fermentation studies and is the normal pathway of behavior in, for example, skeletal muscle.

Pasteur Effect

There have been numerous reports that artery wall does not normally follow the oxidative phosphorylation pathway, but follows the glycolytic pathway even in the presence of molecular oxygen, but more recent work suggests that this is an artifact. The standard biochemical procedure for any metabolic study is to cool the tissue to 4° C, which is supposed to stablize everything. In 1970 Scott and co-workers (2) in Albany, did an experiment in which, instead of precooling the tissue, they kept it at 37° C and found a five or six fold increase in oxygen consumption (2,3,4). It appears that arterial wall is extremely susceptible to what they called "cold shock," and cooling the tissue to 4° C seems irreversibly to damage the oxidative phosphorylation pathway. There have now been several studies in which the artery was maintained carefully at 37° C and some results are

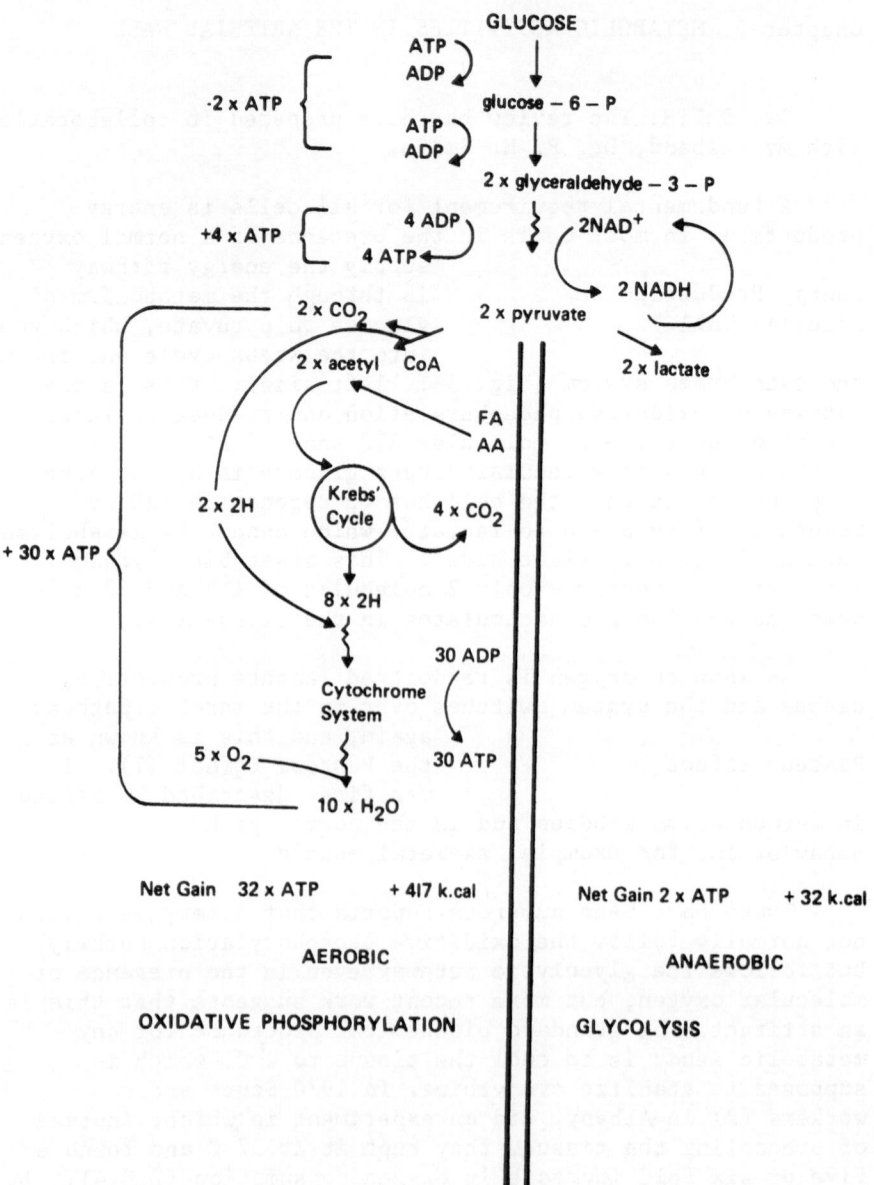

Fig. 5-1: Energy production from glucose.

TABLE 1. Oxygen and glucose utilization by artery

TISSUE	Pre-Treatment	μmol/g wet tissue/hr (37°C) UPTAKE		Lactate produced	
		O_2	Glucose		
PIG AORTA					
Normal (	4°C	1.0	-	5.0	) Scott et al.
(	37°C	5.7	-	11.3	) 1970.(Ref.2)
RABBIT AORTA					
Endothelium intact	37°C	8.7	13.6	3.4	) Morrison, Berwick,
Not intact	37°C	5.1	5.8	5-6	) Orci & Winegrad.) 1976.(Ref.5)
BOVINE	37°				
MESEN-TERIC.	aerobic	-	6	3	) Arnqvist & Lundholm
	anaerobic	-	7	14	) 1976.(Ref.6)

summarized in Table I. It is clear that under these conditions, the artery is utilizing oxygen rapidly and producing relatively small amounts of lactic acid.

Furthermore, Morrison, Berwick, Orci, and Winegrad (5) found that the state of the tissue is extremely important. If they were able to keep the endothelium apparently structurally intact, there was a much higher oxygen uptake than if the endothelium was damaged, although they could see no damage in the smooth muscle cells.

The Pasteur effect has now been demonstrated in artery wall; Table II shows that in arteries maintained at 37° C changing from aerobic to anaerobic conditions increases lactate production four fold. (5,6). In the context of this meeting it is important to notice that lactate production was approximately doubled in stretched artery (6).

Thus it appears that earlier findings indicating primary dependence on glycolysis were probably the result of artifacts. Under normal conditions of oxygen supply ATP appears to be generated by oxidative phosphorylation, and the balance between glycolysis and oxidative phosphorylation depends on oxygen supply, as in other muscles; this raises the question - does the oxygen tension in arterial wall fall to levels at which the glycolytic pathway becomes the major energy source? There seem to be very few studies on the oxygen tension within the wall. Niinikoski et al., (7) measured the O_2 tension in rabbit aorta by passing a very fine electrode through the wall from the adventitia inwards in an intact anesthetized animal (Fig. 5-2, top). The pO_2 remained constant through the adventitia then fell as the electrode approached the central media, then it rose again, and there was a surprisingly large difference of oxygen tension between the blood and the immediate subendothelial area. I have tried to relate these studies on the actual oxygen tension in the wall to Arnqvist and Lundholm's (6) figures for lactic acid production at different oxygen tensions (Fig. 5-2, bottom). In the immediate sub-endothelium the oxygen tension was about 40 mmHg, and at that level there is already significant lactic acid production, but of course the artery is to some extent damaged. In the central media the oxygen tension was about 20 mmHg, and at that level there will be quite a large lactate production. Extrapolation back from the intima (dotted line in Fig. 5-2 top) indicates what might happen in the aorta of a larger animal. This cuts the point of zero oxygen at a distance of about 300 to 350 M from the endothelial surface.

DR. STONE: Does this extrapolation ignore any vasa vasorum of the vessel wall?

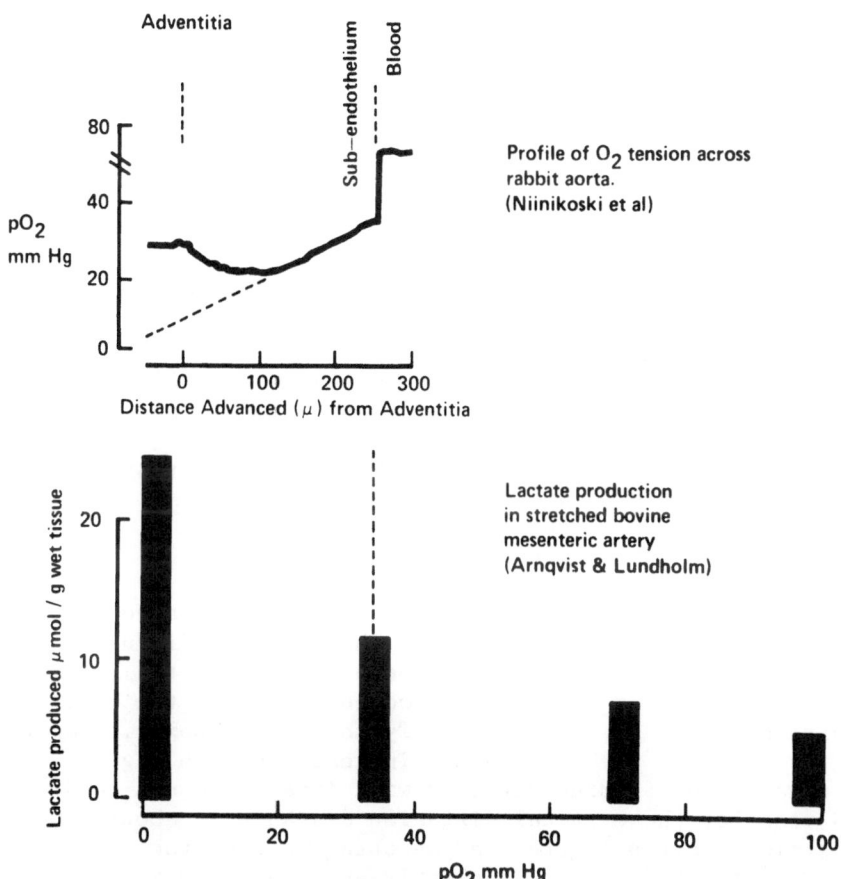

Fig. 5-2: Diagram relating the data of Niinikoski et al., (ref. 7) on oxygen tension within arterial wall with the data of Arnqvist and Lundholm (6) on lactate production in stretched artery at different oxygen levels.

(Reproduced by kind permission of the authors and the publishers of Atherosclerosis).

DR. SMITH: I assume that the vasa stops at the adventitial-
medial junction -- the rabbit does not have a vasa vasorum in
the media.

DR. STONE: What I am saying, your extrapolation to a
larger aorta ...

DR. SMITH: Perhaps you would leave that for the moment,
because I will be talking about it later.

A different approach to the oxygen tension was made by
Kirk and Laursen (8). They took sheets both of pure media and
of intima inner media and measured the diffusion coefficient for
oxygen across these sheets. Surprisingly, the mean coefficient
for intima for both layers tended to increase with age. They
then utilized the equation developed by A.V. Hill for skeletal
muscle (9) to calculate the critical diffusion distance for
oxygen - that is, the greatest depth to which oxygen will
penetrate. This is a function of the diffusion coefficient, the
rate of utilization of oxygen by the tissue and the pO_2.

Greatest thickness to which O_2 penetrates = b = $\sqrt{2ky/a}$ where
  k = diffusion coefficient
  a = rate of oxygen consumption
  y = concentration of oxygen

Using the very low figure for oxygen consumption obtained with
cold-shocked arteries they calculated the critical diffusion
distance of about 900 to 1000 μ
O_2 Diffusion and   which would mean that the wall is
O_2 Requirements   unlikely to become anoxic. However,
                         using instead the much higher
oxygen consumption figures obtained with intact and non-cold
shocked vessels, the critical diffusion distance is about 350 μ
which is close to the figure that we obtained from the extrapolation in Fig. 5-2. This is clearly an area which is extremely
important and in which more data is urgently required on larger
sized blood vessels. Moss et al., (10) found continuous decrease
in pO_2 from adventitia to lumen in the femoral arteries of dogs,
but the diameter of the electrode tip was 125 μ and the authors
state that the area sensed was large in relation to the vessel
wall thickness.

If we now try to relate this to the adult human aortic intima,
and assume from Fig. 5-2 that significant lactate production starts
at a depth of about 100 μ it can be seen in Fig. 5-3, that in
35% of samples of apparently lesion-free intima lactate production
may be increased in the deepest one-third of the tissue, in about
10% in more than half, and in another 10% the deepest layers of
the intima may be totally anoxic.

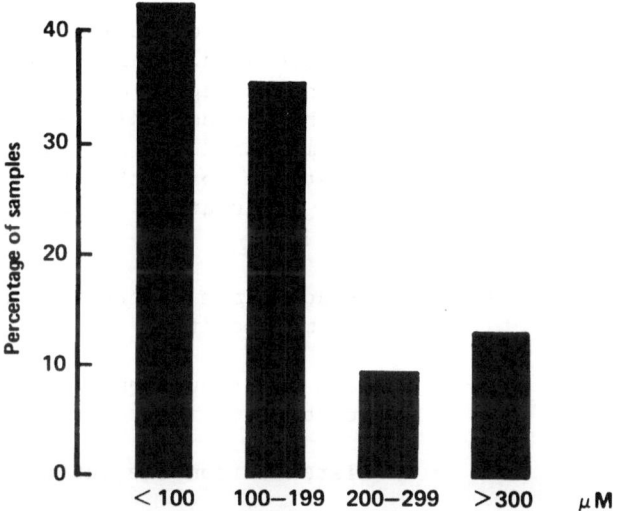

Fig. 5-3: Thickness of apparently normal intima in 54 subjects aged 30-69.

One might postulate that anoxia is pertinent to fibrous
plaque development in the fourth decade. In developing
lesions there must be areas that are totally anoxic. Thus,
these very crude calculations support the concept that
oxygen tension may be a critical factor in atherogenesis,
modifying both the development and regression of lesions.
(11,12,13,14).

Furthermore, haemodynamic factors must have a profound
influence on diffusion of O_2 into the wall; calculations
indicate that in regions of decelerated flow and flow
separation there will be decreased O_2 transport (15).

         One of the major consequences of oxygen deficiency is,
as we have seen, production of lactic acid. Can a significant
                                     amount of lactic acid accumulate
Accumulation of Lactic   in the tissue? Kirk and Laursen
Acid   (8) measured the diffusion
                                     constants for lactid acid, and
A.V. Hill (9) gave an equation for calculating the concentration
of a metabolite in tissue. $y^1 = -ab^2/_{2k} + ab^2/_k + y_0$

                    y^1 =   steady state concentration of
                                   the metabolite

                    a =   rate of production of the
                                   metabolite

                    b =   distance from the surface

                    k =   diffusion constant in the tissue

                    y_0 =   concentration of the metabolite
                                   in the surrounding fluid (plasma)

         In anoxic stretched artery lactate was produced at a
rate of 24 μ mol/g. wet tissue/hour (Table 2); using this
figure the concentration of lactic acid at 300 μ from the
lumenal surface would be 33 milligrams per 100 grams of wet
tissue and at 400 μ which would correspond with an early
gelantinous thickening, it would be nearly doubled to 51 mg.

         So it looks as if significant accumulation of lactic
acid could occur, and this seems to be an area where actual
experimental information is urgently needed.

         At 800 μ the center of a developing fibrous plaque, it
would increase more than three fold to 174 mg/100 g wet
tissue.

TABLE 2. Magnitude of the Pasteur effect

O_2 content	Lactate production	
% of gas mixture	$\mu mol/g.$ wet tissue/hr.	
Resting aorta	1.	2.
95%	3.6	3.3
0%	13.8	13.5

1. Morrison, Berwick et al. 1972.(Ref.5)

2. Arnqvist & Lundholm 1976. (Ref.6)

Stretched aorta	
15%	4.5
10%	7.0
5%	11.5
0%	24.0

15% $O_2 \equiv$ 100mg Hg (pO_2 of arterial blood)

One consequence of increased lactic acid in the tissue is a reduction of pH, and the cell lysosomes seem to be

Effect of Lactic Acid Accumulation on Lysosomes

particularly susceptible to low pH, which increases their fragility or leakiness. The lysosomes contain numerous hydrolases (16), including cathepsins, and B-glucuronidase and hyaluronidase which degrade the glycosaminoglycans. A cathepsin B1 with collagenolytic activity has also been reported (17). In heart muscle there seems to be a population of lysosomes with varying enzyme content and slightly varying density. They may become filled with material such as lipid, detergent or silica which alters their density (16,18).

I could not find any studies on the effects of hypoxia on lysosomes in arteries, but there is a large amount of

DOG Hypoxia

experimental information on infarcted heart muscle. In dog hearts Brachfeld (19) found an increasing lactate concentration within 6 seconds of coronary artery occlusion, and in 5 minutes it had increased 18-fold; pH fell by 0.4 units within 2 minutes. Large intracellular/ extracellular pH gradients have been demonstrated (20,21), intracellular hydrogen ion concentration reaching twice the extracellular level whereas intracellular bicarbonate was only half the extracellular level. The effects of coronary occlusion on the distribution of lysosomal enzymes in heart muscle have been studied by several groups (22,23,24,25) and typical results are shown in Tables 3 and 4. Four hours after coronary occlusion there was significant release of acid phosphatase into the supernatant fraction, so there appears to be a significant increase in lysosomal leakiness. Of course, there are other changes in the cell following myocardial infarction, including a decrease in glycogen (Table 4) but work on isolated lysosomes suggests the pH is one of the most important factors in maintaining lysosomal integrity. Thus, if heart muscle is a valid model for arterial smooth muscle, hypoxia leads to the accumulation of lactic acid, producing a fall in pH which mediates leakage of lysosomal enzymes, which cause general intra- and extracellular damage to arterial tissue.

How do early human lesions seem to tie in with this concept of anoxia as an initiating factor? The early human

Early Lesions and Their Relation to Low Oxygen Tension

lesions fall into two groups: fatty streaks consisting of cells laden with lipid of which the largest single component is cholesterol ester; and

TABLE 3. Activity of lysosomal enzymes in dog left ventricular muscle

	Acid P—ase	β —Glucuronidase
SHAM—OPERATED		
Supernatant fraction	20.1	1.2
Particulate fraction	4.7	0.9
Particulate / supernatant	0.23	0.75
4 HOURS POST CORONARY OCCLUSION		
Supernatant fraction	18.1	1.8
Particulate fraction	2.4*	0.2*
Particulate / supernatant	0.13	0.13

* $p < 0.001$

TABLE 4. Relation between tissue glycogen and pH and lysosomal stability in infarcted heart muscle from dogs

Time after Coronary Occlusion	Glycogen: μg / 100 mg wet tissue	pH	Acid P-ase Activity Ratio: Particulate / Supernatant
Control	60.4	7.0	0.26
I hour	32.9	6.5	0.15
2 hours	17.0	6.4	0.10
4 hours	14.6	6.3	0.06

proliferative lesions which are mounds of thickening of smooth
muscle cells and collagen fibers. These include a wide range
of morphological variants, and in the early stages may contain
very little lipid.

    Looking first at <u>fatty streaks,</u> does it seem reasonable
to postulate that they could be induced by reduced oxygen
                                tension? In our last fifty aortas
Fatty Streaks   I measured the distance from the
                                lumenal surface to the middle of
the main band of fat filled cells in the fatty streaks. Looking
at them macroscopically they appear to be superficial lesions
and this was amply confirmed by microscopic measurement. In
all but one lesion the most superficial fat filled cells lay
immediately under the endothelium; in 40% all the main band
of fat filled cells within 50 μ of the intimal surface (Fig. 5-4)
- in fact, in half of these lesions all fat filled cells were
within 25 μ of the intimal surface. In a further 47% of lesions
the middle of the main band extended to 50 μ. There was just a
small group in which the cells extended deeper, but in all of
these the fat-filled cells also extended all the way to the
surface. In a study on early lesions in cholesterol-fed Rhesus
monkeys, Stary also found that the fat-filled cells were
extremely superficial (26). Increased oxygen consumption in
arteries made atherosclerotic by cholesterol feeding has
been reported (reviewed in references 27,28,29). This is
probably the result of increased fatty acid oxidation and not
increased glucose utilization by the Krebs cycle. There seems
to be no information on the spontaneous human fatty streaks,
and results of metabolic studies in post mortem material are
unlikely to be valid.

    Thus, it seems difficult to postulate that oxygen shortage
could be a factor in the development of fatty streaks, but it
might be a factor in the destruction of the fat-filled cells.
In 18 raised fatty/gelatinous or fatty/fibrous plaques containing numerous scattered fat-filled cells in the cap, no intact
fat-filled cells occurred at a depth greater than about 400 μ.

    However, I think the situation looks different in the
gelatinous and fibrous lesions. Fig. 5-5a shows the
                                gelatinous tail of a developing
Gelatinous and Fibrous   plaque stained with the Verhoeff
Lesions   and Van Gieson stain for elastin
                                and collagen, and it demonstrates
several characteristic features.

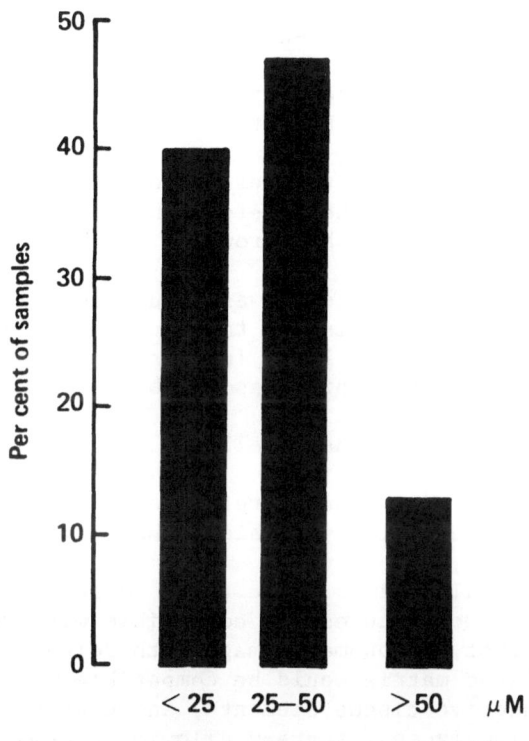

Fig. 5-4: The depth of the centre of the main band of fat-filled cells in fatty streaks from 50 aortas.

There is massive proliferation of smooth muscle cells and
thick collagen bundles rather widely spaced. The lesions
contain large amounts of intact LDL, fibrinogen and other
plasma macromolecules, and in the deep layers what Daria Haust
calls an "area of insudation" can be seen (30,31,32).
Three extreme forms of proliferative lesion are encountered:
closely packed smooth muscle cells with a few thin collagen
strands between, close collagen bundles with few cells
between and the lesions with "loose" collagen bundles shown
in Fig. 5-6. The quantity of plasma macromolecules is roughly
proportional to the looseness of the structure. These
lesions become prominent in the fourth and fifth decades; by
this age there is well developed diffuse intimal thickening
and the deep layers of the intima may be hypoxic.

DR: COLTON: Dr. Smith, before going on give me a typical
dimension or what was there before the lesion developed?
This could tell me what has grown.

DR. SMITH: This lesion was about 1000 in its
maximum thickness. It is the tail end of a fibrous plaque
which was about an inch long. In this age group normal
intima has an average thickness of about 200 μ..

DR. COLTON: Are there cells?

DR. SMITH: Yes, there are. There are variable numbers
of smooth muscle cells lying along the collagen bundles.

The central area of these thick lesions must be hypoxic
and at least two features are compatible with response to
hypoxia. First, lysosomal damage with release of hydrolases
into the tissue matrix would be compatible with separation
of the connective tissue elements, and with slight decrease
in glycosaminoglycans, thereby allowing plasma components to
accumulate (33,34).

DR. COLTON: Is there an identifiable necrosis?

DR. SMITH: I don't know what you mean by 'identifiable
necrosis.' In this higher powered section of the insudation
area Fig. 5-5B the collagen fibers seems to thin out and
disappear. One can interpret this in two ways: Daria Haust
suggests that they are "dissolving" in the insudate, but one
could also postulate that they are growing out of the insudate.
So, I just don't know, one can only speculate (30).

DR. STONE: Dr. Smith, a question. Could this still
be collagen material, young collagen, down here that is not
staining?

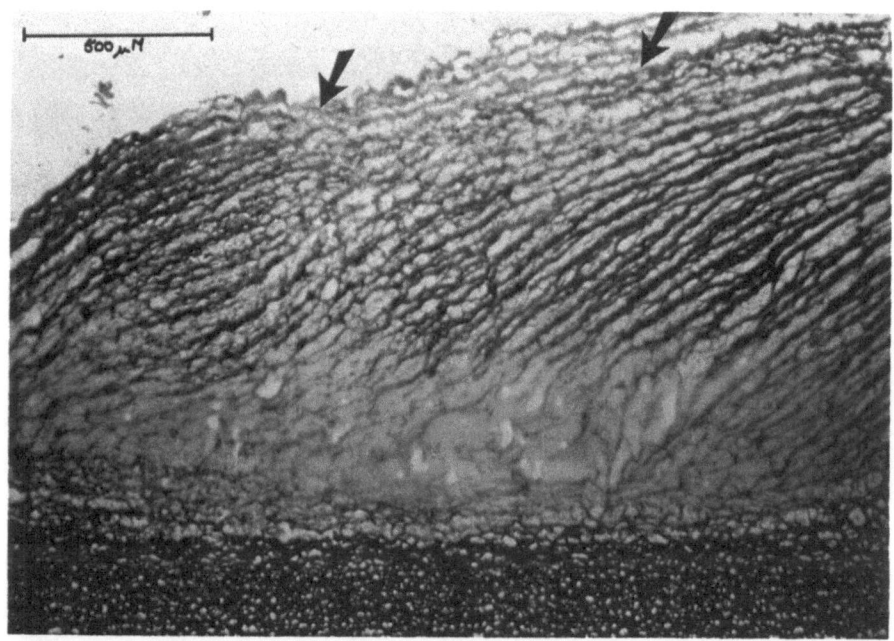

Fig. 5-5: Gelatinous "tail" of a large fibro/gelatinous plaque
from a male aged 58 (sub-arachnoid haemorrhage; aorta obtained
4 hours after death).

A. Low power view of the whole "tail"; two surface layers,
each about 10 uM thick, were peeled off for analysis and their
strip planes are indicated by large arrows. The lesion shows
typical thick collagen bundles with wide spaces between, and
an "area of insudation" in the base. Collagen bundles showed
pale, diffuse sudanophilia, and the cholesterol content was
2.1mg/100mg lipid extracted dry tissue compared with 3.4mg
in adjacent normal intima.

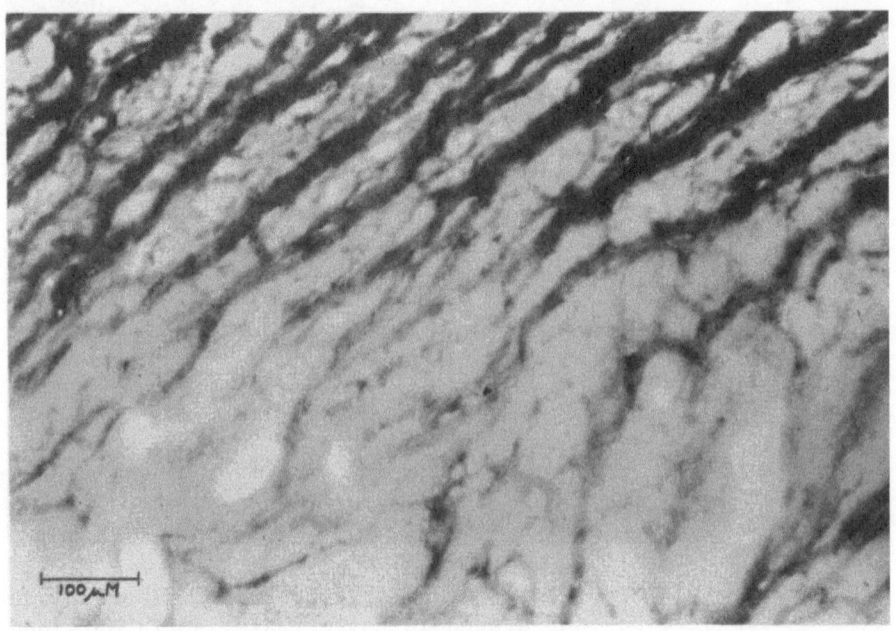

Fig. 5-5: Gelatinous "tail" of a large fibro/gelantinous plaque
from a male aged 58 (sub-arachnoid haemorrhage; aorta obtained
4 hours after death).

   B.   Edge of the insudation area at higher magnification.

THE CONCENTRATIONS OF 'SOLUBLE' AND 'INSOLUBLE' PLASMA DERIVATIVES

(mg / 100mg dry tissue)

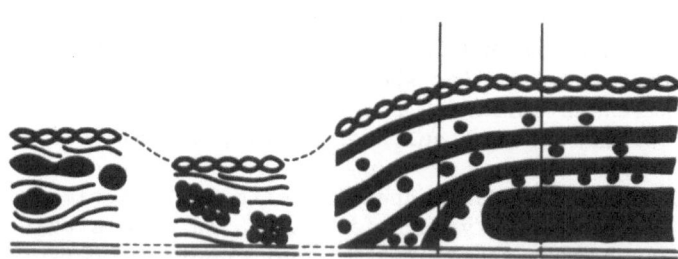

| | Fatty Streak | Adult Normal | Gelatinous 'Tail' | White Plaque | | |
| | | | | Edge | Centre | |
					Cap	Lower
Lipoprotein	1.2*	5.2	13.4*	6.0	2.9	3.7
Fibrinogen	2.5	2.2	6.6*	6.8*	1.4	4.0
'Fibrin'	2.4	2.0	3.5	9.7*	2.1	10.3*
Residual Cholesterol	25.6*	3.8	4.2	27.2*	11.2	97.8*
Immobilized Lipoprotein	1.0	0.8	1.6	—	1.0	5.7

(* Significantly different from normal)

Fig. 5-6: Data from 4 fatty streaks, 12 samples of normal intima, 23 gelatinous "tails" of plaques, 9 plaque edges and 9 central caps, and 37 samples of atheroma lipid from the lower layers of plaques.

DR. SMITH: I don't know. I can't answer that.

DR. STONE: But they would give different reactions with this particular stain. Young and old collagen, as I have heard described.

DR. SMITH: I find very variable staining with the Van Gieson stain. Some collagen bundles stain rather dimly, while adjacent strands are bright pink, and I have no idea what the differences are. Yes, I am quite certain that different collagens in the lesion stain differently but whether they are young collagen or old collagen, or what the differences are, I have no idea. The large amount of collagen is the second feature of these lesions that is compatible with hypoxia and lactate production. There are now at least four studies showing that lactic acid specifically increases collagen, and procollagen proline hydroxylase activity in cell cultures (35,36, 37,38).

It appears to be a specific effect of lactic acid and not of low pH or of oxygen deficiency. In vivo studies on granulomas and wound healing are, however, contradictory (39,40) and this seems to be an area that requires further investigation in terms of smooth muscle cells and the artery wall. Both these in vivo studies indicate that cell protein synthesis HAMSTER is decreased by low oxygen tension and with CHL-F Chinese hamster cells in culture it decreased growth rate (41). Thus, it seems unlkely that hypoxia can be implicated in smooth muscle cell proliferation.

In addition to the risk of hypoxia, the smooth muscle cells are subjected to mechanical stress, which may be a determining factor in Influence of Mechanical their metabolic pattern. I Stress on Proliferation showed a slide from Leung et al., and Synthesis (42) demonstrating the differential development of collagen and elastin in the developing pulmonary and aortic truns (Fig. 2-16). They have also done some elegant culture experiments in which smooth muscle cells were grown on elastin membranes; then some of the membranes were subjected to cyclical stretching; whereas others were agitated in the medium without stretching. Compared with agitation, stretching increased total protein synthesis by 80% and collagen synthesis by 200%, but there was no increase in DNA synthesis (43).

In these experiments Types I and III collagen synthesis were   SHEEP
stimulated to the same degree but in a study on chondrocytes,
those grown in spinner cultures produced a different type of
collagen from monolayers (44). In short-term organ cultures
of pregnant sheep myometrium, R.H. Smith and R. Palmer
studied ^{3}H-proline incorporation and conversion to ^{3}H-
hydroxyproline. In gravid (stretched) areas the ratio
hydro/pro was higher than in unstretched areas, indicating
that a higher proportion of the protein synthesized was
collagen (unpublished observations). So there seems to be a
growing body of information suggesting that mechanical
stresses have a considerable influence on collagen synthesis,
and this may be a self-magnifying system. Stretching increases
collagen synthesis, but it also increases lactic acid production,
and the lactic acid again stimulates collagen synthesis.

A different approach to stress factors has been made
through studies on hypertension. In both spontaneous and
experimental hypertension Wolinsky reports proliferation of
SMCs, and a roughly parallel increase in the amount of
collagen and elastin (45,46). However, in experimental
hypertension produced by renal ischaemia it is possible that
the observed response is to the reninangiotension system and
not to the mechanical factors. In experimental coarctation
of the aorta in dogs Hollander et al., found significant   DOG
increases in sulphated MPS and $^{35}SO_4$ incorporation in the
hypertension segments above the coarctation, significant
decreases below it, and no change in lipid content (47).
Fernandez and Crane (48) examined the very early response of
small arteries rate to constriction of the aorta between the
renal arteries. There was no response in vessels distal to
the constriction, and there was a positive response in
animals subjected to nephrectomy, suggesting that the reninangiotension system was not a primary factor.

By 24 hours, small arteries proximal to the constriction
showed "plasmatic vasculosis," with progressive fragmentation
of elastin, SMC necrosis and deposition of fibrin, but there
was no increase in ^{3}H-thymidine labelling. By 4 days, there
was "florid necrotising arteritis" and a marked increase in
^{3}H-thymidine labelling which continued to increase up to 8
days, (the longest time of observation). Unfortunately the
authors do not report on the large vessels, and made no
comment on them.

Nevertheless, this experiment raises the question of whether the observed response in acute experimental hypertension is truely related to the mechanical factors, or if it is in reality a secondary response to increased insudation of plasma macromolecules, in particular, the increased conversion of fibrinogen to fibrin within the wall. This seems to be an area requiring further elucidation.

Plasma macromolecules seem to enter the intima in relatively large amounts. In normal human intima from the fourth decade upwards in normotensive subjects the concentration, on a crude volumetric basis, of low density lipoprotein (LDL) is approximately the same in the intima and in the plasma, and the concentration of intimal fibrinogen is 1/2 - 1/3 the plasma concentration (59). In the hypertensive individual, intimal LDL may be doubled. The steady state concentration of plasma macromolecules in normal intima seems to be a function of their concentration in the plasma and their molecular weight (50). In a number of samples of normal intima we examined the relative concentrations of LDL (molecular weight 2×10^6), d-macroglobulin (molecular weight 820,000), HDL (molecular weight 200,000) and albumin (molecular weight 68,000). They were quantified in terms of the volumes of the patient's own plasma from which they were derived, to correct for the different concentrations in different subjects.

Taking LDL as a hundred, the retention of the other proteins was calculated as percentage of LDL retention. This gave a linear relation between retention and molecular weight; thus, relative to the plasma concentration, LDL was retained to the greatest extent while there was least retention of albumin (50). This strongly suggests that the accumulation depends on retardation by molecular sieving rather than on specific binding of LDL. In the gelatinous lesions there is also a linear relationship and the slope is steeper; whether that simply depends on the thicknesss, I don't know. The actual concentrations in normal intima are shown in Table 5. where the concentrations in plasma and intima are compared. The figures are for a cube of tissue, so the actual concentration in the extracellular space must be very high. Albumin is still the largest component in intima but relative to its concentration in plasma it is retained to a very small extent. There is a large amount of LDL and fibrinogen (Table 5); fibrinogen is behaving as if it had a molecular weight of about a million.

TABLE 5. Concentration of plasma proteins in normal intima (Volumetric Basis).

	INTIMA	PLASMA
	Mg./100cc	Mg./100ml.
Albumin	725	4,500
LDL	500	500
Fibrinogen	200	325
α_2-macroglobulin	130	285
HDL	90	300

The protease inhibitor, d$_2$-macroglobulin is also present in quite high concentration, thus there is a very interesting mixture in the intima, and this must influence the cells and modify the extracellular matrix to a considerable extent. In the gelatinous lesions the concentrations of LDL and fibrinogen may increase up to three-fold compared with adjacent normal intima, so that the concentration of LDL is substantially greater than the concentration in plasma (49). Thus, these SMCs are in a localized hyperlipoproteinaemic environment even in a subject with normal lipoprotein levels.

DR. CAREW: Would you, just for reference, talk about the concentration....

DR. SMITH: The figure in Table 5 is milligrams total LDL.   Intimal LDL is measured against plasma LDL standards. In normal intima LDL cholesterol is about 30% of the total cholesterol.

DR. COLTON: Okay. So it is protein but in fact what is in the wall could be aproprotein and low cholesterol.

DR. SMITH: No, it is not, because we electrophorese the mobile lipoprotein out of the tissue and stain the immunopeak with a lipid stain; so we are not staining aproprotein which is not carrying lipid.

DR. CAREW: Is it conceivable or certain that this is all intact LDL or fragments or what?

DR. SMITH: On two dimensional electrophoresis it migrates close to the patient's LDL. We did some recovery experiments in which we cut the immuno-peaks out of the agarose gel and measured the ratio of cholesterol to peak area, and compared this for the patient's plasma LDL and the intimal LDL and they came out approximately the same. Now I say this rather guardedly because when we looked at the cholesterol ester fatty acids they were very odd, but then so were the cholesterol ester fatty acids that we recovered from the immunopeaks from the patient's plasma. But it is my impression that this is intact LDL.

I am not going to discuss the effect of cholesterol feeding on atherogenesis in intact animals. There is a vast literature on this type of experimental atherosclerosis, and I do not know whether the atherogenic agent is in fact cholesterol.

Effects of Plasma Fractions
on Aortic Smooth Muscle
Cells in Culture

TABLE 6. Effect of plasma fractions on cell cultures

	Growth	Mitosis	Lipid Uptake
Dzoga et al. (1974) - Primary explants. (51)			
5% hyperlipaemic monkey serum	+ +	+ +	+ +
LDL	+ +	+ +	+ +
VLDL	0	0	0
HDL	0	0	0
Low-lipid infranatant	0	0	0

Ross (1975) - Sub-cultures grown to zero growth in 1%
(52)   normal monkey serum.

Normal monkey serum.	Growth
10% serum	+ + +
5% reconstituted serum	+ +
Low-lipid infranatant	+
LDL + "	+ +
HDL + "	+

Maybe Dr. Werthessen will talk about this later. There
have been a number of studies on the effect of lipoproteins
on smooth muscle cells in culture and some of the results
reported by Dzoga (52) and by Ross (53) are summarized in
Table 6. In primary explants, Dzoga (52) found that compared
with normal monkey serum, hyperlipaemic monkey serum stimulated
growth, mitosis and lipid uptake. In her system, the isolated
LDL seemed to be responsible and there was no stimulation
relative to normal monkey serum by VLDL, HDL or the lipid
poor protein infranatant. Ross (53) seems to get slightly
different results; he works with subcultures, and I don't
know how much difference this makes. They are grown to zero
MONKEY growth in one percent normal monkey serum, the supplements
of monkey serum are added. Serum and reconstituted serum
stimulated growth but he did not get full stimulation without
both LDL and the low lipid infranatent. He suggests that
this contains a low molecular weight protein derived from
platelets which is in fact the stimulating factor. It is,
interesting that Ronnemaa, Juva and Kulonin (54) also found
stimulation of collagen synthesis by the low lipid infranatant
and not by isolated LDL.

How do these cultures relate to the artery wall? I
think this is one of the major questions that we will have
to answer soon. Table 7   shows the concentration of LDL
cholesterol in intima and in the culture medium, and there
is an order of magnitude difference. So either the cultured
cells are very much more sensitive to plasma component or in
the intact intima the cell has some sort of micro-environment
around it which insulates it from the high concentrations of
LP in the whole tissue, or the rate of change of LP level
may be a critical factor.

DR. COLTON: Are you suggesting that people are making
experiments in culture media that is too low in LDL cholesterol?

DR. SMITH: As I understand it, at the concentrations
found in intima the cultures die. I am not suggesting
anything; I am just asking the question, what is the relation
between the cell in culture and the cell in intima?

DR. CAREW: May I comment. We put in a low density
lipoprotein at concentrations upwards of serum concentration
and they don't die in short term. This is a very interesting
problem, though, because we measured degradation rates in
culture of low density lipoproteins which are sufficient to
account for all of the LDL degradation in vivo and serum
concentration or medium concentrations of LDL as low as 1%
plasma.

TABLE 7.   Concentration of LDL cholesterol in intima and culture
medium

        Normal intima   190 mg/100 cc wet tissue

        Gelatinous
        thickenings   380   "   "   "

        Culture Medium   (Dzoga et al., 1974, 52)

        Normal monkey LDL   4mg/100ml.

        Hyperlipaemic LDL   30mg/100ml.

That, of course, raises the question of what is the relationship between the cultured smooth muscle cells and the cells in the artery. I think this is a very important point. I would just like to ask another question which refers back to your previous slide indicating the concentrations of LDL, HDL in the intima and I think these are the data determined from saline extracts and then electrophoresed saline extracts...

DR. SMITH: No, this is from direct electrophoresis actually from the tissue.

DR. CAREW: Well, what is the possibility that not all the LDL comes out of here so that the actual concentration in this tissue is perhaps even considerably larger than this because of that amount which would be collagen or elastin or smooth muscle cell membranes which is not released by the electrophoresis?

DR. SMITH: In normal intima, most of the LP comes out, but in certain lesions a lot more can be released by incubation with proteolytic enzymes, and I will be talking about that shortly.

DR. COLTON: In the normal case could there be more LDL that has not come out? Could it be bound and not liberated by electrophoresis?

DR. SMITH: We get very little more out of normal intima after incubation with chondroitinase or proteolytic enzymes, so in normal intima I don't think there is much more to come out but, as I say, in some of the lesions there is a lot more to come out. I will talk about that later.

DR. SCHWARTZ: Have you added HDL to these tissues to see if in fact you might use that to unblock the LDL binding?

DR. SMITH: No, I haven't.

Studies in vivo on the effects of hyperlipidaemia on collagen synthesis have produced contradictory results (Table 8). Fuller et al., (54) found that in weanling mini-pigs cholesterol feeding stimulated protocollagen proline hydroxylase activity equally in atherosclerotic lesions and in adjacent lesion-free segments of aorta. In contrast, St. Clair et al., in (55) young pigeons found no difference between aortas from controls and cholesterol-fed birds, and no significant difference between lesion-free segments and lesions.

TABLE 8. Effect of hyperlipaemia on collagen synthesis in vivo

Authors.	Species		Lesion	Lesion-free
			Proline hydroxylase activity	
Fuller et. al. 1972 (54)	Pigs	Cholesterol fed	620*	647a
		Control	294*	195⊠
			(* ⊠ Same area, but no lesion)	
St.Clair et al. 1975 (55)	Pigeons Young	Cholesterol fed		
		Fatty streak	5128	4831
		Plaque	5233	
		Control	-	4417
	Old	Spontaneous plaques	3976	4767
			Collagen synthesis.	
McCullagh & Ehrhart 1974. (56)	Dogs	Cholesterol fed	977	187
		Abdominal aorta	977	187
		Femoral artery	1954	186
		Control		
		Abdominal aorta	-	176
		femoral artery	-	97

These preparations included adventitia as well as media, and
as the intima is a very small proportion of the total tissue,
changes occurring there might be obscured; furthermore, the
lesions contained very little collagen. McCullagh and
DOG Erhart (56) measured collagen synthesis in dogs fed semisynthetic
diets supplemented with cholesterol and found up to 10-fold
stimulation of collagen synthesis in the very fibrous lesions,
but no changes in lesion-free segments. Clearly this is an
area that needs further clarification.

       In addition to acting directly on SMCs, plasma macromolecules
may react within the intima with each other, or with the

Interactions between
Plasma and Intimal
Macromolecules

connective tissue components, and
thereby change the extracellular
environment, and thus influence
cellular metabolism. We have
investigated the relation between
soluble fibrinogen and insoluble fibrin, or fibrin-like material
("fibrin") in intima (49). The distribution of "fibrin" is
highly correlated with morphology (Fig. 5-6). In normal
intima there are approximately equal concentrations of
fibrinogen and fibrin, whereas in gelatinous lesions and the
gelatinous peripheries of plaques, there is a very high
concentration of fibrinogen with only a small increase in
"fibrin." At the edge of developed plaques, there is a
consistent and abrupt increase in the concentration of
insoluble "fibrin," suggesting an increase in thrombin
activity in these localized areas. High levels of "fibrin"
are also found in the atheroma lipid pool in the middle of
developed fibrous plaques. I believe that much of this
"fibrin" is derived from fibrinogen which is converted to
"fibrin" within the intima. Fibrinolysis also seems to
occur in some lesions, but it is not clear if this is the
result of plasmin or lysosmal protease activity. In either
case, the activity might be modified by the protease inhibitors,
$_2$-macroglobulin and $_1$-antitrypsin, which are present in
substantial concentrations in intima.

       In answer to the question: Does all the lipoprotein
come out of intima on electrophoresis? Recently we have
found an immobilized lipoprotein fraction that can be released
by incubating the residual tissue, after electrophresis,
with plasmin or crude collagenase (57). The amounts released
after a single incubation with plasmin are shown in Fig. 5-6
(bottom line); in normal intima and low lipid gelatinous
lesions the lipoprotein released is only 10-15% of the
mobile lipoprotein fraction, and is not increased by repeating
the incubation.

It is present in highest concentrations in areas of maximum
extracellular lipid accumulation; in these areas more lipoprotein
is released on repeating the incubation with plasmin, and
its total concentration may be two or three times greater
than the concentration of mobile LP. This suggests that
immobilization of the LP may be a first step in the irreversible
disposition of lipid from plasma LDL. Incubation with
chrondroitinase ABC releases only small amounts of lipoprotein,
and maximum release is obtained with plasmin; the simplest
explanation of these findings is that lipoprotein is in some
way bound to fibrin (57,58). This idea receives some support
from the work of Camejo et al. (59). who have found a lipoprotein
protein complex in intima-medial extracts

Lipoproteins form ionic complexes with glycosaminoglycans
(GAG) in vitro and it has frequently been suggested that
this also occurs within the intima (60,61,62); our data on
the relation between molecular weight and relative retention
(50)does not really support the concept that this is the
mechanism of LP accumulation in intima. Fibrinogen can also
form complexes with GAG (63) and GAG - fibrinogen - lipoprotein
complexes have been described. There is no definite proof
that any of these complexes actually exist in the wall.

Thus, there are high concentrations of LDL and other
plasma macromolecules in normal intima, and in the gelatinous
precursors of fibrous plaques

Stimulation of Smooth Muscle Cell Proliferation in Intima

the concentrations are subtantially
higher than in plasma. It seems
reasonable to postulate that, as
in cultures, (52) this will
stimulate the smooth muscle cells to proliferate and accumulate
lipid. Unfortunately, there does not seem to be any constant
relationship either between intimal lipoprotein concentration
or proliferation of intracellular lipid accumulation. This
is clearly demonstrated in Table 9 which compares the concentration
of lipoprotein in normal intima and adjacent gelatinous
thickenings in three patients with different levels of serum
cholesterol and blood pressure. In all patients the lesion
contained twice as much lipoprotein as adjacent normal
intima, but there was more lipoprotein in the normal intima
of Patient 2 than in the lesion of Patient 1. Patient 3 had
a high serum cholesterol and hypertension, and his normal
intima contained more lipoprotein than the lesion of Patient
2, and twice as much as the lesion in Patient 1. None of
the lesions contained a significant number of cells with
intracellular fat droplets.

TABLE 9. "Lipoprotein-bound" cholesterol in normal intima
and early fibrous lesions

Subject sex & age	Serum cholesterol mg/100ml	Blood Pressure	Intimal lipoprotein Cholesterol mg/100mg dry tissue	
			Normal	Lesion
1) F.32y	130	$\frac{130}{80}$	1.3	3.2
2) M.61y	267	$\frac{130}{80}$	3.8	6.2
3) M.49y	332	$\frac{260}{130} - \frac{220}{120}$	6.4	12.5

Thus, a high concentration of intimal lipoprotein does not in itself constitute a lesion: possibly it provides a stimulating environment for proliferation of smooth muscle cells that are already altered in some way, or possibly the high level found in gelatinous lesions is secondary to pre-existing proliferation, and not an initiating factor.

Large, raised lesions with massive proliferation of smooth muscle cells and collagen but not significant increase in cholesterol are frequently found in human arteries, (64.65,32); thus cholesterol accumulation is not an obligatory factor in lesion development. Recently, Benditt and Benditt (64) have made a very important contribution to the problem of smooth muscle cell proliferation by suggesting that the fibrous plaque is comparable to a benign tumor, and the cells are transformed. As a result of X-chromosome inactivation in some heterozygous Negro women, the tissue consists of a mosaic of cells in which the X-chromosome is derived from either the father or the mother. Using the A or B iso-enzymes of glucose - 6 - phosphate dehydrogenase (G-6PDH) as cellular markers, Benditt showed that normal intima contained both isoenzymes but fibrous plaques contained only one iso-enzyme (either A or B), suggesting that they are monoclonal in origin. These findings have been confirmed and extended by Pearson et al. (66) and the combined results from the two groups are summarized in Table 10.

In normal intima 97% of the samples contained both A and B isoenzymes. In the fibrous plaques 85% of the samples examined were monoclonal and they were equally divided between A and B isoenzymes; most fatty streaks have an AB configuration and are not monoclonal lesions. It is difficult to integrate this idea into our present concepts of atherosclerosis. But it is an idea that we cannot dismiss and that we must try to reconcile with existing information.

Benditt has commented that the risk of transformation by agents such as viral or chemical mutagens is increased where there is increased rate of mitosis. In a gelatinous lesion there may well be an increased rate of mitosis; and it also contains an enormous amount of low density lipoprotein which might carry a mutagenic steroid. Thus one can postulate that cells are undergoing increased mitosis in a micro-environment which is greatly enriched in LDL carrying the mutagen. I will leave it to Dr. Werthessen to tell us what sort of mutagenic steroid might be involved; Lee, Werthessen and co-workers (67) have isolated an extremely atherogenic fraction from cholesterol, and increased mitotic activity is an early response to cholesterol feeding (67,68,69).

TABLE 10. Distribution of isoenzymes of glucose-6-phosphate dehydrogenase in samples of aortic intima from heterozygous women

| | | ISOENZYME DISTRIBUTION | | | | |
| | | Number of samples | | | Percentage | |
	No. of patients	AB	A	B	AB	A or B
Lesion-free intima	20	156	1	3	97.5	2.5
Fibrous plaques	12	9	25	25	15.3	84.7
Fatty streaks	11	23	2	3	83.2	17.8

Combined data of Benditt & Benditt (1973) (64), and Pearson et al. (1975) (66).

In the centers of fibrous plaques that have accumulated a pool of extracellular atheroma lipid it appears there is either irreversible precipitation of LDL or the apoprotein has been degraded or split off the lipid. There is also loss of cells, decrease in the concentration of GAG, and loss of the architecture of the collagen bundles, although it is not clear if there is a quantitative decrease.

Effect of Cellular Enzymes Components of the Extracellular Environment

In preliminary studies we have found a rapid loss of intact LDL from the amorphous lipid centers of plaques that have been minced, and then incubated; the level falling to about a quarter of the control level in 3-4 hours incubation (70). Increased activities of lysosomal enzymes, particularly -glucuronidase, have been reported in atherosclerotic aortas (71). Increased cathepsin D has been reported by several authors (reviewed by Zemplenyi (72) and there seems to be little doubt that lysosomal enzymes, released as a result of increased lactic acid production, or of cell death in the hypoxic centers of larger plaques, play an important role in the later stages of plaque development.

THE ACCUMULATION OF LIPID IN THE FAT-FILLED CELLS OF FATTY STREAKS

One reason that I have hardly mentioned lipid metabolism is that it has been covered in several recent and expert reviews (27,28,29). There are also other reasons: first, and most important, I do not now believe that the primary factor in the genesis of occlusive atherosclerotic lesions in humans is disordered lipid metabolism of the artery wall. Second, most of the studies of arterial lipid metabolism have been made on cholesterol-fed animals and I question if the response to this acute cholesterol stress is really relevant to the average human subject. It may be relevant to subjects with familiar Type II hypercholesterolaemia, but according to Oliver's calculations (73) in Britain these patients account for only one in every 400 coronary deaths. An example of this acute cholesterol stress is given by Day and Proudlock (74) who found increased cholesterol esterifying activity in aortas of rabbits fed cholesterol for only three days. RABBIT During the three days, serum cholesterol rose from 78 - 415mg/100 ml. It is difficult to imagine any situation in which a patient's cholesterol could increase more than 5-fold in three days.

Irrelevance of Induced Hypercholesterolaemia

The lesions that do appear to be primary disorders of arterial SMC lipid metabolism are fatty streaks.

Fatty streaks in children and adolescents consist of clusters
of cells filled with lipid, of which cholesterol ester is the
major component. All the evidence
Intracellular Lipid   suggests that most of the cholesterol
Accumulation in Fatty   comes from plasma lipoprotein, but
Streaks   the ester that accumulates is not
like plasma cholesterol ester, so
either the cells take up only free cholesterol and esterify it -
mainly with oleic acid - or they take up whole lipoproteins,
hydrolyse the cholesterol esters and re-esterify them.

There is now very detailed information on the metabolism
of cholesterol and LDL by fibroblasts and SMCs in culture
and also by macrophages. Goldstein and Brown (75) have
recently summarized their extensive studies on lipoprotein
uptake, and discussed them in relation to the intracellular
lipid accumulation in fatty streaks.

It is clear that the results still do not explain what
is happening; indeed, the data from the cultures suggest
that all the cells in the body should be filled with cholesterol
ester. The problems of translating from cultures to intact
animals are further emphasized by Weinstein, Carew and
Steinberg (76) who calculate that the rate of degradation of
LDL protein per kg smooth muscle is 120 times greater in
cultures than in the whole animal. The fat-filled cells of
fatty streaks consistently deplete their immediate vicinity
of lipoprotein reducing it to about a quarter of the concentration
in adjacent normal (Fig. 5-6) (31,32). Possibly they are
behaving more like cells in culture, and have somehow
escaped a control that is acting on adjacent cells.

If, as seems possible, smooth muscle cells and fibroblasts
constantly degrade LDL protein without accumulating cholesterol,
then cholesterol must be transported
Reverse Transport of   out of cells as well as into them,
Cholesterol   and failure of this "reverse
transport" may account for
cholesterol ester accumulation. There have been several
studies showing transport of cholesterol out of cells and
HDL or derivatives of HDL seem to be particularly effective
cholesterol receptors. (76,77,78,79).

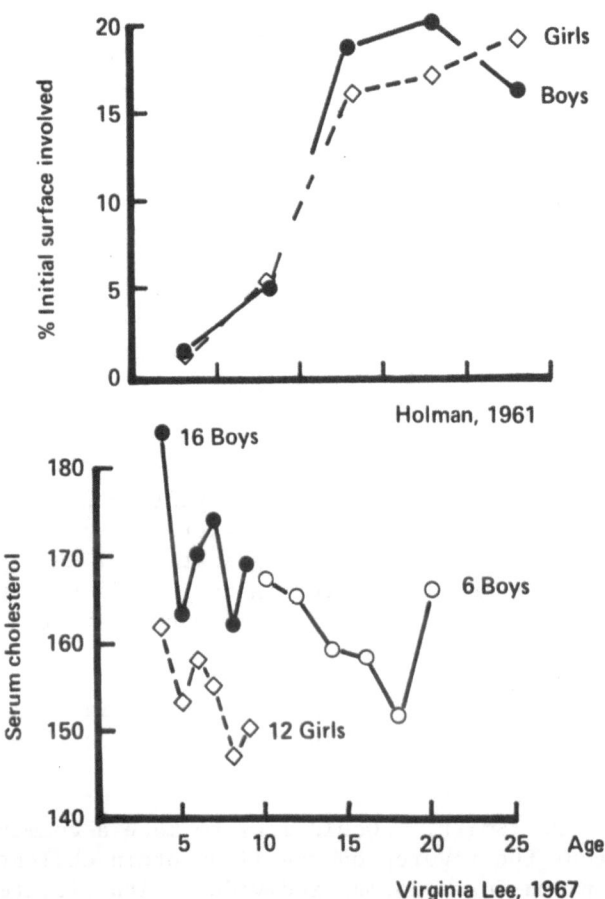

Fig. 5-7: Comparison of data from Holman (80) on the extent of fatty streaking with data from Lee (81) on serum cholesterol levels in three groups of children studied longitudinally over several years.

When one considers the relation between accumulation of intracellular cholesterol and plasma cholesterol levels, the idea of a failure to transport cholesterol out of the cells appears particularly attractive. Figure 5-7 combines the data from Holman on the percent of the intimal surface involved in fatty streaking in young people (80) which the data of Virginia Lee on serum cholesterol levels followed longitudinally in children (81). These are groups of children in which she measured the cholesterol every six months for five or ten years. The extent of fatty streaking was lowest when serum cholesterol was highest. During the 8 - 18 age span, when fatty streaking was increasing at the maximum rate, these childrens' cholesterol was drifting down. At the end of the adolescent growth spurt when the normal adult rise in serum cholesterol starts, the fatty streaking has levelled out. I think this diagram is worth pondering by anybody who is thinking of feeding cholesterol to rabbits.

EDITORIAL NOTE: From evidence developed since this colloquium the angiotoxic properties of oxydation products of cholesterol, notably 25 hydroxy cholesterol have been established and newly developed data indicate that the oxygenated sterols, normally present in very small concentration in man, perform a regulatory function through negative feedback of cholesterol synthesis.

Kandutsche A.A., Chen H.W., Heiniger, H.G., Biological Activity of some Oxygenated Sterols. Science: 201: 498-501, 1978.

DR. DEWEY: Dr. Smith, I would like to make a comment relative to one of the figures on the lipoprotein cholesterol levels in the intima for a normal individual with elevated blood cholesterol, also the one with elevated cholesterol and the one with hypertension. One of the characteristics of the hypertensive state is that the excursion between systolic and diastolic pressure goes up more proportionally with blood pressure. The significance of this effect depends on a lot of things including the potential effects of trans-endothelial transport during the cardiac cycle according to the mechanism that Dr. Kenyon suggested yesterday. When we are comparing a hypertensive and a normal tensive individual and their propensity to exhibit disease, I think that the pressure excursion as well as the absolute pressure level are important.

DR. SMITH: Unfortunately, I have not looked at the data in terms of systolic-diastolic differences.

The hypertensives always have more lipoprotein in the
intima than normals and the average is just about double.
But whether this is a direct result of the hypertension or
whether it is because the hypertension does something to the
wall, so that the wall retains more, I have no idea.

DR. COX: I have a question about the points that you
made with regard to the collagen synthesis and its relationship
to stretch. I want to comment on
some work being done in our
laboratory by Dr. Grace Fisher.
She is currently studying the
differences in collagen and
elastin synthesis in vitro using segments of thoracic and
aortic arch in normal rabbits and rabbits fed one of those
non-acceptable high cholesterol diets. Basically, what she
has found in vitro is that both collagen and elastin synthesis
are elevated in the cholesterol fed rabbit, within, both
instances, a higher rate of synthesis in the arch compared
with the thoracic aorta. This, however, was done in vitro
in which there was no stretch on the vessel. The question
with regard to the studies that you mentioned, is it possible
that these cells have memory in the sense that having been
subjected to elevated stretch, do they still retain the
characteristics of higher rates of collagen synthesis or do
they turn off quickly? My question basically relates to the
time course of response of collagen synthesis both in the
uterus and in these cultured smooth muscle cells. Is there
any information that you know of?

Collagen and Elastin
Synthesis Increased in
Cholesterol-fed Rabbit

RABBIT

DR. SMITH: I don't think there is any information on
this, and it is the sort of information that is required. I
suppose that the stretch induces proline hydroxylase synthesis,
but how rapid this is and how long the additional proline
hydroxylase lasts, I didn't find any data on this.

DR. COX: One might expect in the aortic arch compared
to the thoracic aorta, a larger stretch over the cardiac
cycles associated with pulse pressure. If there is memory
in the form of a protein or something of that sort, one
might expect to see this difference in the arch and in the
descending aorta.

DR. SMITH: I suppose it depends on the turnover rate
of the enzyme.

DR. COX: The other comment I had was in making this connection to neurohumoral control in regard to your suggestion about this hypoxic or anoxic zone beyond 300 μ in the arterial wall. Activation of smooth muscle cells to produce a contraction in blood vessels, would be expected to increase the thickness of the arterial walls so that the fraction of the wall that is "within a hypoxic zone" would increase through muscle activation.

DR. SCHWARTZ: I enjoyed Dr. Smith's presentation very much and I have several very brief questions and comments. One relates specifically to lactate accumulation; could Dr. Smith say just where this lactate is, what level of pH change would result, and what evidence have we that lactate might interfere with the lysosomal stability. I notice that the pH values you gave are in fact not nearly as low as the pH optima for the lysosomal enzymes.

DR. SMITH: I don't know if there is really any adequate reply to this. As far as I can see from the literature on myocardial infarction, not of course, on aorta, progressive loss of lysosomal stability occurs, below about pH 7. Probably, as you say, this is not down to the pH optimum for the enzymes but then they have significant activity even at pH 6 or so. So I think this is an area that requires a lot of further work. I think it is a very interesting area. The calculated concentration of lactic acid in a plaque at 800 μ from the surface is 175mg/100ml. At this concentration, in 25% serum the pH was 4.8 and in 50% serum it was 5.9. With 50mg/100ml lactic acid - the calculated concentration in an early thickening of 400 μ - the pH in 25% serum was 6.9, and in 50% serum was about 7.4.

DR. SCHWARTZ: Going back quite a few years, I recall some studies on the effect of hypercholesterolemia on oxygen transport. I am not sure what the current status of this work is, but it is my understanding that under certain circumstances hypercholesterolemia may modify oxygen transport across membranes. Is this being re-examined, and furthermore, is A.V. Hill's theoretical data applicable in the hypercholesterolemia situation?

DR. SMITH: In the only papers that I managed to find the results seemed very equivocal, and I did not really understand what they were telling us. I did not find any clear and convincing data on what hypercholesterolemia is doing to oxygen transport but one's guess would be that it wouldn't improve it.

DR. SCHWARTZ: Concerning the apparent discrepancy
between data from Russell Ross and Dr. Dzoga's group
in Chicago it is my understanding that the Chicago group
have shown that LDL prepared without any platelet contamination
still produces smooth muscle cellular proliferation.

DR. SMITH: I did forget to make a comment there that
this monkey hyperlipemic LDL is not really a large amount of   MONKEY
normal LDL, it is a highly abnormal molecule containing a
gross cholesterol overlay, and I think one might think of it
as being like a floating beta of a type III hyperlipidemia -
it is not a normal LDL.

DR. WOLF: Relating to the lactic acid concentration
and the evidence of hypoxia, do we have evidence that the
collagen excess or increase is real collagen or is it defective
collagen in some way? And I am reminded of a note or page
25 volume I of our Lindau Conference in which it was pointed
out that Stetten had shown that the synthesis of hydroxyproline
requires the presence of molecular oxygen and the suggestion
was made that abnormal collagen was being synthesized in the
presence, if indeed there was a presence of low oxygen
tension (82).

DR. SMITH: This idea that hydroxyproline could only be
synthesized at a high O_2 tension has been shown by Langness
and Udenfriend (36) to be untrue.

DR. LEE: This is just a short comment on the G-6-PD
studies. Dr. Benditt of Seattle reported that one out of
                              three or four black families
Benditt's Neoplastic   is heterozygous and has two
Theory of Atherogenesis   variants, A and B, of G-6-PD
                              while black males and all other
non-black people are homozygous and have only one variant,
A or B, of G-6-PD.   He found that atherosclerotic lesions
of these heterozygous black females showed only one variant
of G-6-PD and concluded that atherosclerotic lesions develop
from a single cell, thus monoclonal in origin (64). A group
at Johns Hopkins carried out a similar study in heterozygous
females and confirmed that well developed fibrous lesions
had one variant of G-6-PD (83). However, they found both
variants of G-6-PD in fatty streaks and concluded that
fibrous lesions and fatty streaks have different origins.
We have been interested in this subject for the past couple
of years and studied a large number of aortas from autopsied
black females.

Essentially, we confirmed the findings of the Seattle and
Baltimore groups but came to a somewhat different conclusion.
When we examined very small lesions, we found both variants
A and B, of G-6-PD but well developed lesions showed one
variant, A or B. It seems to us that when a lesion begins
to develop smooth muscle cells multiply in a random fashion
until it reaches a certain size. At this stage, the lesion
will show both variants of G-6-PD. After the lesion reaches
a certain size, the fittest cell would dominate within the
lesion and multiply faster than other cells, as in a bacterial
culture; and at a later stage the lesion will consist of
this particular type of cells. At this stage, the lesion
will show one variant. Thus, a well developed lesion will
show a monoclonal pattern. Our conclusion is that an atherosclerotic lesion begins to develop from cells in a random
fashion but it takes a monoclonal pattern after it reaches a
certain size.

DR. COLTON: According to Benditt's theory there is
high mitotic activity in those regions that have been looked
at from a fluid mechanic viewpoint such as near bifurcations.
The blue regions also have high mitotic activity. So we can
add another speculative hypothesis which in fact totally
bypasses fluid mechanics.

DR. DEWEY: I think it would be interesting to do a
quantitative calculation of the rate at which one would need
to increase the mitotic activity of one particular cell type
so that over a substantial period of time, the net volumetric
growth of lesion material would exhibit a preponderance of
the hyperactive cell type. If there already is a substantial
amount of growth and turnover activity in the tissue under
normal circumstances, we may be talking about the small
difference between two large numbers, which does not strike
me as being the same as cancerous-type mitotic activity.

DR. STONE: What is the critical oxygen concentration
for the vessel wall and what is the answer to my question
about the vasa vasorum.

DR. SMITH: I was showing you the thickness of normal
intima in the human aorta; normal intima may be anything up
to 300 microns; the media in the human is about 1100 M in
thickness and the vasa are supposed to penetrate only the
outer third of the vessel. So, in a human aorta you have
theoretically a large block that could pretty well be anoxic.
The vasa go in about 350 M.

DR. STONE: Let me make sure. Are you saying "anoxia" or "hypoxia."

DR. SMITH: Hypoxia, and I think if the Hill calculation is correct there will be a quite definitely anoxic area. We require a repetition of the oxygen probe data in a dog, or better still, in a bovine or something with a thick vessel. Those were two studies that I put together myself. One was the study on the oxygen tension across the rabbit aorta in vivo; that was the top curve (Fig. 5-2). And the other was in vitro work on the effect of different oxygen tensions on lactic acid production.

COW
RABBIT

DR. COX: You have to be careful about the vasa vasorum because they are very variable. There are reports in the literature that the vasa vasorum extend all the way to the intimal-medial junction in some places, especially in the main pulmonary artery and in the ascending aorta of man. There could be a lot of variability.

DR. MANSFIELD: I think we have to be very careful in terms of extrapolating from a pO_2 value as to the viability of the tissues that we are talking about. If in the dog or cat, you excise a segment of the aorta so it is totally separated on the ends, sew it back and encapsulate it in an absolutely non-porous backing, you will find that all the exterior wall is dead up to about 500 microns from the intima. Now if you take fibroblasts and line the inside of a non-porous tube, thrombus deposits on this and when that thrombus reaches the level somewhere between 500 and 800 microns, the fibroblasts will die and you can show cell death at that time. So these are two indications that we are in the ball park in terms of the limits of diffusion depth which leads to cell death. We do not see that in the human normal aorta, regardless of what your pO_2 values are, it is unlikely that anoxia is occurring or we should see the histological changes of cell death and destruction. Rather there may be various degrees of hypoxia depending on what the oxygen requirement is within the wall itself. I think it is very important that we are cautious in terms of saying, "What is going on in the cell?" When the cell is obviously alive, and even though it may be quite removed from either side of lining of the vessel wall itself.

DOG OR
CAT

DR. SMITH: I quite agree with you, and I never seem to see medial necrosis.

DR. SCHWARTZ: Just a very brief comment to remind us of Seymour Glagov's important work, which indicates that approximately 20 medial lamella can occur without any vasa vasorum, a finding which suggests that diffusional nutrition is of considerable importance in the inner media (84).

DR. COLTON: With regard to those tabulations one must be very careful. Hill's calculation assumed zero order kinetics. The available evidence suggests that oxygen uptake kinetics follows a Michaelis-Menten form. When pO_2 is low enough to become first order, the rate is not constant but decreases as the pO_2 decreases. One needs to know what is the critical pO_2 at which necrosis occurs. I don't think there are good data for this.

DR. KENYON: There is always interesting speculation on the effects of increased demand due to mechanical stressing on the wall and I think that in the arch of the aorta and especially with unusually large pressure differences there are large dynamic strains which could produce anoxia. This could be quite important because the smooth muscle cells presumably are attempting to synthesize the material and any additional barrier to diffusion you may get could be a self-destructive mechanism.

DR. LEE: Of course, we do not see necrosis in a normal vessel no matter how thick the vessel is, for example the aorta. However, when lesions develop and the thickness of the intimal lesion exceeds the thickness of the media we begin to see necrosis in the center of the lesion. I was told some years ago that one simple reason to have central necrosis in these thick lesions is that the distance to the center of the lesion is too great for efficient supply of oxygen. I don't know whether that is true or not.

DR. SMITH: Well, I don't know that they expect an answer. When I was looking at the depth of the fat filled cells from the surface in Mixed Lesions   fatty streaks I also had a number of mixed lesions which I called mixed lesions. They were proliferative lesions in which there were also fat filled cells in the cap of the lesion, and I noticed that there seemed to be a critical depth below which fat filled cells deeper than about, I think, three to four hundred microns from the surface seemed to disappear and I think it is possible that these fat filled cells come to grief once they get to a certain critical depth, and disintegrate.

DR. BJORKERUD: We have not emphasized the fact that
mechanical factors and injury could be beneficial in some
situations and function as feed-
Growth Factors of   back mechanism. If we assume, for
Arterial Tissue   instance, that a segment of an
                                 artery is mechanically insufficient
the mechanical factors may injure the wall. The injury will
promote entry of nutrients or other factors will stimulate
growth in the tissue. The growth will reinforce the wall so
that injury no longer occurs. What I would like to ask is:
Is it really that clear, what factors we have stimulating growth
of the arterial tissues? Because as far as I can understand
there are many factors.

DR. SCHWARTZ: I can't really make any definitive comments,
but let me respond at least superficially to some aspects of
cell growth. There are many factors which appear to enhance
cell growth or proliferation in tissue culture. Gospodarowicz
has reviewed this field (85); growth factors include insulin,
pituitary factor, a platelet factor described by Russel Ross
of Seattle, (86) low density lipoprotein, and prostaglandin,
F_{zx} to mention but a few. It will, I believe be some time
before we are in a position to place specific factors into a
pathological perspective.

DR. BJORKERUD: I think the notion in some of Benditt's
work that the fibrous plaque might be similar to a benign
tumor might be unnecessarily specific. It would be quite
enough if the control of growth by one of these factors was
lost.

EDITORIAL NOTE: Thomas and associates at Albany (W.A. Thomas,
J.M. Reiner, R.A. Florentin, K. Janakidevi and K.T. Lee: Arterial
Smooth Muscle Cells in Atherogenesis: Births, Deaths and Clonal
Phenomena, Proceedings of IVth Inter'l Symposium on Atherosclerosis
in Tokyo, Japan, 1976) have offered an alternate to Benditt's
monoclonal or neoplastic theory of the origin of atherosclerotic
plaques. They observed that the monotypism (a simple variant of
the G-6-PD) gene in fibrous arteriosclerotic lesions of heterozygous women) was characteristic only of the very thick lesions.
The presence of both variants in thinner fibrous plaques in the
same vessel led them to the inference that there was not an
original cell transformation but rather a selection process that
endowed the progeny of one variant with greater survival capability
than the other. Hence one variant would appear exclusively in
older lesions. In experiments on pigs they were able to strengthen
their evidence that diet-induced lesions were of multiple cell
origin but that one or anther cell type often showed superior
survival over several generations of mitosis.

Secondly, in connection with the oxygen concentration in the tissue it has been shown in cultured smooth muscle cells, that they lose, some of their capacity to cope with LDL when cultured at low oxygen pressure. This seems to be a very important observation. Finally, I think Colin Adams showed that a certain degree of intimal thickening, some figures indicate 100-200 microns, the underlying cells seem to be injured (87).

DR. SMITH: I seem to visualize it as a mid-medial loss, but you think it was as near the surface as 100 microns.

DR. BJORKERUD: Yes, I might be wrong but Benditt disusses that.

DR. SMITH: We really do not have accurate information on the pathways of energy production in artery. It looks as if the earlier results indicating primary dependence of glycolysis are probably artifacts, and that under normal conditions of oxygen supply ATP is generated by oxydative phosphorylation, and that balance between glycolysis and oxydative phosphorylation depends on oxygen supply as in other muscles.

However, the results may also indicate that artery is abnormally sensitive to damage, and switches over to glycolysis and lactic acid production in response to rather minor injury. Thus, although the endothelium was damaged in Morrison, et al's., preparation (5) they could see no evidence of damage to the smooth muscle cells, which suggests that minor disturbance of the endothelium may influence the metabolism of the whole wall.

BIBLIOGRAPHY

1. Lehninger, A.L.   Biochemistry. Worth Publishers,
        N.Y., 1970.

2. Scott, R.F., Morrison, E.S. and Kroms, M.: Effect of
        cold shock on respiration and glycolysis in swine
        arterial tissue. Am. J. Physiol. 219, 1363-1365,
        1970.

3. Scott, R.F., Morrison, E.S., and Kroms, M.: Aortic
        respiration and glycolysis in the pre-proliferative
        phase of diet-induced atherosclerosis in swine.
        J. Atheroscler. Res. 9, 5-16, 1969.

4. Morrison, E.S., Scott, R.F., Kroms, M., and Frick, J.:
        Glucose degradation in normal and atheroslerotic
        aortic intima-media. Atherosclerosis 16, 175-184,
        1972.

5. Morrison, A.D., Berwick, L., Orci, L., and Winegrad, A.I.:
        Morphology and metabolism of an aortic intima-media
        preparation in which an intact endothelium is
        preserved. J. Clin. Invest. 5, 650-660, 1976.

6. Arnqvist, H.J. and Lundholm, L.: Influence of oxygen
        tension on the metabolism of vascular smooth muscle;
        demonstration of a Pasteur effect. Atherosclerosis
        25, 245-253, 1976.

7. Niinikoski, V., Heughan, C. and Hunt, T.K.: Oxygen
        tensions in the aortic wall of normal rabbits.
        Atherosclerosis 17, 353-359, 1973.

8. Kirk, J.E. and Laursen, T.J.S.: Diffusion coefficients
        of various solutes for human aortic tissue, with
        special reference to variation in tissue permeability
        with age. J. Gerontol. 10, 288-302.

9. Hill, A.V.: The diffusion of oxygen and lactic acid
        through tissues. Proc. Roy. Soc. (London) Ser. B.,
        104, 39-96, 1928-29.

10. Moss, A.J., Samuelson, P., Angell, C. and Minken, S.L.:
        Polarographic evaluation of transmural oxygen
        availability in intact muscular arteries. J. Atheroscler.
        Res., 8, 803-810, 1968.

11. Kjeldsen, K., Wanstrup, J. and Astrup, P.: Enhancing
        influence of arterial hypoxia on the development
        of atheromatosis in cholesterol-fed rabbits.
        J. Atheroscler. Res. 8, 835-845, 1968.

12. Kjeldsen, K., Astrup, P., and Wanstrup, J.: Reversal of
        rabbit atheromatosis by hyperoxia. J. Atheroscler.
        Res., 10, 173-178, 1969.

13. Vesselinovitch, D., and Wissler, R.W.: Experimental
        atherosclerosis in rabbits - the effect of oxygen
        and/or cholestyramine on its reversibility.
        Circ. 38, Suppl. VI, 198, 1968.

14. Vesselinovitch, D., Wissler, R.W., Dzoga, K., Hughes, R.H.,
        and Dubien, L.: Regression of atherosclerosis in
        rabbits; Pt. 1, Treatment with low-fat, hyperoxia
        and hypolipidemic agents. Atheroclerosis 19,
        259-275, 1974.

15. Zemplenyi, T.: In: The Smooth Muscle of the Artery
        (Eds. S. Wolf & N.T. Werthessen) . Advan. Exp. Med.
        Biol. 57, 302, 1975.

16. Peters, T.J.: Lysosomes of the cardiovascular system.
        Prog. in Cardiol. 4, 151-164, 1975.

17. Burleigh, M.C., Barrett, A.J. and Lazarus, G.S.: Cathepsin
        B1: a lysosomal enzyme that degrades native
        collagen Biochem. J. 137, 387-398, 1974.

18. de Duve, C., and Wattiaux, R.: Functions of lysosomes.
        Ann. Rev. Physiol., 28, 435-492.

19. Brachfeld, N.: Maintenance of cell viability. Circ.
        Suppl. 4, Vols. 39-40, 202-214, 1969.

20. Robin, E.D., Wilson, R.J., and Bromberg, P.A.: Intra-
        cellular acid-base relations and intracellular
        buffers. Ann. N.Y. Acad. Sci. 92. 539-546, 1961.

21. Reijngoud, D.J., and Tager, J.M.: Measurement of
        intralysosomal pH. Biochem. Biophys. Acta.
        297, 174-178, 1973.

22. Ravens, K.G. and Gudbjarnason, S.: Changes in the
     activities of lysosomal enzymes in infarcted canine
     heart muscle. Circl. Res. 24, 851-856, 1969.

23. Ricciutti, M.A.: Myocardial lysosome stability in the
     early stages of acute ischaemic injury. Am. J.
     Cardiol. 30, 492-497, 1972.

24. Ricciutti, M.A.: Lysosomes and myocardial cellular
     injury. Am. J. Cardiol. 30, 498-502, 1972.

25. Welman, E.: Lysosomal changes during anoxia in guinea-
     pig heart. Biochem. Soc. Trans. 2, 746-748.

26. Stary, H.C.: Coronary artery fine structure in Rhesus
     monkeys: the early atherosclerotic lesion and its
     progression. Primates in Medicine 9, 359-395, 1976.

27. Whereat, A.F.: Atherosclerosis and metabolic disorder
     in the arterial wall. Exp. Mol. Path. 7, 233-247,
     1967.

28. Portman, O.W. and Illingworth, D.R.: Arterial metabolism
     in primates. Prim. Med. 9, 145-223.

29. St. Clair, R.W.: Metabolism of the arterial wall and
     atherosclerosis. Atherosclerosis Revs. 1, 61-117,
     1976.

30. Haust, M.D.: The morphogenesis and fate of potential
     and early atherosclerotic lesions in man. Hum.
     Pathol. 2, 1-29, 1971.

31. Smith, E.B. and Slater, R.S.: Lipids and low-density
     lipoproteins in intima in relation to its morphological
     characteristics. In: Atherogenesis: Initiating
     factors. Ciba Symp. No. 12 (NS) 39-52, 1973.

32. Smith, E.B. and Smith, R.H.: Early changes in aortic
     intima. Atherosclerosis Revs. 1, 119-136, 1976.

33. Smith, E.B.: Acid glycosaminoglycan, collagen and
     elastin content of normal artery, fatty streaks and
     plaques. In: Arterial Mesenchyme and Atherosclerosis
     (Eds. W.D. Wagner and T.B. Clarkson) Advan. Exper.
     Med. & Biol. 43, 125-138, 1974.

34. Lindner, J.: Regressive und progressive arterielle
     Reaktionen bei Atherosklerose: 5. Veranderungen
     im extracellularen Kompartment. Verh. Dt. Ges.
     inn. Med. 78, 1166-1175, 1972.

35. Green, H. and Goldberg, B.: Collagen and cell protein
     synthesis by an established mammalian fibroblast
     line. Nature. 204, 347-349, 1964.

36. Langness, U. and Udenfriend, S.: Collagen proline
     hydroxylase activity and anaerobic metabolism.
     In: Biology of fibroblast (E. Kulonen &
     J. Pikkarainen) Academic Press, 373-377, 1973.

37. Levene, C.I. and Bates, C.J.: The activation of
     protocollagen proline hydroxylase and its effect
     on collagen synthesis in culture 3T6 fibroblasts.
     Ital. J. Biochem. 24, 36, abs. 1975.

38. Schwarz R., Colarusso, L. and Doty, P.: Maintenance of
     differentiation in primary cultures of avian
     tendon cells. Exp. Cell Res. 102, 63-71, 1976.

39. Chvapil, M., Hurych, J. and Mirejovska, E.: Effect of
     long-term hypoxia on protein synthesis in granuloma
     and in some organs in rats. Proc. Soc. Exp. Biol.
     Med. 135, 613-617, 1970.

40. Hunt, T.K. and Pai, M.P.: The effect of varying ambient
     oxygen tensions on wound metabolism and collagen
     synthesis. Surg. Gyn. Obs. 135, 561-567, 1972.

41. Bedford, J.S. and Mitchell, J.B.: The effect of hypoxia
     on the growth and radiation response of mammalian
     cells in culture. Brit. J. Radiol. 47, 687-606,
     1974.

42. Leung, D.Y.M., Glagov, S., Clark, J.M. and Mathews, M.B.:
     Mechanical influences on the biosynthesis of
     extracellular macromolecules by aortic cells.
     In: Extracullular Matrix Influences on Gene
     Expression. (Eds. H.C. Slavkin & R.C. Greulich).
     Academic Press 633-645, 1975.

43. Leung, D.Y.M., Glagov, S., and Mathews, M.B.: Cyclic
     stretching stimulates synthesis of matrix components
     by arterial smooth muscle cells in vitro. Science
     191, 475-477, 1976.

44. Norby, D.P., Malemud, C.J. and Sokoloff, L.: Modulation
     of phenotypic expression of collagen synthesis by
     lapine articular chondrocytes in spinner and mono-
     layer cultures. Fed. Proc. 35, 714 (abs) 1976.

45. Wolinsky, H.: Effects of hypertension and its reversal
     on the thoracic aorta of male and female rats.
     Circulation Res. 28, 622-637, 1971.

46. Wolinsky, H.: Long term effects on hypertension on the
     rat aortic wall and their relation to concurrent
     aging changes. Circulation Res. 30, 301-309, 1972.

47. Hollander, W., Kramsch, D.M., Farmelant, M. and Madoff, I.M.:
     Arterial wall metabolism in experimental hypertension
     of coarctation of the aorta of short duration.
     J. Clin. Invest. 47, 1221-1229, 1968.

48. Fernandez, D. and Crane, W.A.J.: New cell formation in
     rats with accelerated hypertension due to partial
     constriction. J. Path., 100, 307-316, 1970.

49. Smith, E.B., Alexander, K.M. and Massie, I.B.: Insoluble
     "fibrin" in human aortic intima: quantitative studies
     on the relationship between insoluble "fibrin" soluble
     fibrinogen and low density lipoprotein. Atherosclerosis
     23, 19-39, 1976.

50. Smith, E.B. and Crothers, D.C.: Interaction between plasma
     proteins and the intercellular matrix in human aortic
     intima. Protides of the Biological Fluids, 22,
     315-318, 1974.

51. Fisher-Dzoga, K., Chen, R. and Wissler, R.W.: Effect of
     serum lipoproteins on the morphology, growth and
     metabolism of arterial smooth muscle cells. Advan.
     Exp. Med. Biol., 43, 299-311, 1974.

52. Ross, R.: The smooth muscle of the artery. Advan. Exp.
     Med. Biol. 57, 64-79, 1975.

53. Ronnemaa, J., Juva, K., and Kulonen, E.: Effect of
     hyperlipidemic rat serum on the synthesis of collagen
     by chick embryo fibroblasts. Atherosclerosis, 21,
     315-324, 1975.

54. Fuller, G.C., Miller, E., Farber, T. and Vanloon, E.:
     Aortic connective tissue changes in miniature pigs
     fed a lipid-rich diet. Connective Tiss. Res.
     1, 217-220, 1972.

55. St. Clair, R.W., Toma, J.J. and Lofland, H.B.: Proline
     hydroxylase activity and collagen content of pigeon
     aortas with naturally-occurring and cholesterol-
     aggravated atherosclerosis. Atherosclerosis, 21,
     155-165, 1975.

56. McCullagh, K.G. and Ehrhart, L.A.: Increased arterial
     collagen synthesis in experimental canine atherosclerosis
     Atherosclerosis, 19, 13-28, 1974.

57. Smith, E.B., Massie, I.B. and Alexander, K.M.: The
     release of an immobilized lipoprotein fraction from
     atherosclerotic lesions by incubation with plasmin.
     Atherosclerosis, 25, 71-84, 1976.

58. Smith, E.B.: Arterial wall and lipoproteins - steady state
     aspects. Proc. IV International Symposium on
     Atherosclerosis, Tokyo, 1976. In Press.

59. Camejo, G., Lopez, A., Vegas, H., and Paoli, H.: The
     participation of aortic proteins in the formation of
     complexes between low density lipoproteins and
     intima-media extracts. Atherosclerosis, 21, 77-91,
     1975.

60. Tracy, R.E., Dzoga, K., and Wissler, R.W.: Sequestration
     of serum low density lipoproteins in the arterial
     intima by complex formation. Proc. Soc. Exp. Biol.
     Med., 118, 1095-1098, 1965.

61. Bihari-Varga, M. and Vegh, M.: Quantitative studies on
     the complexes formed between aortic mucopolysaccharides
     and serum lipoproteins. Biochem. Biophys. Acta., 144,
     202-210, 1967.

62. Srinivasan, S.R., Dolan, P., Radhakrishnamurthy, B. and
     Berenson, G.S.: Isolation of lipoprotein-acid
     mucopolysaccharide complexes from fatty streaks of
     human aortas. Atherosclerosis, 16, 95-104, 1972.

63. Anderson, A.J.: The formation of chondromucoprotein-
     fibrinogen and chondromucoprotein-B-lipoprotein
     complexes. Biochem. J., 88, 460, 1963.

64. Benditt, E.P. and Benditt, J.M.: Evidence for a
    monoclonal origin of human atherosclerotic plaques.
    Proc. Nat. Acad. Sci. U.S.A., 70, 1753-1756, 1973.

65. Panganamala, R.V., Geer, J.C., Sharman, H.M. and
    Cornwell, D.G.: The gross and histologic appearance
    and the lipid composition of normal intima and
    lesions from human coronary arteries and aorta.
    Atherosclerosis, 20, 93-104, 1974.

66. Pearson, T.A., Wang, A., Solez, K. and Heptinstall, R.H.:
    Clonal characteristics of fibrous plaques and fatty
    streaks from human aortas. Am. J. Pathol., 81,
    379-387, 1975.

67. Lee, K.T., Imai, H., Werthessen, N.T., and Taylor, C.B.:
    Necrogenic agent obtained from cholesterol used in
    dietary experiments. In: Atherosclerosis III
    (Eds. G. Schettler and A. Weizel) 344-347, 1974.

68. Florentine, R.A., Nam, S.C., Lee, K.T., Lee, K.J.,
    and Thomas, W.A.: Increased mitotic activity in
    aortas of swine. Arch. Path., 88, 463-469, 1969.

69. Stary, H.C. and McMillan, G.C.: Kinetics of cellular
    proliferation in experimental atherosclerosis.
    Arch. Path., 89, 173-183, 1970.

70. Smith, E.B. and Massie, I.B.: Destruction of endogenous
    low density lipoprotein in incubated intima.
    Atherosclerosis. In press.

71. Miller, B.F. and Kothari, H.V.: Increased activity of
    lysosomal enzymes in human atherosclerotic aortas.
    Exp. Mol Path., 10, 288-294, 1969.

72. Zemplenyi, T.: Vascular enzymes and the relevance of
    their study to problems of atherogenesis. Med. Clin.
    of North Amer., 58, (no.2), 293-321, 1974.

73. Oliver, M.F.: Dietary cholesterol, plasma cholesterol
    and coronary heart disease. Brit. Heart J., 38,
    214-218, 1976.

74. Day, A.J. and Proudlock, J.W.: Changes in aortic
    cholesterol-esterifying activity in rabbits fed
    cholesterol for 3 days. Atherosclerosis, 19,
    253-258, 1974.

75. Goldstein, J.L. and Brown, M.S.: Lipoprotein receptors,
     cholesterol and metabolism and atherosclerosis.
     Arch. Pathol., 99 181-184, 1975.

76. Weinstein, D.B., Carew, T.E. and Steinberg, D.:
     Uptake and degradation of low density lipoprotein
     by swine arterial smooth muscle cells with inhibition
     of cholesterol biosynthesis. Biochim. Biophys. Acta,
     424, 404-421, 1976.

77. Stein, Y., Glangeaud, M.C., Fainaru, M. and Stein, O.:
     The removal of cholesterol from aortic smooth muscle
     cells in culture and Landschutz ascites cells by
     fractions of human high density apolipoprotein.

78. Brown, M.S., Faust, J.R. and Goldstein, J.L.: Role of
     the low density lipoprotein receptors in regulating
     the content of free and esterified cholesterol in
     human fibroblasts. J. Clin. Invest., 55, 783-793,
     1975.

79. Werb, Z. and Cohn, Z.A.: Cholesterol metabolism in the
     macrophage, III. Ingestion and intracellular fate
     of cholesterol and cholesterol esters. J. Exp. Med.,
     135, 21-44, 1972.

80. Holman, R.L.: Atherosclerosis - a pediatric nutrition
     problem? Am. J. Clin. Nutr., 9, 565-569, 1961.

81. Lee, V.A.: Individual trends in the total serum cholesterol
     of children and adolescents over a ten-year period.
     Am. J. Clin. Nutr., 20, 5-12, 1967.

82. Stetten, M.R.: Some aspects of metabolism of hydroxyproline,
     studied with aid of isotopic nitrogen. J. Biol.
     Chem. 181, 31, 1949.

83. Pearson, T.A., Wang, A., Solez, K., and Heptinstall, R.H.:
     Clonal characteristics of fibrous plaques and fatty
     streaks from human aortas. Am. J. Path. 81, 379-387,
     1975.

84. Wolinsky, H., Glagov, S.: A lamellar unit of aortic
     medial structure and function in mammals. Circ.
     Res., 20:99-111, 1967.

85. Gospodarowicz, D., Moran, J.S.: Growth factors in
    mammalian cell culture. Ann. Rev. of Biochem.
    45:531, 1976.

86. Ross, R., and Glomsett, J.A.: The pathogenesis of
    atherosclerosis. N. Eng. J. Med. 295-369, 1976.

87. Adams, C.W.M. and Bayliss, O.B.: The relationship
    between diffuse intimal thickening, medial enzyme
    failure and intimal lipid deposit in various human
    arteries. J. Athero. Res., 10:327, 1969.

Chapter 6 TRANSPORT OF PROTEIN AND LIPID INTO THE ARTERIAL WALL

DR. COLTON:* We have recently carried out experimental measurements of the distribution of labeled albumin and of labeled low density lipoprotein (LDL) across the rabbit thoracic aorta in vivo following intravenous injection (1,2). We have also developed a theoretical model of labeled protein transport across the arterial wall, and we have begun to use it to analyze our experimental results (3). In this mini-review, I shall first discuss our experimental procedures and then summarize our results. Next I will discuss the basis for the mathematical model we have developed. Since our efforts in this area are still in progress, I will provide some representative examples of comparison between theoretical prediction and experimental data, and I will conclude with a brief discussion of the kind of insights this type of analysis provides.

The experimental procedures employed are illustrated in Fig. 6-1. LDL was isolated from freshly drawn human blood plasma and was iodinated with Na^{125}I using the iodine mono- chloride method. Free iodine was removed by ultracentrifugation followed by three sequential dialyses against saline containing EDTA. The integrity of the labeled LDL was verified by a variety of techniques. The labeled LDL was filtered and injected intravenously into normal conscious New Zealand White rabbits, (3.5 to 5.0 kg). The fraction of label in the injectate which was precipitable by trichloroacetic acid (TCA) averaged about 99% for albumin and 97% for LDL. A blood sample was taken about five minutes after injection and at specified times thereafter for plasma radioactivity and total cholesterol determinations. Plasma lipoproteins were isolated by ultracen- trifugation and assayed for radioactivity at the end of several experiments. The animals were sacrificed after 10 min., 30 min., 4 hr., 24 hr., or 67 hr., and the descending thoracic aorta was immediately excised, opened longitudinally, rinsed, and frozen to prevent further diffusion. The time from sacrifice to freezing was 3 to 6 min.

Experimental Procedure

Samples of frozen aorta were sectioned (20 μm thickness) parallel to the intimal surface on a refrigerated microtome.

* The work reported here was done in collaboration with R.L. Bratzler, K.A. Smith and R.S. Lees.

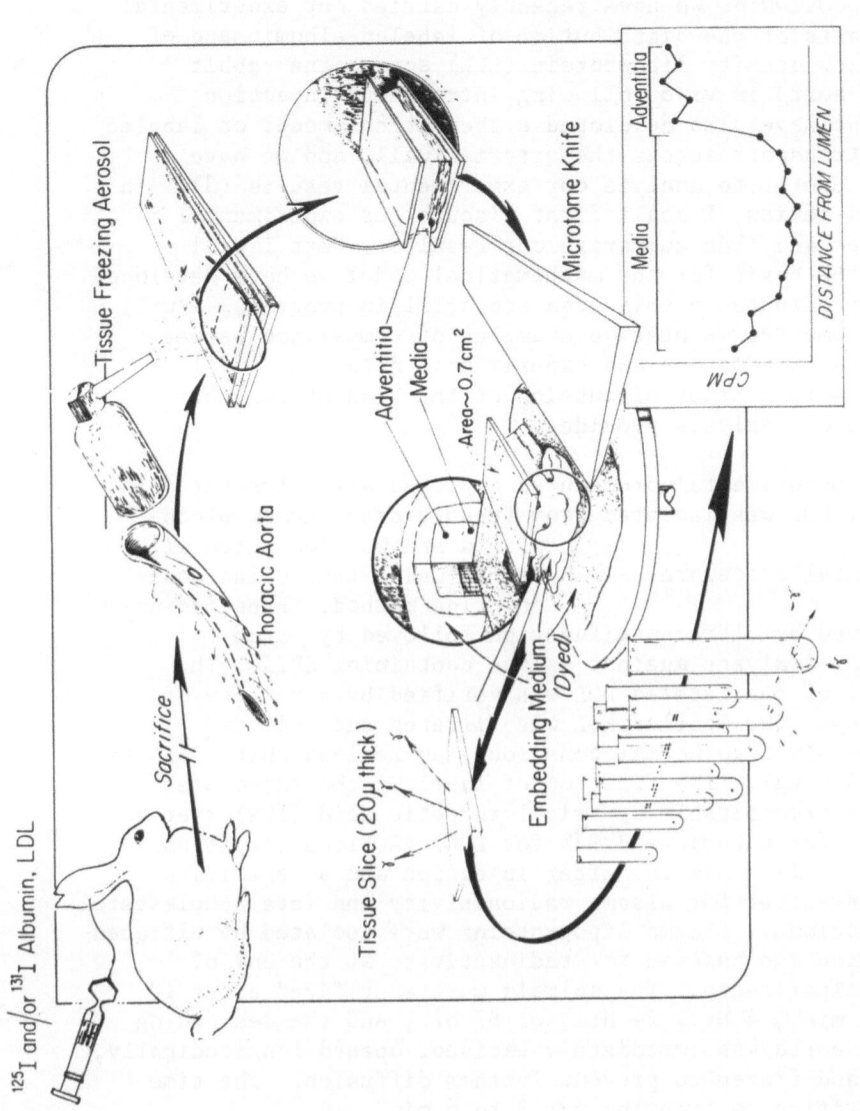

Fig. 6-1: Illustration of experimental procedure used to measure the distribution of ^{125}I-labeled proteins across the rabbit thoracic aorta <u>in vivo.</u>

Slicing proceeded from the adventitial side. After every
slice, the upper and lower edges of the knife blade were
cleaned with absorbent paper to prevent radioactive contamination
of subsequent sections. Each slice and the associated paper
were placed in 10-mm diameter, precooled test tubes and set
aside for radioassay. Slices exhibiting visible blood
contamination were discarded. Positions of the intimal
surface and the medial-adventitial border were noted, and
the total thickness (L) between them was estimated to within
$+ 20 \mu$m. Similarly, the distance (x) from the intimal
surface to the midpoint of each tissue slice was noted and
the location of the slice designated by x/L. The volume of
each slice was estimated from its known thickness and measured
cross sectional area. We have measured aortic wall thickness
as a function of applied pressure when the aorta is stretched
to its normal in vivo dimensions. The medial thickness in
the related state (in which it was frozen for this study)
was 2.4 times greater than under in vivo conditions. Each
tissue slice, injectate, and plasma sample was extracted at
least twice with 10% (w/v) TCA to remove non-protein-bound
radioactivity before radioassy in a gamma counter. All
slices were counted for 10 min., and almost all had counting
rates in excess of 10 cpm above the background rates, which
ranged between 40 and 70 cpm. Virtually identical procedures
were employed using ^{125}I-albumin prepared from rabbit serum
albumin obtained commercially.

Figure 6-2 contains two graphs which show the concentrations
of labeled albumin and labeled LDL in plasma, divided by
their initial values, as a

Results   function of time. The initial
                                       rapid decay and subsequent slower
decline for each solute could be fitted well with a double
exponential function. The concentration of plasma label
dropped to about 45% of its initial value after 24 hours
with albumin, whereas LDL decreased to about 25%. After 67
hours, the relative plasma concentration for LDL was about 5
to 10%.

Figures 6-3 and 6-4, taken from reference (2), compare
the concentration profiles and the mean concentration in the
media as a function of time for both ^{125}I-albumin and
^{131}I-LDL. The results obtained with ^{131}I-LDL were qualitatively
similar to those obtained with ^{125}I-albumin. Up to 4
hours, transmural concentration profiles of TCA-precipitable
radioactivity for both solutes had steep gradients near the
intimal surface, moderate gradients near the medial-adventitial
border, and were relatively flat in the middle of the media.

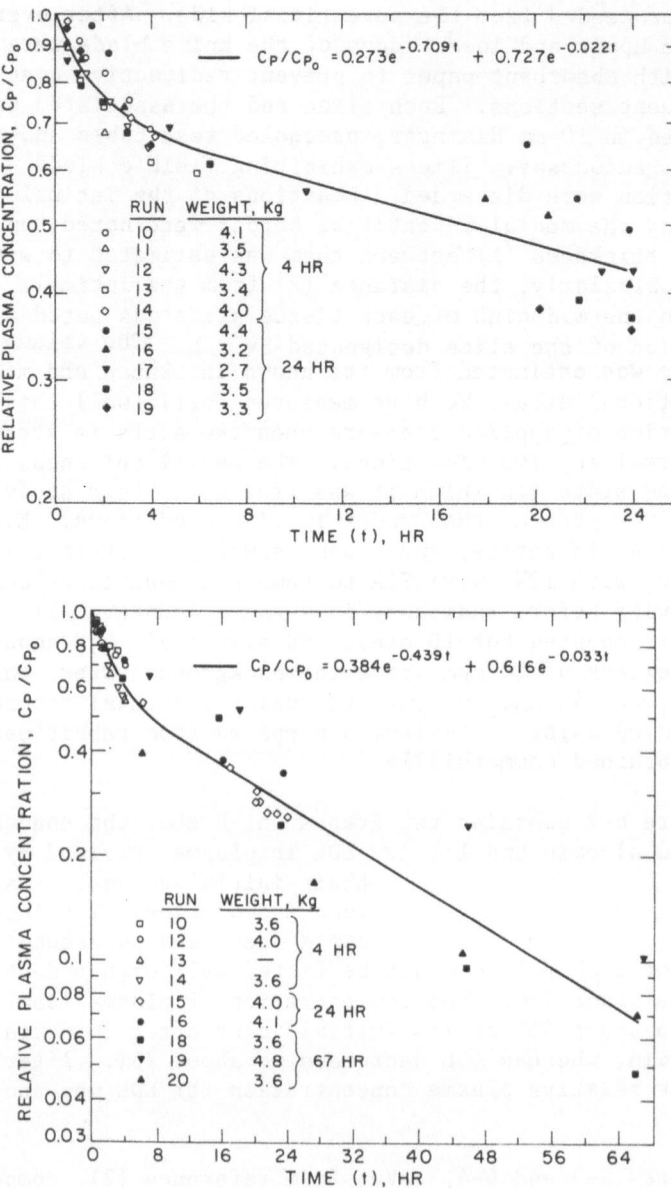

Fig. 6-2: Relative TCA-precipitable ^{125}I-labeled protein concentration in plasma as a function of time following injection
of labeled albumin (uppergraph) and LDL (lower graph). C_p is the
TCA-precipitable plasma concentration (counts/min per cm³ plasma),
and C_{p_o} is the value about 5 minutes after injection. Sold
curves were fitted to data by nonlinear regression analysis.
(Composite figure taken from references 1 and 2).

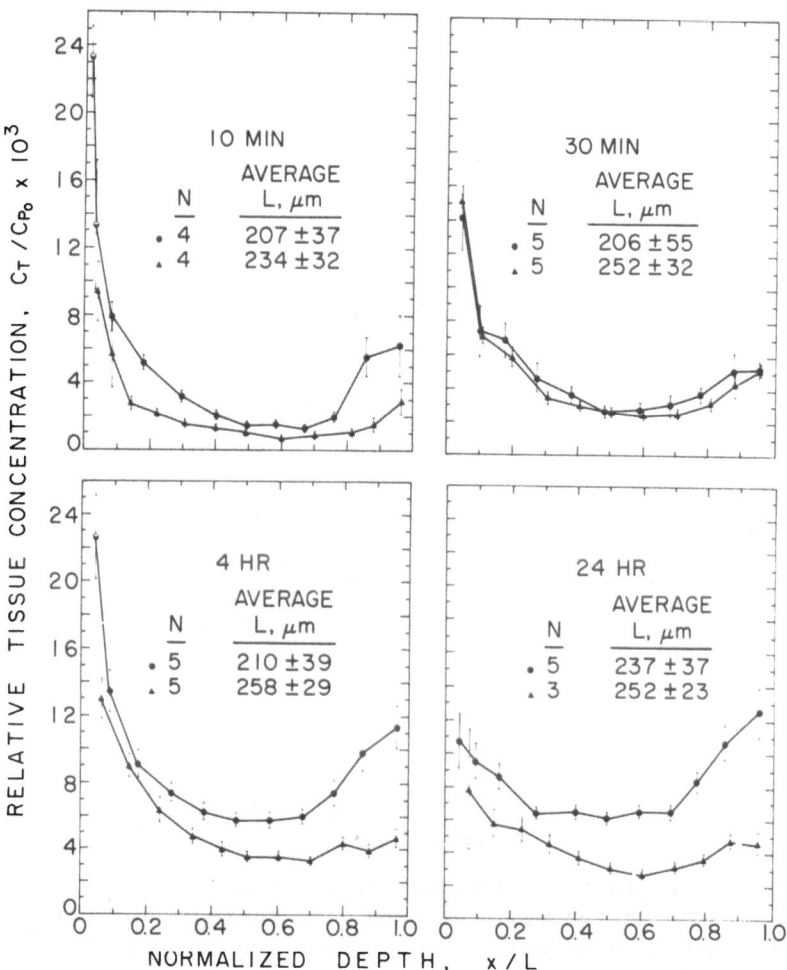

Fig. 6-3: Comparison between profiles of relative tissue con-
centration, C_T/C_{p_o}, for ^{125}I-LDL ($\triangle$) and ^{125}I-albumin (O) for
10-min, 30-min, 4-hr, and 24-hr experiments. C_T is the con-
centration of TCA-precipitable tissue radioactivity (counts/min
per cm^3 wet tissue). C_{p_o} is the TCA-precipitable plasma concentration (counts/min per cm^3 plasma) 5 minutes after injection.
x is the distance from the intimal surface to the midpoint of the
tissue slice, and L is the distance between the intimal surface
and the medial-adventital border. Error bars represent standard
error of the mean. N is the number of rabbits studied (Taken
from reference 2).

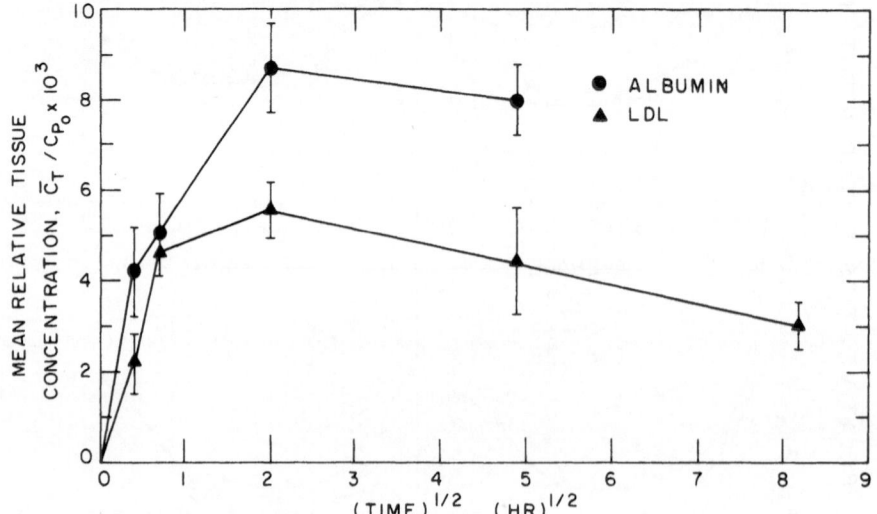

Fig. 6-4: Mean relative labeled LDL and labeled albumin
concentrations in the media at each time period. The values
were obtained by numerical integration of the data in Fig. 6-3.
(Taken from reference 2).

The results were consistent with entry of ^{131}I-labeled protein into the media from both the luminal and adventitial sides. After 24 hours, the steep intimal gradient disappeared. Concentration levels were otherwise comparable to those at 4 hours. TCA-soluble tissue radioactivity slowly increased with time, suggesting that some labeled protein may have been catabolized to TCA-soluble fragments by aortic tissue. The rate of accumulation of TCA-precipitable radioactiviy was initially rapid (measurable concentrations of both solutes were found throughout the media after only 10 minutes) and decreased with time. The relative concentration levels and the rate of influx was greater for labeled albumin than for labeled LDL, thereby suggesting that the transport mechanism(s) involved may be in part dependent upon molecular size. The very low values for relative tissue concentration are noteworthy. The concentration of ^{131}I-LDL in tissue ranged from 10^{-3} to 10^{-2} times its initial concentration in plasma; the mean value reached a maximum of about 5×10^{-3} at four hours following injection.

We have begun to develop theoretical models of the arterial wall to aid in the interpretation of experimental data. To date, these models have been compared only with the LDL data. These models

Theoretical Models

are based on fundamental mass transport principles and, at different levels of complexity, incorporate mechanisms believed relevant to transport of LDL into the wall. The physical basis for the theoretical models is presented schematically in Figure 6-5. The description is applicable to the transport of LDL in rabbit aorta; it may also apply to other plasma proteins and to other large blood vessels as well. It is likely that plasma LDL is capable of penetrating intimal endothelium by transendothelial vesicular transport. Diffusion and/or convection of LDL through the junctions between endothelial cells is possible but not likely under normal conditions. Both mechanisms are included in the model for the sake of generality. Another possible route of LDL entry into the aortic media is by transport across capillary endothelium present in the adventitia. LDL which has gained access to the media will diffuse in a direction consistent with its local concentration gradient. Since there exists a pressure difference across the rabbit aortic wall, a, filtration flow may also affect LDL movement by convecting entrained solutes radially toward the adventitia. LDL transport across the arterial wall may also be influenced by interactions with components of the wall. For example, LDL will likely bind to components of the tissue, such as glycosaminoglycans elastin, and collagen.

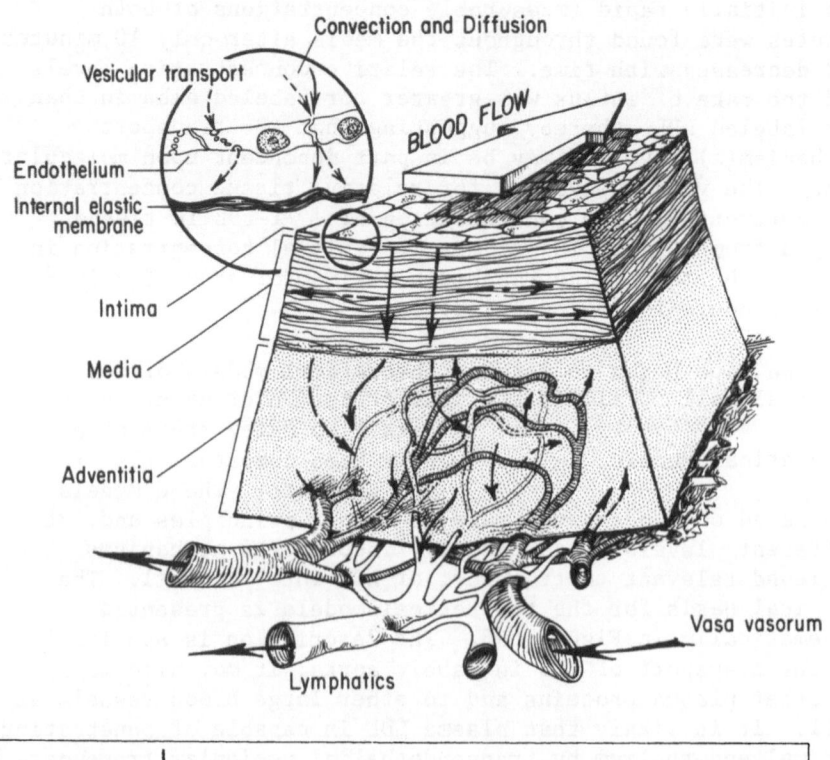

Fig. 6-5: Conceptual illustration of arterial wall showing modes
of LDL transport and reaction believed to occur in the rabbit
thoracic aorta.

Evidence from tissue culture studies suggests that aortic
smooth muscle cells may be capable of interiorizing and
degrading LDL. Thus, smooth muscle cell metabolism may be
an important determinant of LDL removal rates. Another
mechanism for clearance from the arterial wall is drainage
into the lymphatic system. In short, the concentration of
LDL in the arterial wall is likely to be effected in a
complicated fashion by the plasma LDL concentration, the
transport properties of both intimal and capillary endothelium,
and the rates of diffusion, convection, binding, and cellular
uptake and reaction within the arterial wall, as well as
transport into the lymphatic vessels.

    The partial differential equations which describe
transport in the media are summarized in Figure 6-6. We
have assumed that the media can be represented by a continuum
so that species conservation equations can be derived for
transport of labeled solute. Transport across the intimal
endothelium, and between the media and the capillaries and
lymphatic vessels in the adventitia, is represented by the
boundary conditions shown in Figure 6-7. This represenation
is physically reasonable for rabbits because the "vasa
vasorum" are contained solely within the adventitia and do
not penetrate the media itself. In many larger mammals,
including humans, the vasa vasorum penetrate well into the
media, for which case the analysis would have to be extended.

    Within the media, labeled protein can be found in at
least three forms: (a) in the extracellular fluid in a
freely diffusible state; (b)

Transport of Labeled
Protein

in the extracellular fluid but
bound to the wall components
(e.g., glycosaminoglycans and
cell surfaces); and (c) within the cells. The latter category
may itself represent a variety of forms. We have assumed that
the binding reaction is reversible and that it leads to
formation of a non-diffusible complex. The total concentration
of TCA-precipitable labeled protein is the sum of the concentrat-
tions of each of the various forms. The species conservation
relation is obtained by applying a material balance for
freely diffusible labeled protein over a differential volume
element within the media. The various terms within that
relation represent accumulation of free and bound solute,
convection of free solute, diffusion of free solute, and
permeation of free solute into the cells. Separate conservation
relations are also written for accumulation of bound and
intracellular solutes. The kinetics of the binding reaction
are assumed to be linear.

$$D \frac{\partial^2 C_f}{\partial x^2} - \frac{V}{\varepsilon_f} \frac{\partial C_f}{\partial x^2} - \frac{Pa\varepsilon_i}{\varepsilon_f}(C_f - \frac{\varepsilon_f}{\varepsilon_i} C_i) = \frac{\partial C_f}{\partial t} + \frac{\partial C_b}{\partial t}$$

diffusion   convection   permeation   free   bound
                           into cells $\underbrace{\hspace{3cm}}$
                                            accumulation

$$\frac{\partial C_b}{\partial t} = k_1(C_f - \frac{k_2}{k_1} C_b)$$

binding reaction
(reversible)

$$\frac{\partial C_i}{\partial t} = -k_3 C_i + \frac{Pa\varepsilon_i}{\varepsilon_f}(C_f - \frac{\varepsilon_f}{\varepsilon_i} C_i)$$

intracellular   permeation
degradation   into cells

C_f, C_b, C_i = concentration (moles/unit volume of media) of solute

   (f) free in extracellular space
   (b) bound in extracellular space
   (i) intracellular

   $C_T = C_f + C_b + C_i$

ε_f, ε_i = volume fraction (diffusion space/unit volume of media) available to solute in (f) extracellular and (i) intra-cellular phases

k_1, k_2 = rate constants for binding to extracellular components

k_3 = rate constant for intracellular degradation

D = effective diffusion coefficient in media

V = superficial fluid velocity in media

P = diffusive permeability (length/time) of medial cell membran

a = specific surface area (cell surface area/cell volume) of medial cells

t = time

x = spatial coordinate

Fig. 6-6: Conservation of species relationships which describe transport of a tracer solute in the media.

$x = 0$ (Intimal Endothelium)

$$VC_p(1 - R_E) + K_E(C_p - \frac{C_f}{\epsilon_f}) = \frac{VC_f}{\epsilon_f} - D\frac{\partial C_f}{\partial x}$$

| transport across junctions | vesicular transport | convection in media | diffusion in media |

$x = L$ (Medial-Adventitial Border)

$$\frac{VC_f}{\epsilon_f}(1 - R_L) + K_L(\frac{C_f}{\epsilon_f} - C_L) + K_C(\frac{C_f}{\epsilon_f} - C_p) = \frac{VC_f}{\epsilon_f} - D\frac{\partial C_f}{\partial x}$$

| transport across junctions (lymphatic) | vesicular transport to lymphatics | vesicular transport from capillaries | convection in media | diffusion in media |

$t = 0 \qquad C_p = C_{p_0}$

$\qquad\qquad\quad C_L = C_{L_0}$

$t > 0 \qquad C_p = C_p(t)$

K_E, K_L, K_C = apparent mass transfer coefficients (length/time) for vesicular transport across (E) intimal endothelium, (L) lymphatic, and (C) capillary endothelium cells

$\qquad K$ = $N v \kappa$, where N = vesicle flux [number/(time x unit intimal surface area)], v = vesicle volume, κ = partition coefficient

R_E, R_L = phenomenological rejection coefficients for simultaneous convection and diffusion across junctions of (E) intimal endothelium and (L) lymphatics.

C_p, C_L = tracer concentration in (p) plasma and (L) lymphatic vessels

Fig. 6-7: Boundary conditions and initial conditions for transport of a tracer solute across rabbit arterial wall following injection of tracer.

The permeation rate into the smooth muscle cells is assumed
to be a linear function of the concentration difference.
Finally, a linear kinetic expression is assumed for the rate
of disappearance of protein label by catabolic processes
within the cells. These hypotheses are reasonable for the
case of tracer kinetics which applied to our experiments.

The boundary conditions at the intimal endothelium are
derived from a balance which equates convective and diffusive
(including pinocytotic) transport across the endothelium to
similar processes in the immediately adjacent media. We
have combined convective and diffusive phenomena in the
intracellular junctions and have expressed the transport
rate therein in terms of an effective rejection coefficient.
A comparable relation holds at the medial-adventitial interface;
it includes both convection and diffusion into the lymph but
only diffusion from the capillaries. By considering diffusion
as the dominant mode of transport between capillaries and
lymphatic vessels, we have implicitly assumed that lymph
formation in the adventitia results from the sum of transmural
volume flow and from a very small difference between a large
local fluid filtration and an almost equally large fluid
reabsorption, either in the same capillary or in different
capillaries. Although this assumption may not be valid, the
predicted profiles are not sensitive to this aspect of the
boundary condition at the medial-adventitial border.

The equations to be solved are shown in dimensionless
form in Figure 6-8. Among the independent dimensionless
parameters, the most notable are the Fourier number, which
is a measure of the elapsed time following injection divided
by the relaxation time for diffusion in the media; the
Peclet number, which is a measure of the relative rates of
convection and diffusion in the media; three Biot numbers,
each of which is a measure of the diffusive mass transfer
resistance in the media divided by the diffusive resistance
at a specific boundary; two Thiele moduli, each of which is
a measure of the relaxation time for diffusion in the media
divided by the relaxtion time for a specific reaction; and
an internal permeation-diffusion modulus which is a measure
of the relaxation time for diffusion through the media
divided by that for permeation into smooth muscle cells.
By use of Laplace transforms, we have obtained an analytical
solution to the general problem when all parameters are
assumed to be independent of position. We have also obtained
an analytical solution for the case when plasma concentration
changes with time, through the use of Duhamel's superposition
integral, as shown in Figure 6-9.

DIMENSIONLESS RELATIONS

$$\frac{\partial^2 \theta_f}{\partial \eta^2} - Pe\frac{\partial \theta_f}{\partial \eta} - \frac{\Omega}{\nu}(\theta_f - \nu\theta_i) = \frac{\partial \theta_f}{\partial \tau} + \frac{\partial \theta_b}{\partial \tau}$$

$$\frac{\partial \theta_b}{\partial \tau} = \phi_b(\theta_f - m\theta_b)$$

$$\frac{\partial \theta_i}{\partial \tau} = -\phi_i\theta_i + \frac{\Omega}{\nu}(\theta_f - \nu\theta_i)$$

$\eta = 0$
$$Pe\theta_p(1 - R_E) + B_E(\theta_p - \frac{\theta_f}{\epsilon_f}) = \frac{1}{\epsilon_f}\left[Pe\theta_f - \frac{\partial \theta_f}{\partial \eta}\right]$$

$\eta = 1$
$$\frac{Pe\theta_f}{\epsilon_f}(1 - R_L) + B_L(\frac{\theta_f}{\epsilon_f} - \theta_p) + B_C(\frac{\theta_f}{\epsilon_f} - \theta_p) = \frac{1}{\epsilon_f}\left[Pe\theta_f - \frac{\partial \theta_f}{\partial \eta}\right]$$

$\tau = 0$
$$\theta_p = 1$$

$$\theta_f = \theta_b = \theta_i = \theta_L = 0$$

$\tau > 0$
$$\theta_p = \theta_p(\tau)$$

<u>Dimensionless Parameters</u>

Concentration	$\theta_j = \frac{C_j}{C_{p_o}}$ $\genfrac{}{}{0pt}{}{j=f,b,i}{L,p}$	Internal Permeation-Diffusion	$\Omega = \frac{Pa_L^2}{D}$
Time (Fourier No.)	$\tau = \frac{Dt}{L^2}$	Binding Equilibrium	$m = \frac{k_2}{k_1}$
Distance	$\eta = \frac{x}{L}$	Volume Fraction Ratio	$\nu = \frac{\epsilon_f}{\epsilon_i}$
Peclet No.	$Pe = \frac{VL}{D\epsilon_f}$	Biot Nos.	$B_j = \frac{K_j L}{D\epsilon_f}$ $j=E,L,C$
Thiele Moduli	$\phi_j = \frac{k_n L^2}{D}$ $\genfrac{}{}{0pt}{}{j=b,i}{n=1,3}$	Rejection Coefficients	R_E, R_L

Fig. 6-8: Equations from Figs. 6-6 and 6-7 expressed in terms of dimensionless parameters.

$$\theta_p = 1, \quad \text{all } \tau$$

$$\psi(\eta,\tau) = \theta_f + \theta_b + \theta_i = f(\eta, \tau, \dots)$$

$$\theta_p = \theta_p(\tau)$$

$$\theta_T(\eta,\tau) = \frac{C_T}{C_{P_0}} = \psi(\eta,\tau) + \int_0^\tau \psi(\eta,\tau-\xi) \frac{d\theta_p(\xi)}{d\xi} d\xi$$

$$\overline{\theta}_T(\tau) = \frac{\overline{C}_T}{C_{P_0}} = \int_0^1 \theta_T(\eta,\tau)d\eta$$

Fig. 6-9: For a step change in plasma concentration, the solution to the equations in Fig. 6-8 is given by $\psi(\eta \tau)$. Integration across the wall provides the solution for the mean concentration in the wall, $\overline{\theta}_T(\tau)$.

This permits us to analyze the effect of the time-varying
plasma concentration levels which actually occurred in our
experiments (Figure 6-2), thereby permitting comparison
between theoretical prediction and experimental data.

Even though many simplifications were made in deriving
this theoretical model, it is nevertheless complicated and
contains many adjustable parameters. A wide range of these
parameter estimates have been investigated in order to find
one or more combinations which yield reasonable agreement
between theoretical prediction and experimental data.
Specific combinations of parameters for three illustrative
examples are tabulated in Figure 6-10. Two of these are
compared with data from the 10-min and 30-min LDL experiments
in Figure 6-11. Theoretical prediction is plotted for cases
1 and 2 which are based upon the occurence of only diffusion
and convection (no metabolic phenomena) in the media. Near
the intimal surface, the predicted profiles for case 1
approximate the experimental data nicely, but agreement is
less satisfactory for case 2. Prediction for case 2 compares
favorably with experimental data in the center and outer
media but not near the intima where the measured concentration
gradient is much steeper than that predicted by theory.
Numerous parameter combinations have been tried to improve
the correspondence between prediction and data. However, it
was not possible to fit the data precisely over the entire
thickness of the aorta with a single set of parameters. The
two values of the LDL diffusion coefficient in cases 1 and
2, which differ by a factor of about 6 and may bound the
true value, are approximately a factor of 100 lower than the
diffusion coefficient in solution. Such a large reduction
may not be surprising in view of the microporous and heterogenous
nature of the arterial wall.

At times longer than 30 minutes, the concentration
profiles cannot be described by any single combination of
parameters which includes diffusion and convection only, as
shown in Figure 6-12. The predicted profiles for case 2 are
clearly unsatisfactory at 4 hours and longer. Conversely,
when binding, cellular permeation, and intracellular degradation
are included in the model (case 3), the agreement between
theoretical prediction and data is much better. These findings
suggest strongly that metabolic phenomena play a very important
role in the transport of LDL in the arterial wall.

	Example Cases		
Variable Parameters	1	2	3
D (cm^2/sec)	1.2×10^{-9}	7.5×10^{-9}	7.5×10^{-9}
K_C (cm/sec)	1.1×10^{-8}	3.3×10^{-8}	3.3×10^{-8}
K_L (cm/sec)	4.1×10^{-7}	3.3×10^{-6}	3.3×10^{-6}
Pe	0.1	0.1	0.1
ϕ_b	0	0	0.3
ϕ_i	0	0	10
Ω	0	0	10
m	0	0	0.2
B_E	0.3	0.05	0.05
B_L	8	10	10
B_C	0.2	0.1	0.1
τ 10 min	0.0075	0.05	0.05
30 min	0.0225	0.15	0.15
4 hr		1.2	1.2
24 hr		7.0	7.0
67 hr		19	19

$\underbrace{\qquad\qquad\qquad\qquad}$ Diffusion and Convection Only

$\underbrace{\qquad\qquad}$ Binding, Cellular Permeation, and Intracellular Degradation Included

Fixed Parameters:

$$L = 96\ \mu m \qquad \varepsilon = 0.42 \qquad \nu = 1 \qquad C_L = 0$$

$$K_E = 1.6 \times 10^{-8}\ \text{cm/sec} \qquad R_L = 0 \qquad R_E = 1$$

Fig. 6-10: Parameter values used in illustrative examples.

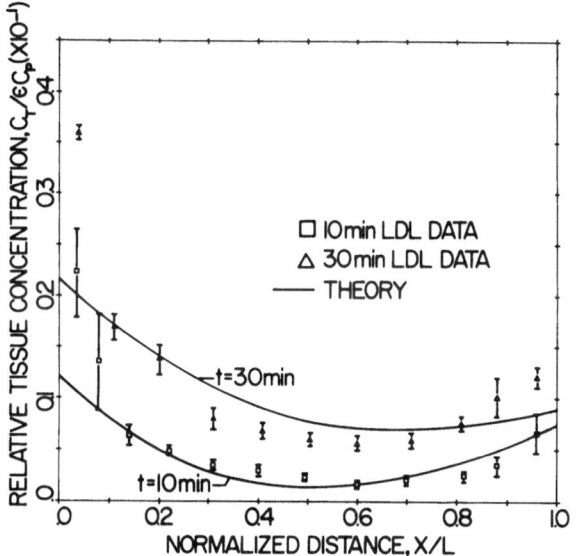

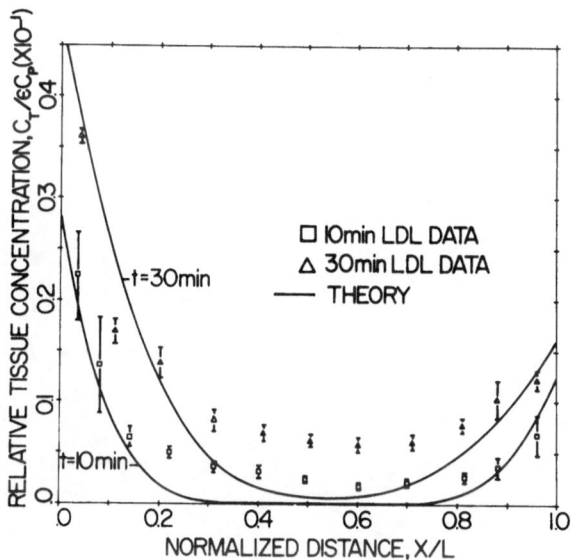

Fig. 6-11: Comparison between theoretical prediction and experimental data for ^{125}I-LDL distribution in rabbit thoracic aorta. Theoretical prediction includes diffusion and convection only. Parameters of case 1 (Fig. 6-10) are used on the lower graph; parameters of case 2 apply to the curves on the upper graph.

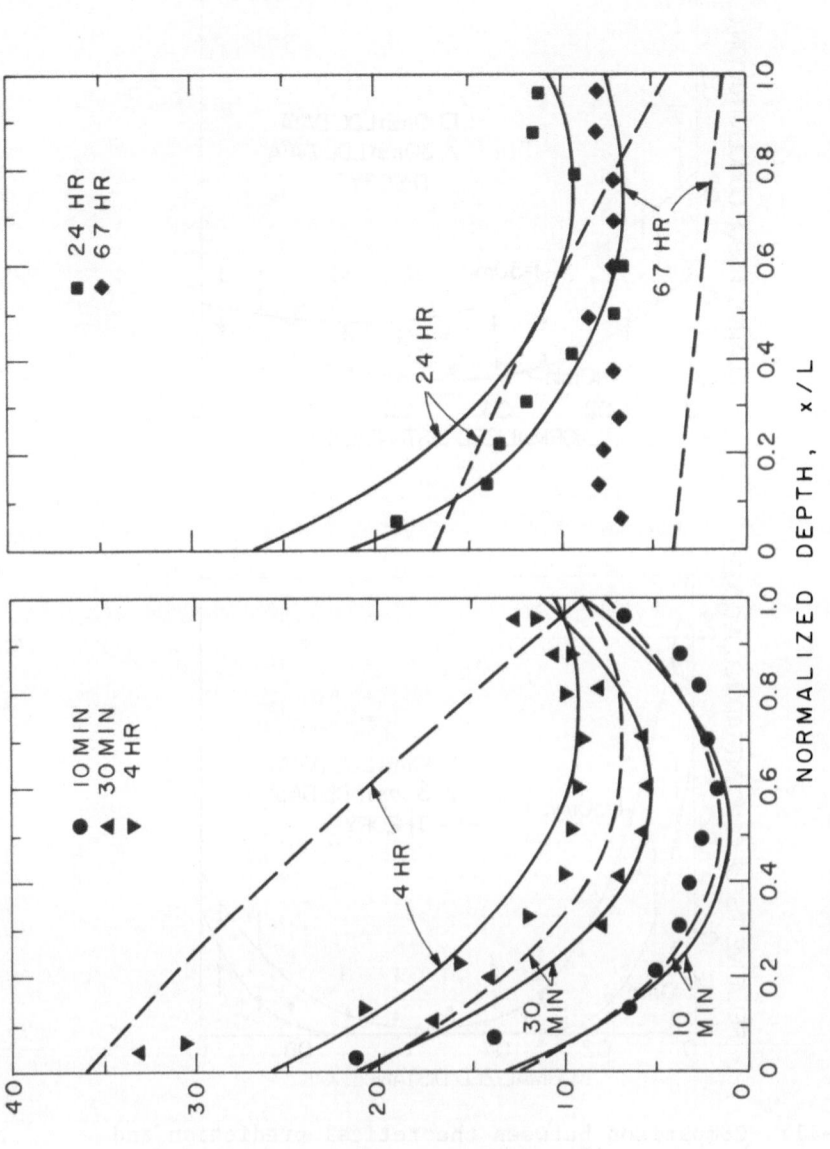

Fig. 6-12: Comparison between theoretical prediction and experimental data. _____ diffusion and convection only (case 2); _____ binding, cellular permeation, and intra-cellular degradation also included (case 3).

Further analysis and refinement of the model parameters is underway. Nevertheless, even at this early stage we have been led to several important findings with respect to the transport of ^{131}I-LDL in the arterial wall of normal rabbits, First the endothelium is the dominant barrier to transport, and permeation rates across it are consistent with uptake solely by vesicular transport. Secondly, the solute concentration profiles demonstrate a predominatly diffusive, rather than convective, character. Although it appears not to play a major role in transendothelial transport in normal rabbits, convection may play some role in the removal of LDL from the media to the lymphatic vessels. Quantitative estimation of transport parameters showed that the mass transfer resistance of the endothelium may be as much as 20 times larger than that of the entire media, despite the fact that the thickness of the endothelial lining is less than one percent of the medial thickness. Thus, a very large concentration drop occurs across the layer of normal endothelial cells, even under steady state conditions. These findings suggest that, to a first approximation, the LDL concentration to which medial smooth muscle cells are exposed in the normal rabbit is less than five percent of their plasma concentration. An increased permeability of the endothelial barrier could therefore lead to a major change in the milieu of the medial smooth muscle cells in terms of the concentration of LDL and other plasma constituents to which they are exposed.

DR. DEWEY: I want to bring everybody's attention to some recent work by Dr. Michael Gimbroni. His group, at the Peter Bent Brigham Hospital in Boston, has been studying various kinds of chemical synthesis processes in the endothelial cell itself (4). One of the findings that I am not in a position to evaluate but I think is very interesting, is that the angiotensin level in the endothelial cell is governed by chemical processes which are occurring primarily in the cell itself and are not determined by the circulating levels in the blood. If that is true, it means that there may be vaso-active compounds which do, in fact, locally control the state of the endothelial cell and its properties and by inference, also control transport to the subendothelial space. I can conceive that if you upset the balance of the angiotensin by increasing its plasma concentration, that you could, in the initial instance, change the character of the endothelial barrier. After some time, the cell itself and the autonomous chemical processes in the cell could then compensate for this change.

Local Control of Cellular Functions

But in the initial instance when you change the angiotensin concentration in the plasma, you would have essentially a wave of infusion of material across the endothelial barrier which would, in fact, appear as a "bump" at a later time after the autonomic processes took over the restored ordinary transport across the endothelial cell. If the barrier to diffusion were broken down on a short time scale, on the order of minutes, there would be a large transendothelial infusion after which other processes would have taken over which would produce a lower concentration at the surface but produce the high concentration observed further into the arterial wall.

DR. SCHWARTZ: Could there be an interaction of epinephrine with angiotensin in these frightened animals?

DR. COX: Yes, as a matter of fact, the effects of angiotensin are mediated in part by augmenting the effects of circulating catecholamines. Interaction of Angiotensin That is one of their actions with Circulating Catholamines as well as their direct action. In addition, there are liberated catecholamines and these certainly produce further augmentation of any kind of a response.

DR. BJORKERUD: Rabbits are rather specific in this respect. You can induce medial sclerosis just by taking the animal and putting it in an upright position or turning it upside down. They are very sensitive to stress, so a number of things could happen by rather trivial manipulation as e.g. blood sampling. We sampled blood each hour in a series of rabbits and many of the animals developed severe medial sclerosis.

DR. STONE: What anesthesia did you use on those rabbits?

DR. COLTON: Sodium pentobarbitol.

DR. STONE: The anesthesia may add a further complicating factor. It will potentiate a norpinephrine effect.

DR. CAREW: I would like to come back to your challenge to the tissue culturists. Being a tissue culturist, I would suggest conversely that there are certain methodologic things which we have been able to get a handle on in tissue culture which are a little bit more difficult to handle in the other situation.

And that is the question of how good tracer either the I-131 labeled albumin or the iodide labeled LDL is? It is a difficult thing to test, how good a tracer is? If it is not an adequate

Problems of Isotopic
Labeling

tracer, if it is bound in either greater or lesser quantities than is the tracee, then all of the suppositions with regard to what are the dominating factors may be influenced. I would cite, particularly, some evidence -- I can't remember the author at the moment - but, having looked at I-131 labeled albumin uptake by macrophages, he found that in halogenated albumin preparations, uptake of the albumin was enhanced many fold over that which was apparently more physiologically labeled. In our own studies on labeled LDL, what we do is present low density lipoprotein at a given concentration to cells and then vary the ratio of labeled/ unlabeled and make sure that the tracer is an adequate tracer and in most cases that is the case. But there are occasional cases where apparently the labeled material is denatured and it is taken up to a considerably lesser degree than the unlabeled material. So I would just offer that as a caution, I am not sure that I have an answer as to how it could be tested in the in vivo situation.

DR. COLTON: We have exercised great care to ensure that our labeled LDL was not denatured. Chromatography of labeled LDL on Sepharose 4B and on Sephadex G-200 resulted in a single radioactive peak, indicating that neither aggregates nor smaller labeled molecules were present. Immunoelectrophoresis, double immunodiffusion and paper electrophoresis also failed to indicate the presence of any contaminating proteins. Extraction into chloroform-methanol indicated that less than 4% of the TCA-precipitable radioactivity in the injectate was associated with lipid.

DR. WERTHESSEN: I would like to take the Chairman's prerogative here to make a comment. I suggest that you use a built in isotope when you use a tracer. A very good one is Carbon 14, biologically and chemically synthesized into the desired molecules. This can be very easy to do if you don't mind using a lot of 14 C acetate.

Popjacks' classic method of the 40's to make labeled cholesterol by feeding an egg laying hen labeled acetate has often been repeated. A good hen can lay a dozen eggs and also provide a liver containing labeled lipids (5).

DR. COX: Most often our animals are humans.

DR. WERTHESSEN: Well, it becomes more difficult in
your case. But in your tissue culture work, you can use
tissue in vitro to build the tracer you want. And you can
get very high counts via these preparations.

DR. COLTON: You are talking of building it into what
part of the molecule?

DR. WERTHESSEN: Just let the appropriate tissue build
the tracer that you want from an appropriately labeled
substrate.

DR. COLTON: We have been interested in developing a
double label which has ^{125}I on the apoprotein and 14 C on the
cholesterol ester so as to avoid the artifactual results
associated with exchange of free cholesterol, by sequentially
contacting the LDL with red cells. We have succeeded in
doing this in vivo, and produced 99+% of the label on the
cholesterol ester. The problem is that the yield is low and
the cost is prohibitive for the large amounts needed in our
experiments.

DR. SCHWARTZ: I think that Dr. Carew's comment is
really very timely. One has to be cautious with the isotopic
cholesterol as a lipoprotein label, not only because of
unesterified and cholesterol exchange, but also because of
the possibility that cholesterol esters might also exchange.

DR. CARO: We have Ralph Dell with us at the moment
from Columbia University, and he has reported the same
problem, studying the uptake of radioactively labeled albumin
by rabbit vessels in vivo. His results suggest that denatured
label and free iodine are interfering very significantly.

DR. WEINBAUM: We have done, as you might guess, a lot
of modeling. I want to describe how we are going to use the
vesicle data that Colin Schwartz
Steady State Vesicle   and Dr. Palade's group have
Diffusion Model   collected. Those of you who are
interested in the details of the
theoretical model are referred to our recent paper in the
Journal of Fluid Mechanics (6). Fig. 6-13 is a schematic of
the mathematical model . A typical transendothelial diffusion
distance is about 3200 Å. The vesicle diameter is 700 Å.
The vesicle diffusion problem is complicated by the two
features which I mentioned yesterday. When a vesicle comes
near a wall it undergoes a strong hydrodynamic interaction.

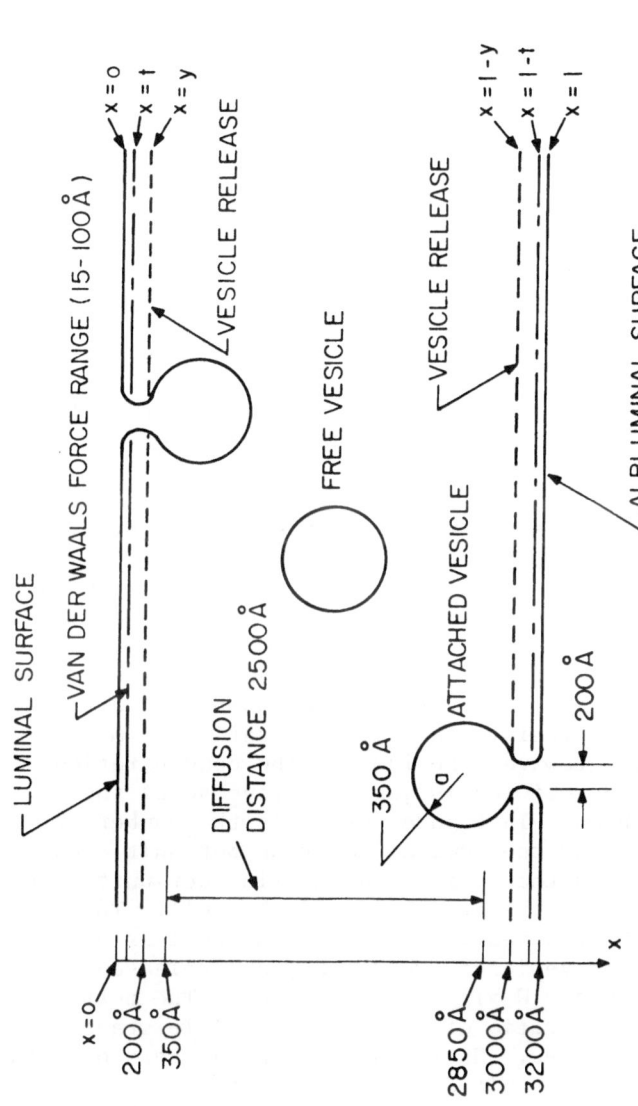

Fig. 6-13: Schematic illustration of mathematical model for the Browncain diffusion of a plasmalemma vesicle across an endothelial cell. Dashed line plane of releases; unequal dashed line effective range of Van der Waals forces. From Weinbaum and Caro (4-1)

The effective hydrodynamic resistance is a sensitive function of
its spatial position within the endothelial cell. The Van der
Waals force on a vesicle as it approaches the plasmalemmas has
been treated as the sum of all binary interactions between
molecules distributed over the surface of the plasmalemma and
the vesicle. In this first paper, we consider only the steady
state problem. This corresponds to an in vitro experiment with
no disturbances present. The key result one wishes to obtain
from the steady state model is the ratio of the time a vesicle
stays attached to the plasmalemma to the time it takes to
diffuse model. The diffusion time can be determined from
time-dependent vesicle diffusion experiments by looking at
labeled vesicle density profiles at short time intervals after
fixation. The attachment time is then determined from the
ratio provided by the steady state theory. Figure 6-14 shows
the steady state vesicle concentration profile near the plasmalemma for vesicles released 200 Å from the luminal surface.
This is the length of a typical vesicle neck. Note that the
vesicle concentration rapidly approaches zero for small
spacings. The attractive Van der Waals force very quickly draws
the vesicle toward the plasmalemma for small fluid gaps.

Figure 6-15 shows the vesicle concentration profile in
the interior of the cell for vesicles released at the luminal
surface. There are several different curves each one corresponding to a different effective range of the Van der Waals
forces. The number of free vesicles is the area under each
of the curves. The crucial data that we need to determine
from the EM studies is the ratio of the number of attached
to free vesicles. Vesicles are also migrating from the
abluminal surface towards the lumen. The concentration
profile for these vesicles is just the reverse of the
curves I have shown. In Figure. 6-15, is the number of
vesicles released at the luminal membrane per unit area
per second. $\emptyset$ R is the vesicle number flux per unit area per
second that cross to the other side of the cell. The
probability $\emptyset R/\emptyset$ of a vesicle crossing the cell is a function
of the size of the vesicles, where they are released, and
the effective Van der Waals force distance. The next
result t_a/t_D is the ratio of how long a vesicle stays attached
to how long it is free. N_a and N_g are the numbers of attached
and free vesicles per unit endothelial surface. F is the
interaction function obtained from the theory. The ratio
t_a/t_D depends on N_a, N_f and F.

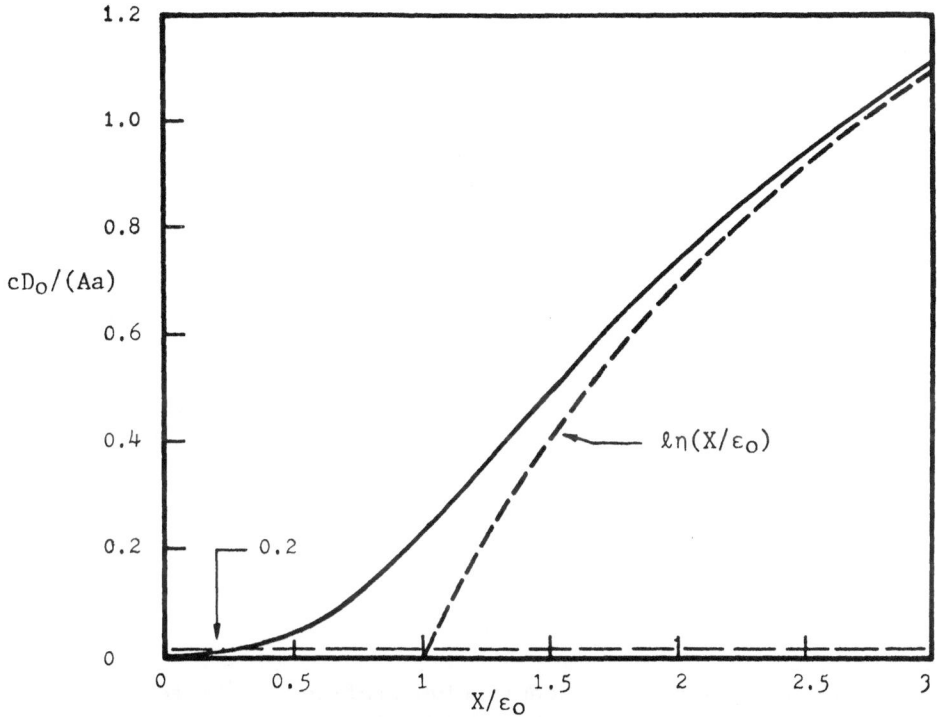

Fig. 6-14: Dimensionless vesicle concentration profile cD_O/Aa near plasmalemma in region where Van der Waals forces are important. ε_O effective Van der Waals force range X/ε_O scaled normal coordinate. Dashed curve concentration profile if no Van der Waals forces present; solid curve concentration profile modified by Van der Waals forces. Theory in Weinbaum and Caro (4-1).

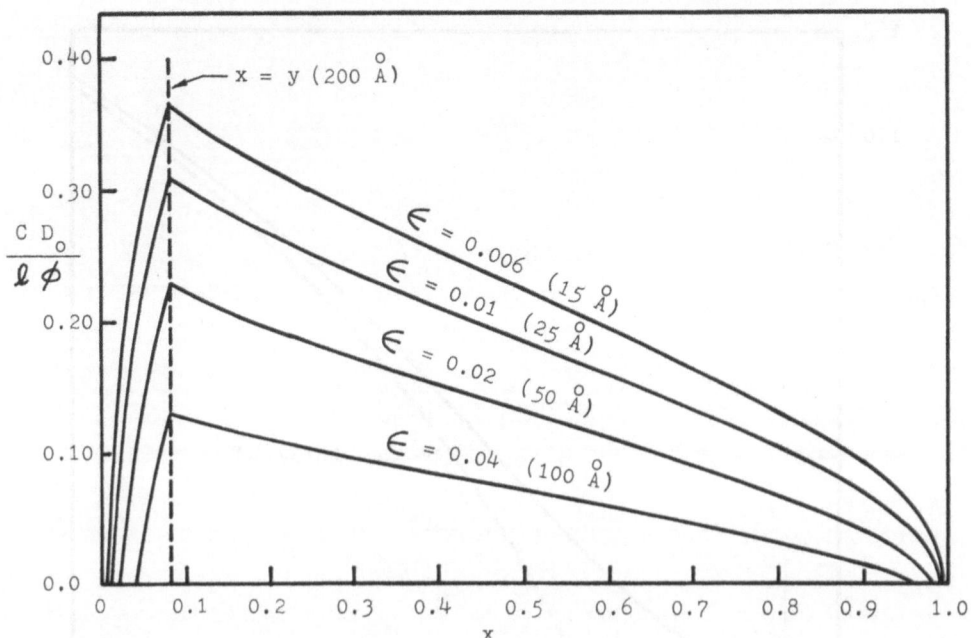

Fig. 6-15: Dimensionless concentration profile $cD_0/\ell\phi$ for free
vesicles outside of region of Van der Waals force interaction.
X = Y plane of vesicle release and Van der Waals cut off distance
defined in Weinbaum and Caro (4-1). X normal coordinate scaled
relating to transendothelial diffusion distance ℓ. Curves shown
are for vesicles released at luminal surface. Curves for vesicles
released at albuminal plasmalemma are a mirror image.

Based on capillary data for Na and N_f and the effective Van der Waals force range between roughly 75 and 15 angstom units, I obtained ratios of t_a/t_D somewhere between 1/10 and 1/14. Thus, for capillaries the diffusion time is roughly four to ten times as long as the attachment time. I believe that the values of Na and Nf are very different for arterial endothelium. Thus, the ratio t_a/t_D will be substantially different.

DR. WERTHESSEN: Which way?

DR. WEINBAUM: I think the attachment time is going to be much longer, that is why when we look at freeze fracture EMs, you see such a high density of attached vesicles. I think you will find many more attached vesicles than free.

DR. SCHWARTZ: My impression is that one normally sees considerably more free vesicles than caveolae. The relative numbers may depend on whether one is looking at enface preparations or transfer sections.

DR. WEINBAUM: We are going to have to do extensive number counts in the future for Na and Nf in arterial endothelium. The other thing which we have already done is to combine the diffusion model, just described, with the model for the underlying tissue. This is an alternate way of obtaining the value of t_D. The first approach which I have already mentioned is to use time dependent EM tracer studies for vesicle labeling. These studies would be more reliable, however they are not yet available. We have developed a model for the underlying tissue which is very much like the one Dr. Colton has already described in detail. In Figure 6-16 I will describe the basic differences between the models. Dr. Colton's model corresponds to an in vivo situation where the correct boundary condition at the adventitial surface is very complicated and one also has to worry about the vasa vasorum. For these reasons we have treated the simplest experimental situation an in

An In Vitro Model   in vitro isolated artery segment

with an outer bathing solution at essentially zero concentration. The model assumes a homogeneous distribution of interstitial fluid with a dispersed cellular phase of smooth muscle cells. The volume fraction of each phase was determined by measuring with a polar planimeter, the area actually occupied by smooth muscle cells as compared to interstitial fluid cross-sectional area.

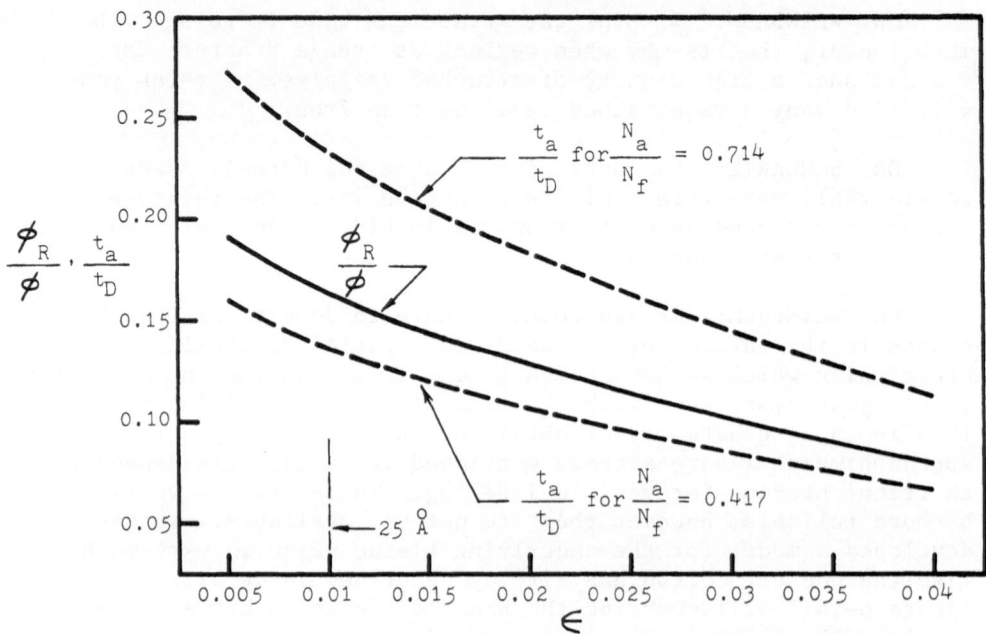

Fig. 6-16: Solution for fraction ϕ_R/ϕ of vesicles released at luminal front that cross cell and attach at abluminal plasmalemma. t_a/t_D ratio of vesicle attachment to diffusion time. Na/Nf ratio of the member of attached to free vesicles. Numbers based on capillary endothelium. ϵ Van der Waals cut off distance. From Weinbaum and Caro 4-1.

DR. COLTON: Do you have estimates for the volume fraction of smooth muscle cells in the arterial wall?

DR. WEINBAUM: I do have those numbers. They are in the paper I mentioned before (6).

DR. CARO: Bill Keating, and I haven't got the reference, says that his results showed a marked variation of the ratio of interstitial to extracellular volume proceeding from the intima toward the adventitia in an artery. The volume of the ratio increases proceeding radially (7).

DR. WEINBAUM: It varies. The cellular area can be as high as 85% in some regions of the intima and can decrease to 60% in the media. One of the things that we plan to examine more carefully is the spatial density distribution of smooth muscle cells. Dr. Colton's model is very general. It introduces many phenomenological coefficients which have to be determined experimentally. Convection is not present and the complicated in vivo boundary condition at the adventitial surface is eliminated. It is only a three parameter model. One is the volume fraction of the two phases just discussed, and the other two are the dimensionless transport coefficients. Now this was very appealing to me becaue I could immediately use uptake experiments available in the literature like Dr. Fry's (8) or Siflinger, Parker and Caro's (9).   To determine the two transport coefficients you need two sets of data, one for the normal artery and the other for an artery specimen with the endothelium removed. Unfortunately in these in vitro experiments, we don't have concentration profiles like those Dr. Colton has obtained in his in vivo studies (1) This is something we shall want to do in the future. Dr. Harold Weyland at Cal. Tech. has been measuring the interstitial fluid diffusion coefficient using other techniques than those discussed here. These measurements provide an independent check on one of the two transport coefficients determined by curve fitting the theoretical model results to Dr. Fry's or Dr. Caro's data. The values obtained are in rather good agreement.

DR. MALLIANI: The electrostatic charges which are on the walls of the vessel may be changing continuously. As far as I know, the electro-Electrostatic Charges static charges are dependent also on the electrogenic activity of the contractile elements. Thus, in vivo, the active muscle tension, which is also modulated by reflexes, may modify these electrostatic properties.

DR. WEINBAUM: We are going back to the very simplest
possible experimental situation to try and understand the
dynamics of vesicle motion. The things that you mention
that happen in vivo may well be more important than anything
that happens passively. I don't know.

DR. MALLIANI: The point is that the wall of a vessel
which undergoes active contractions may attract more vesicles,
or less vesicles. In short, the electrostatic properties may
change in a more complicated manner with respect to what can
be simulated in vitro.

DR. WEINBAUM: The capillary experiments are all, by the
way, in vivo experiments. This includes most of the previous
work done by Casley-Smith, Palade, Shea and Karnovsky, and by
all of these other people who have been doing EM studies on
vesicle transport.

DR. DEWEY: One very brief comment. It is indeed a
problem to get diffusion coefficients for large molecules
through various solutions like interstitial fluid. There is
a technique which has been developed over the last few years
which has been quite successful in obtaining this type of
data and that is using a Laser-Doppler technique to measure
Browning diffusion, thereby obtaining the diffusion coefficient.
Assuming that one could extract the interstitial fluid it
should be possible to get accurate numbers -- certainly
within a factor of two -- for those diffusion coefficients.

DR. STONE: May I add a comment to that. There are
data similar to that if you will accept one small possible
difference. Guyton and Kurt Winderhelms have used implanted
plastic balls to obtain tissue pressure measurements
(10). The fluid inside the ball has been shown to be very
representative of interstitial fluid.

DR. COLTON: The parameter one wants is not the diffusion
coefficient in interstitial fluid which should be very close
to the value in water -- rather, one would like to have the
value in the extracellular space in the presence of collagen,
elastin, and glycosaminoglycans. For that kind of situation
the Laser-Doppler technique would run into problems because
in that technique one would observe the movement of all the
macromolecules at the same time, including those which make
the extracellular matrix.

I also have a comment for Dr. Weinbaum. Even in the in vitro experiments with albumin, there is the possibility that intracellular degradation plays a role. Our data suggest it occurs in vivo and significantly influences the concentration profiles four hours after injection.

DR. WEINBAUM: The experiments that we have done so far have lasted roughly, at most, two or three hours. Professor R. Pfeffer, my colleague
Kinetic Model   at City University, has been looking into development of kinetic models which are almost identical to the ones Dr. Colton talked about. The reason I was worried about the comparison with the Evans blue dye experiments is that we know that the dye does not stay attached to the albumin molecules and a kinetic model is needed to describe this reaction. The albumin itself is inert. I discussed this with Derek Bergel and he felt that it was a reasonable assumption.

DR. SCHWARTZ: I just want to make a point to Dr. Weinbaum, because it could be helpful. A number of people have done fairly thorough stereomorphometric studies on the vessel wall. Ross Gerrity, one of my colleagues at McMaster University has done this with respect to the rat aorta (11). These data permit one to define the relative volumes of all the components present. I suspect this would give one a better approximation for theoretical transport studies rather than to assume a totally homogeneous media for diffusion.

DR. SCHWARTZ: Now I should like to review some aspects of endothelial structure and function, with particular reference to permeability.
Endothelial Structure   There are a number of processes
and Function Regarding   involved in transport; one that
Permeability Transport   is particularly interesting is the likely possibility that particles of differing size are taken up in plasmalemmal vesicles and then transported bi-directionally across the vessel, some being discharged on the albuminal surface of the cell. This process has been termed vesicular transport. Siminescu, Siminescu and Palade (12) have demonstrated that vesicles may coalesce to form a continuous patent channel across the endothelium, providing a variation on the theme of vesicular transport.

Another mechanism may combine both vesicular and junctional transport. The overall importance of junctional transport, however, remains uncertain. Junctional transport is theoretically feasible, as demonstrated by the passage of horseradish peroxidase, but the extent of intercellular transport of this probe appears to depend not only on dose, but duration of exposure. Simple diffusion of molecules across the endothelium may also occur. If this process is important, it is likely to be restricted to small molecules such as ions and water. These and other aspects of transport have been recently reviewed in some detail elsewhere (13).

I would like to further discuss aortic permeability, employing the Evans Blue model to illustrate selected facets. When the protein-binding azo
Evans Blue Model   dye Evans Blue is injected
                                     intravenously, the dye exhibits
a specific uptake pattern in the aorta in and around the intercostal ostia and the main brachiocephalic branches, and on the flow dividers at the aortic trifurcation. If one studies radioiodinated albumin uptake at two hours, for example, in blue versus white areas, there is a significantly greater uptake of the ^{125}I-albumin into aortic tissue from blue as distinct from white areas. Additionally there is indeed a significantly greater ^{125}I-albumin uptake in the thoracic part of the aorta relative to the upper or lower abdominal segments (14).

Interestingly, if one studies the distribution of the isotope across the aortic wall, activity is greatest in the innermost intima and media and least in the outer media. With albumin this transmural gradient exhibits a biphasic curve, with a "secondary" peak at some $500\,\mu$ from the endothelial surface. At all levels across the aortic wall isotopic activity is greater in blue than in white areas.

DR. WEINBAUM: Where are the vasa vasorum in the last figure?

DR. SCHWARTZ: This is an interesting point. The vasa vasorum are probably not all that far from the secondary peaking and in all likelihood about $500\,\mu$ from the endothelium.

DR. CARO: Also, at what time...

DR. SCHWARTZ: Those were two hour studies.

DR. FRY: Did you pressure rinse these animals to clear the capillary beds in the outer media of the residual radiolabeled plasma?

DR. SCHWARTZ: No. These were not pressure rinsed, so there could be some vasa vasorum contamination. The serial sections were rinsed carefully, however.

DR. CHIEN: Were these uptake measurements made at physiologic pressures?

DR. SCHWARTZ: These were all <u>in vivo</u> studies.

Essentially similar data emerged for fibrinogen. We used fibrinogen as a convenient and much larger molecule. Again the studies were conducted on a 2-hour period. Fibrinogen probably behaves like a molecule 1×10^6MW although its actual molecular weight is much less. It is interesting that the transmural gradient of fibrinogen is very much steeper than that of albumin with no tendency to the secondary peak.

Transmural Gradients for Fibrinogen and Albumin

DR. CARO: Again at two hours?

DR. SCHWARTZ: Again at two hours. I would be interested in your comments on why we should get this difference in the slope of the transmural curves for albumin and fibrinogen. Isotopic cholesterol also exhibits a distinct transmural gradient with the activity greatest in the intima and least in the outer media. The cholesterol distribution probably does not to any great extent reflect lipoprotein movement across the vessel, but rather a physico-chemical exchange of unesterified cholesterol. Approximately 80 to 90 percent of the label across the aortic wall is associated with unesterified cholesterol and only 10% of the label is associated with cholesterol ester. Additionally, it is interesting that the gradients are associated with unesterified cholesterol, the transmural distribution of cholesterol ester activity showing no slope differences across the aortic wall.

DR. DEWEY: Inasmuch as the gradient is so dramatic at the luminal side, and it is well understood that these are difficult sections to do, it might be that in certain of these experiments the gradient prior to sectioning is in fact even steeper than shown in these pictures.

DR. SCHWARTZ: Yes, this is possible.

DR. DEWEY: Another way of saying it is that the penetration from the luminal side may be incredibly small.

DR. SCHWARTZ: On the contrary, the data suggest that penetration from the lumen is greater than entry from the adventitia. We did another set of experiments to examine the possible problem of non-specific binding to the endothelial surface. The endothelium was removed by doing Hautchen preparations. With fibrinogen, only 5% of the total activity of that particular area was removed with the endothelial monolayer, leaving in excess of 90% of the label in the underlying media.

DR. CAREW: I have two questions really. First, a methodological question -- how was the cholesterol presented?

DR. SCHWARTZ: The cholesterol in these experiments was presented initially by adding the isotopic cholesterol in a very small volume of ethanol to a large volume of plasma, mixing, and allowing the mixture to stand for 60 minutes. By this time the cholesterol had exchanged with the plasma lipoprotein cholesterol; so the cholesterol was in fact introduced as lipoprotein cholesterol. Particulate cholesterol was not present in the preparation, as the mixtures were filtered prior to injection. Isotopic cholesterol was also introduced by mouth. The resulting uptake patterns were similar to those obtained by intravenous administration.

DR. CAREW: The next question probalby relates to Dr. Dewey's question that it is surprising that the gradient appears steeper with time. Do you have any explanation for its being steeper between the first and second sections?

DR. SCHWARTZ: I have no explanation. I would certainly be interested in any comments you may have on these data

DR. FRY: The concentration gradient as measured by this technique might be expected to rise with time in the subendothelial region particularly in the presence of an intact endothelial and basement membrane barrier. The gradient as measured is proportional to the difference in the average concentration of radiolabeled substance between successive tissue sections. Since the initial concentration distribution across the wall would be very nonlinear with the distance (x) across the wall, i.e., very convex toward the x axis, and only gradually assume a more linear configuration with the approach to the steady state, the average concentration in the first slice will increase with time more rapidly than in the second slice.

Accordingly the difference in the average concentration between the two successive slices (the measured gradient) will increase with time while the true gradient may in fact be decreasing with time.

DR. CHIEN: The gradient is shown here on a linear scale. In order to make a fair comparison of different slopes, one should really make semilogarithmic plots.

DR. SCHWARTZ: That is a good point.

DR. CHIEN: If a semilog plot is made, I don't think there is that much difference in gradients.

DR. SCHWARTZ: To recapitulate, in the normal, healthy, six to eight week old pig one can identify areas of spontaneously differing aortic permeability to proteins with recourse to perfusion with a trypan blue dye (Evans blue). Areas of greater permeability, or blue areas, show a variety of fine structural features (15). The endothelium is relatively cuboidal, and the intercellular junctions tend to be short and abut end to end without any interdigitations. The subendothelial space is considerably thickened and edematous, and contains many cells, many of which are undifferentiated. In the subendothelial space there is copious scattered elastin and collagen, with a floccular matrix or low electron density.

By contrast, areas of lesser permeability to the blue dye (white areas) differ significantly. The subendothelial space is thin and inconspicuous containing some floccular material. Cells are present in the subendothelium, most of which have the appearance of smooth muscle cells, while only a few are undifferentiated. In the white areas, the endothelial cells are characteristically thinner and elongated with long interdigitating intercellular junctions. Cell death or cell injury is seen more frequently in blue relative to white areas, the dead cells occurring with a frequency of 2.9 in blue and 0.7% in white areas, respectively (15).

DR. SMITH: In the very young endothelium do you get this cuboidal type of cell? I am wondering whether there is a rapid turnover in the blue area so that, in a sense, there is young endothelium. Would that account for the thicker cells or not?

DR. SCHWARTZ: I think it could, Elspeth. Generally speaking, younger cells tend to be more rounded and larger.

Whether the turnover difference is sufficient to account for
the consistent morphologic differences observed between blue
and white areas is, I think speculative. It is more likely
that the more rounded, less polarized endothelial cells of blue
areas are reflective of altered hemodynamic stress in these
areas (15).

DR. LEE: It is interesting to note that in the blue area
endothelial cell death or injury occurs more frequently than
in the white area.

DR. SCHWARTZ: This is one of the important questions
which has not yet been resolved. I will come back to permeability
data in terms of ultra-structure in a minute. We obviously
considered the possibility that cell death might provide the
ultrastructural basis for an "ultra large pore" which could
contribute significantly to the observed permeability differences.
We have not been able to obtain evidence that these sites of
injury, death or ablative loss are indeed areas of increased
permeability. It is possible that platelets and proteins
which adhere to the surface may provide an impenetratable
barrier, thus preventing influx at these sites. At present
we have no evidence pro or con the "ultra large pore" resulting
from cell injury or death.

DR. LEE: We denude the artery by removing the endothelial
cells by mechanical means to accelerate the development of
atherosclerosis in various vessels. We presume that denuding
endothelial cells and thus removing the barriers between the
bloodstream and subendothelial space results in increased
diffusion of blood constituents and acceleration of development
of atherosclerosis.

EDITORIAL NOTE: Platelet adhesion to the endothelium --
free surface has been observed. The platelet "mytogenic
factor" or "growth stimulating factor" described by Ross and
others may be involved in this process (16).

DR. SCHWARTZ: Over these spontaneously-occurring sites
of cell death or cell loss, we sometimes find an attenuated
degranulated platelet. How these platelets will influence
permeability at these sites is unknown.

DR. BJORKERUD: I think there is some evidence that
these are large pores, or super-large pores. I am referrring
to perfusion staining experiments with markers.

If a solution of uncomplexed Evans blue is used, we can
actually see that the cells that take up Evans blue also
pass Evans blue into the media. This indicates that injured
cells represent large "pores." I am also referring to
Shimamoto's experiments with coal particles in suspension
where he could see that coal particles actually pass into
sub-endothelial space at places with more frequent dead
cells.

DR. SCHWARTZ: With scanning electron microscopy, white
area endothelium exhibits regular contours, with a significant
degree of polarity in the direction of blood flow (Fig. 6-17)
Blue area endothelium on the other hand, exhibits a less
discrete polarity (Fig. 6-18). The cells appear more cuboidal
and raised into the lumen. Their surface is distinctly rougher
with many projections and blebs. These differences are entirely
consistent with the silver-stained Hautchen preparations of
endothelium derived from areas of spontaneously-differing
permeability.

Another striking difference between blue and white
areas relates to the surface coating or glycocalyx over the
endothelium. Blue area endothelium stained with Ruthenium
Red reveals a dense inner glycocalyx layer closely applied
to the plasma membrane and a somewhat fibrillary, less dense
layer luminal to this. Ruthenium-staining material is present
in some but not all the plasmalemmal vesicles. This surface
coat is some 2-5 times thicker over the endothelium of white
areas. The role of the glycocalyx is of considerable interest.
It has to be part of any theoretical consideration of the way
in which molecules come into contact with the cell surface.
It may present a simple chemical barrier, or it may function
like a gel and thus modify the ways in which molecules are
oriented at the surface. The glycocalyx may also control
entry to vesicles and may have a significant role in
determining the nature of receptor sites, or immunologic
reactions at the cell surface.

DR. CARO: Dr. Schwartz, does this also lie in a similar
thickness over cell junctions?

DR. SCHWARTZ: It is certainly present in the outer part
of the junction.

DR. CARO: What I had in mind is that it is going to
present a barrier there to the transport of small molecules
into the intercellular junctions. They would have to get
through that barrier.

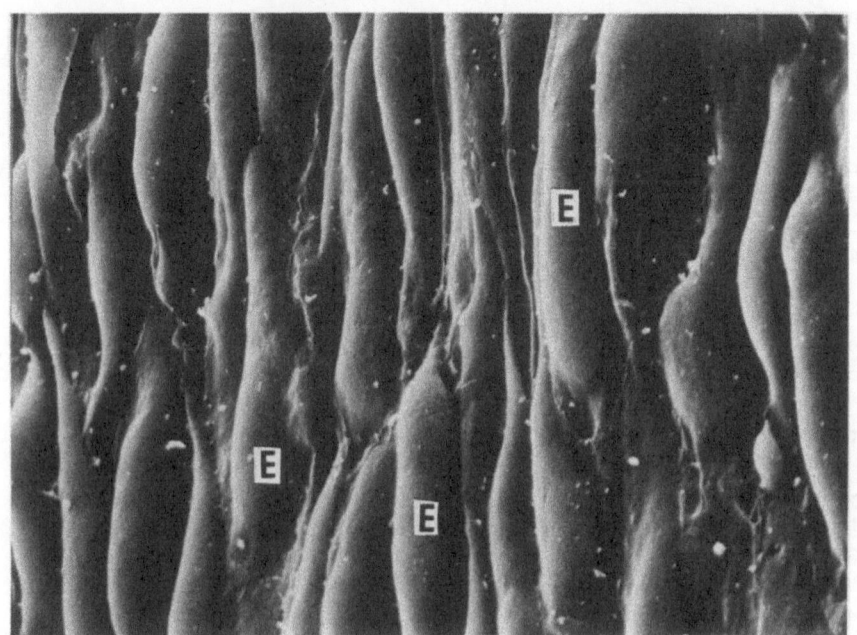

Fig. 6-17: Scanning electron micrograph of the endothelial
surface of a white area in the aortic arch of a normal six-week-
old pig. Endothelial cells (E) are ovoid in shape, with smooth
outlines and few surface projections, and exhibit a distinct
polarity in the direction of blood flow. Compare with Fig. 1-16.
X 2,000.

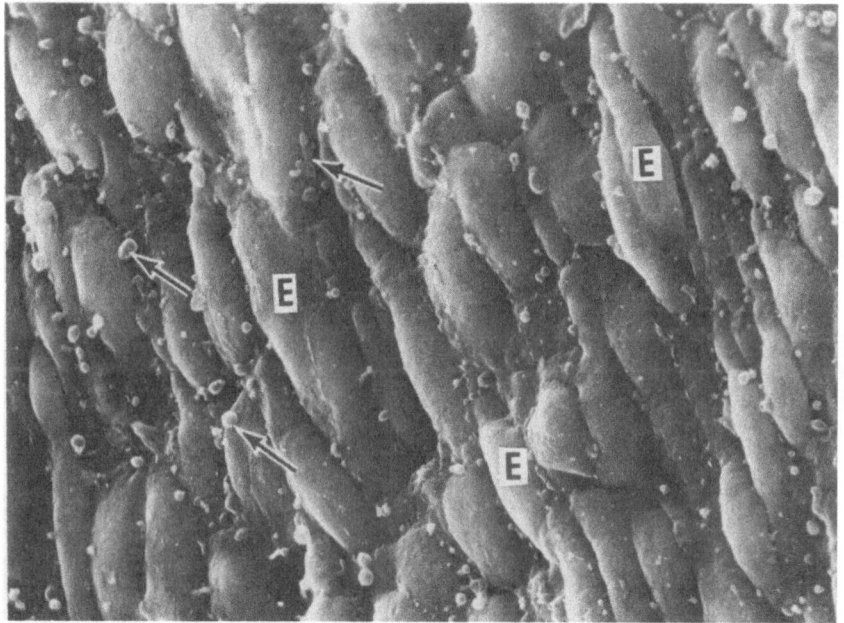

Fig. 6-18: Scanning electron micrograph of a blue area from the
aortic arch of a normal six-week-old pig. Endothelial cells (E)
are more cuboidal and raised than in white area, with less
distinct polarity (compare Fig. 1-15). Numerous surface
projections are visible (arrows) which are not as frequent in
white areas. X 2,000.

DR. SCHWARTZ: We ask ourselves questions about junctions
in terms of transport phenomena. Now I would like to show
you a little of the recent data that is being obtained in our
laboratory on the transport of ferritin particles across
arterial endothelium. We have examined ferritin transport
at one, five and fifteen minutes after a single intravenous
pulse in the young, healthy pig. Transport of this particulate
probe is, in the aorta, exclusively vesicular, and there is
no evidence of transendothelial junctional transport.
Preliminary quantitative results of these studies are now
available. We have examined both blue and white areas, and
have quantitated the number of plasmalemma vesicles per
square micron of endothelium in cross-section, the percentage
of vesicles that contain ferritin, and the average number of
ferritin grains per vesicle. Blue-white differences in the
transendothelial transport of ferritin appear to be due to
the number of active vesicles. In terms of the Evans Blue
model a valid question could relate to the nature of the
biological control mechanisms for vesicular transport.

DR. DEWEY: Dr. Schwartz, I would like to ask you if
there are any chemical mechanisms that you or other people
have identified that would cause the transformation of the
endothelial cells from the type that you see in white areas
to the conformation you observe in blue.

DR. SCHWARTZ: Could you repeat the question? Are you
referring to the shape of the cells?

DR. DEWEY: You mentioned that they were in the two
different areas, either cuboidal or spear-like and this
difference in shape is clear from the scanning electron
microscope and all the other evidence. But are there any
chemical substances which would cause this?

DR. SCHWARTZ: The reason for moving to a particulate
probe and not to horseradish peroxidase specifically in this
set of experiments is explicit. We wanted to be able to
precisely quantitate at an ultrastructural level where the
probes are going, at one minute, before there is any significant
back diffusion, and at 5 and 15 minutes after injection. A
time sequence set of studies such as this is a reasonable
way to construct a dynamic picture of transport ultrastructurally.
We have avoided horseradish peroxidase for another reason,
namely the histamine release which accompanies this probe in
some species.

DR. DEWEY: I have already referred to the work of Dr. Michael Gimbroni who found evidence for very substantial chemical activity within the endothelial cell itself. There is more than one vasoactive substance being produced, and the list includes factors like angiotensin. To the extent that chemical activity might be influenced by fluid shear stress mechanisms or whatever you want to evoke, the chemical activity in itself might cause the shape changes. So this might be an indirect effect of some chemical variation.

DR. BJORKERUD: If the Evans Blue-albumin complex is transported through vesicles, then you are showing the same parameter with ferritin as an object for transendothelial transport.

That is, blue areas might be blue because of a larger vesicular transport of Evans Blue-albumin complex which may also apply to ferritin in your blue areas.

DR. MEYER: Are there some structural differences in the internal elastic membrane between the white and blue areas or some other structural differences in light micrography?

DR. SCHWARTZ: I am unable to say if there are any structural differences.

DR. SMITH: My comment really fits in with that quite well; coming back to the gradient, in the blue area you have a very thick subendothelial layer. Now if you plot your gradient in terms of where the internal elastic lamina comes, it is going to come in a different position in the blue areas than in the white areas. And I wonder how that will affect the gradient. And thinking again along the lines of this thickness, if you have an endothelial cell which is twice as thick and you have the same number of vesicles taking the same length of time, in a thick cell won't you have, at any given moment, twice as many loaded vesicles actually visible in the cell? In the thin cell they would have got across and discharged where as in the thick cell they would only have got half way across. Or is that not true? In terms of the data that are involved at this point of time. Because the number of vesicles with or without particles is the same in both blue and white areas.

DR. SCHWARTZ: Well, that is not true.

DR. SMITH: Oh, I see. So the total number of vesicles in the whole cell is the same, not just the same number on the surface.

DR. SCHWARTZ: In terms of the data we have, the number of vesicles with or without ferritin grains is similar in both blue and white areas.

DR. CAREW: You may have just answered part of the question I was going to ask. It basically relates to whether all vesicles are the same. You mentioned that you made a distinction between vesicles and inclusions and I was wondering if you could give us some size distribution of the types of vesicles versus inclusions that you see.

DR. SCHWARTZ: After preliminary observation it became apparent that it would be wise to separate the large vacuole from the smaller vesicle and this we have done. I have already commented also on the fact that some but not all vesicles contain Ruthenium Red-staining material.

DR. CAREW: Is that your only criterion?

DR. SCHWARTZ: No, there are other possible distinctions. It is just possible, for example, that some of the larger vesicles or vacuoles are lysosomal, or that they are formed from the fusion of pinocytotic vesicles. We have ultrastructural evidence for the latter. The larger vacuoles can be five to ten times the diameter of the vesicles.

Some Large Vesicles or Vacuoles may be Lysosomal

DR. CAREW: Because much of the discussion has been focused on the idea that all vesicles are identical, I really wonder whether all parts of the cell membrane are alike and in that regard there is some preliminary evidence from Dr. Norman Miller in our laboratory in La Jolla. His evidence suggests that the internalization of low density lipoprotein and sucrose may, in fact, be independent of one another, indicating that there may be some specificity for certain types of endocytic processes to the exclusion of non-specific types.

Possible Specificity for Certain Types of Endocytic Processes

DR. SCHWARTZ: This is a very important observation. If you look closely at, say, Ruthenium Red staining, you will note that not all vesicles contain glycocalyx-type material. One could speculate that perhaps the amount or nature of the surface containing glycoproteins may have something to do with whether certain vesicles take up certain types of macromolecules or not.

DR. CARO: What was the thickness of your sections? Is the endothelial cell a large fraction of any one section, or only a very small fraction?

DR. SCHWARTZ: The first section was one hundred microns thick and thereafter sections were cut at 200 microns.

DR. CARO: So really whether the cell is fat or thin makes very little difference.

DR. SCHWARTZ: Certainly. The first section comprises endothelium, SES, and inner media.

DR. CARO: You showed a very nice slide of ferritin.
                                I anxiously looked to see
Ferritin   whether it was held up in
                                the subendothelial space.

DR. SCHWARTZ: Yes. I doubt if endothelial thickness per se will account for the gradient differences.

DR. CARO: I asked because in my unpublished studies with 14 C sodium acetate, in the isolated perfused dog common carotid artery, the transport rate was about two orders of magnitude higher than for proteins. It may well be that a structure beyond the subendothelial space provides a substantial barrier for low molecular weight materials, whereas the endothelium provides the main barrier for higher molecular weight materials. A preliminary account of these experiments is contained in Caro, 1973 (17) The fact that you don't see Ruthenium Red in all the vesicles could just possibly be explained by the fact that some vesicles unload again. They have been equilibrating with the fluid in the subendothelial space and not with the luminal fluid.

DR. SCHWARTZ: Not specifically being held up in the subendothelial space but rather within cells in the intima; what we have found are significant differences in the blue and white areas in the rate at which the subendothelial cells phagocytose the ferritin particles. Not all the subendothelial cells are phagocytic, and there may be more than one cell type in the subendothelium.

DR. COLTON: I would like to second Dr. Caro's idea concerning barrier properties of the subendothelial space. In some uptake experiments in vitro with denuded aorta, we have seen the kind of growth of the concentration on the surface which would only be consistent with surface resistance, one whose magnitude is much smaller than the endothelium but nevertheless significant.

DR. CHIEN: I will go over very quickly some of the
ultrastructural studies we have done on the common carotid
                                    dog. Scanning electron
Ultrastructural Studies   microscopic pictures of the
on Common Carotid Artery   common carotid artery fixed at
                                    zero transmural pressure (done
with collaboration of Dr. Mary Lee at Columbia) show many
parallel grooves inside the artery along its longitudinal
axis. (Fig. 6-19). Endothelial nuclei can be seen along the
grooves. Sometimes, the endothelial surface has a velvety
appearance, with very tiny foldings. Pictures taken with
the artery fixed at 100mm Hg transmural pressure gradient
show that grooves are no longer visible, but the nuclei are
still present. The comparison between the zero pressure and
the 100mm Hg pressure indicates that the surface geometry of
the arterial lumen, as seen by scanning electron microscopy,
varies considerably with the transmural pressure.

We have performed some preliminary studies on the
uptake of ^{125}I labelled albumin by isolated canine common
carotid arteries at different transmural pressures. We
determine the arterial uptake of ^{125}I-albumin following 15
minutes of incubation with labeled serum. The result of
radioactivity per unit artery weight was calculated as a
ratio to the serum activity. The uptake at 100mm Hg was
higher than at zero mm Hg by approximately 60%, and this
difference is statistically significant. If the uptake
results are expressed in terms of activity per unit inner
area of the arterial lumen, then the data between the two
pressure levels are more comparable.

Now I would like to mention some of our studies on
transmission electron microscopy (done in collaboration with
                                    Dr. Kung-ming Jan), which agrees
Transmission Electron   with Dr. Schwartz's results. The
Microscopy   transmission EM pictures show a
                                    large number of plasmalemma
vesicles in the endothelial cell (Fig. 6-20). There are
many vesicles facing the intercellular junction. Thus, in
agreement with what Dr. Schwartz said, materials may be
transported by the vesicle and discharged into the intercellular
junction. With the use of horseradish peroxidase, Dr. Jan
showed their uptake into the plasmalemma vesicles of the
carotid artery endothelium. Wherever there are filaments in
the endothelium the vesicles are not present. Hence, macromolecular movements to the basal side of these filaments probably
are achieved by vesicle transport via adjacent areas.

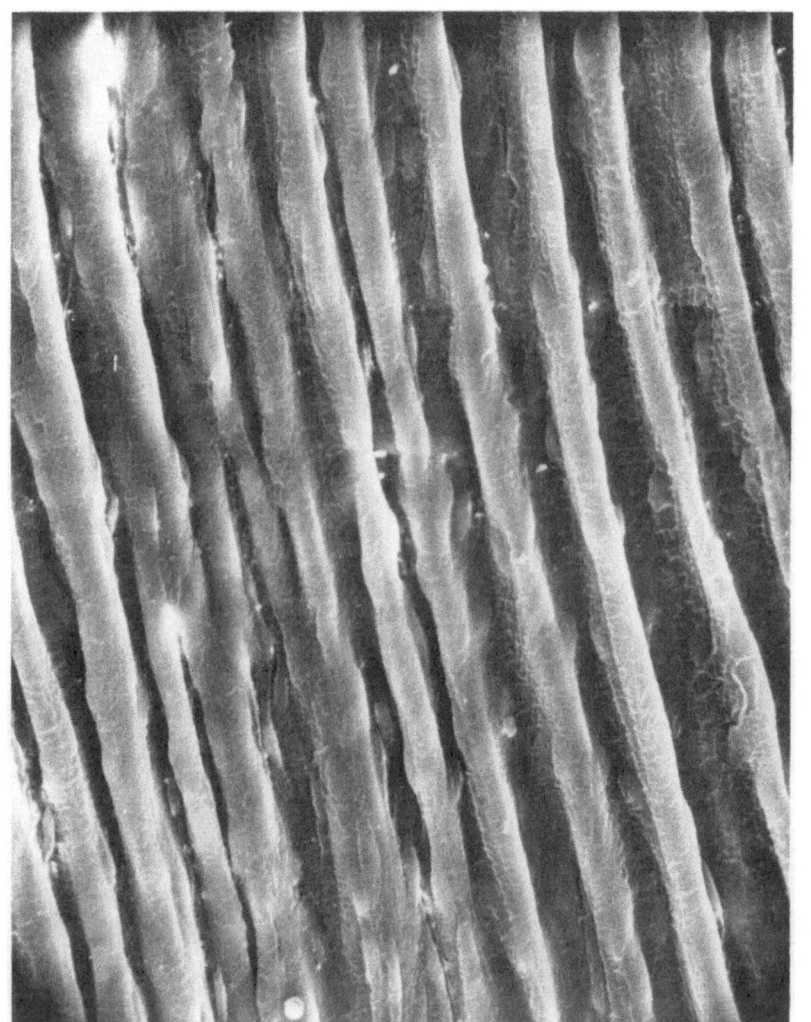

Fig. 6-19: Scanning electron micrograph of luminal surface of canine common carotid artery fixed at zero transmural pressure (M.M.L. Lee and S. Chien, submitted to Anat. Rec. for publication) (800x) (Reduced 40% for purposes of reproduction.)

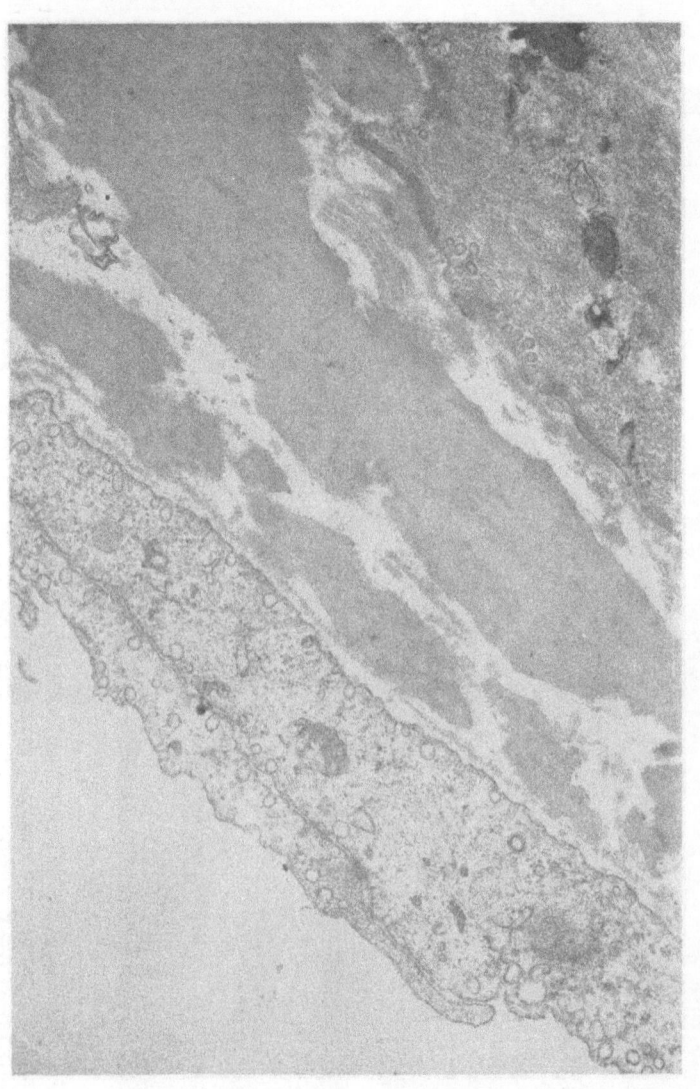

Fig. 6-20: Transmission electron micrograph of canine common carotid artery showing endothelial cells, internal elastica and smooth muscle cell. The internal elastica has a dark appearance because of tissue treatment with low molecular weight galloylglucose (tannic acid) after osmication. Note the vesicles in the endothelial cells and also in the smooth muscle cell. 40,000x (Courtesy of Dr. Kung-ming Jan.) (Reduced 40% for purposes of reproduction.)

Dr. Jan has performed freeze fracture studies on carotid endothelium with Dr. Maia Simionescu in Dr. George Palade's laboratory at Yale University.

Freeze Fracture Studies   By freezing the specimen and then fracturing it, one can expose the interior of the endothelial plasmalemma membrane just underlying the luminal surface. The vesicles can appear as either a protrusion or a depression, depending upon where the fracture plane is. The fractured surface is nearly covered with tremendous numbers of vesicles. (Fig. 6-21). Other pictures also show large numbers of these vesicles everywhere in the endothelial surfaces, except at the intercellular junction. Although the intercellular junction has many vesicles at the cell-to-cell interface, it is essentially devoid of vesicles at either the luminal or basal surface. These vesicles can also be seen in the smooth muscle layer underneath. The extremely high vesicle density in the artery endothelium has significant implications in the transport of macromolecules across the arterial endothelium, as discussed by Dr. Schwartz in his excellent overview.

DR. DEWEY: Is it possible that the low temperatures and the vacuum in which these tissues were prepared could produce artifacts that appear as vesicles?

DR. CHIEN: We can apply the same technique to other kinds of tissue, for example, red blood cells and many other cells and you would not see this number of vesicles. Besides, one also sees this high vesicle density in the en face picture that Dr. Schwartz showed, where low temperature freezing was not performed.

DR. NEREM: You show albumin data and you mention that, if you put these data on the basis of surface area, the numbers for pressures of 100 millimeters of mercury come closer together.

DR. CHIEN: That is correct.

DR. NEREM: Do the data then become statistically the same? In other words, is the statistical significance of any difference then absent?

DR. CHIEN: Yes, it disappears.

DR. COLTON: All the slides you showed, were they of surface attached vesicles? Secondly, did I detect an orderliness in the array, that is uniform spacing around each row of vesicles?

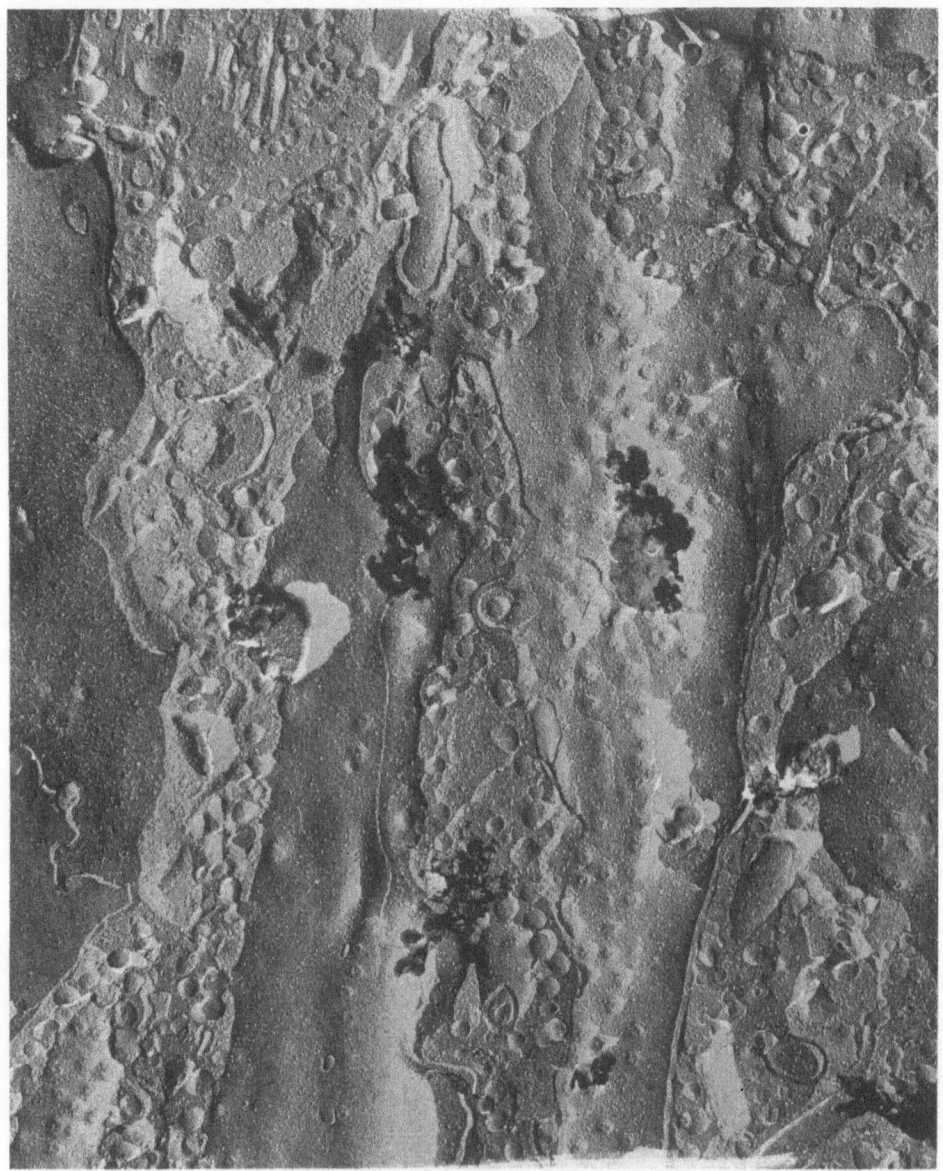

Fig. 6-21: Freeze fracture of rat mesenteric artery showing plasmalemmal vesicles in the endothelium. (43,000x) (Courtesy of Drs. Maia and Nicholae Simonescu.) (Reduced 30% for purposes of reproduction.)

DR. CHIEN: In the freeze fracture picture, these are surface attached vesicles. In the transmission E.M. sectioned normal to the surface, one sees both free and attached vesicles. As to the arrangement of vesicles, the density is so high that it's really hard to picture any particular pattern. It is probably random.

DR. COLTON: Is it possible to freeze fracture through the cell and see the distribution of vesicles that way?

DR. CHIEN: The freeze fracture will split through the hydrophobic layer of the membrane near the surface. It is more difficult to get to the inside.

DR. STONE: The data that you showed when you distended the vessel to 100mm Hg pressure, are they in vivo or in vitro?

DR. CHIEN: These are in vitro studies using the method of Caro and Nerem (18). The common carotid artery of the dog was isolated and mounted on an in vitro apparatus and incubated at 37 degrees C for 15 minutes with the ^{125}I-albumin.

DR. STONE: Both you and Dr. Schwartz are saying that the vesicular movement through the central core of the endothelial cell may be impeded by the filaments in the nucleus. Is this correct?

DR. CHIEN: Correct, yes.

DR. STONE: Then what you are inferring is that the cytoplasmic flow is around this area. Is that a correct assumption?

DR. CHIEN: Yes, you can see horseradish peroxidase in vesicles in the peripheral zone just outside this area (i.e., toward the intercellular junction), where marker-filled vesicles are present through the whole thickness of the endothelial cells. Then you also see the horseradish peroxidase accumulating in the subendothelial cell layer, where there is a resistance to macromolecular diffusion. It is possible that the macromolecules traversing the peripheral zone via vesicles to reach the subendothelial space can then return by vesicles into the endothelial cell or by diffusion back into the intercellular junction.

DR. CARO: This is where timing becomes very important.

DR. CHIEN: That is correct.

DR. WEINBAUM: The other thing that I wanted to emphasize
here, which I think is of interest to the fluid mechanics
people, is related to the effect
Interaction of Shearing   of shearing stresses and their
Stresses with Membrane   interaction with the membrane
Surface   surface. I was very pleased to
see the flacid appearance of the
upper endothelial surface in the scanning E.M., taken at
magnifications of two to three thousand. If the numerous
enfoldings in the plasmalemma are not artifacts it is obvious
that the membrane will deform extremely readily to whatever
fluid mechanics is going on above it. The whole surface
seems to be rippled, but these dimensions of these ripples
are large compared to the 700 angstrom vesicles. These
ripples have dimensions of several thousand angstoms or more
and are present over the entire surface both at zero pressure
and 100 millimeters pressure.

DR. SCHWARTZ: In one of the lovely pictures you showed
there were no vesicles along the junction. I wonder if you
would comment on whether all junctions have vesicles, and
what indeed determines the distribution of vesicles along
the junctions? Why also should there be vesicles on junctions.

DR. CHIEN: We have not done a sufficiently large
number of specimens to be really sure as to what the answer
is. From what we have seen so far I wou..d say that on the
external surface of the endothelium, the junction area is
devoid of vesicles as demonstrated by the freeze fracture
pictures. But if you go deeper, then the junction area has
a lot of vesicles, which is shown by the transmission E.M.

DR: BJORKERUD: I have two questions. One, do you
know anything about the distribution of intermembraneous
particles? Second, could the marginal zone on the intercellular
junctions devoid of vesicles correspond to the so-called
muffling zone of growing cells? Do you have any idea about
this?

DR. CHIEN: These specimens were all taken from adult
animals. So as you pointed out, they were probably not
growing except for repair. So I don't think really that the
membraneous foldings represent an extra surface area which
is available for the arteries to form new cells.

They have this extra surface area so you can redistribute
the surface area for different regions of the artery. In
this way, you can achieve deformation and flow inside endothelial
cells, As to the intra-membrane distribution of vesicles,
this is one of the things we want to study, but this requires
a large number of countings and I cannot give you a definitive
figure at this moment. We hope to get that in the near
future.

DR. COLTON: In respect to Colin Schwartz's question,
we have been doing some E.M. lately and have seen there
phenomena of vesicles attached to junctions and they seem to
appear whenever there is significant overlap of two cells
such that the junction is almost horizontal. It is as if one
cell is over the other. The cells apparently just don't
know. Their normal top and bottom behaves as it would
whether or not there was another cell under it. On the
other hand, when the junction is more verticle, that is...

DR. SCHWARTZ: End to end.

DR. COLTON: Right. There is not much projected area,
not nearly as much, and in those cases we don't seem to get
quite the same super density, in other words it is a short
junction. When cells grow so that there is a significant
overlap that seems to be when you get the higher circulation.

DR. STONE: Is there a relationship between vesicles
and systemic arterial pressure?

DR. CHIEN: We have not done enough specimens to allow
us to give you an answer that is supported by statistics,
but the first impression is that there is not, but we have
to do more work.

DR. DEWEY: I emphasize that we are trying to achieve some
kind of constructive synthesis which will not only identify
where we are today in understanding the Dynamics of Arterial
Flow, but perhaps more importantly we are trying to suggest
how, as engineers, physiologists, lipid chemists and people
who work more than one side of the fence, we may achieve even
more accelerated progress in the future.

This is not an easy task because the demands of the interdisciplinary field are very great and they certainly tax our
abilities to evaluate the information that is relevant to
arterial disease as we design our own programs and try to
further this understanding.

I personally feel a substantial amount of optimism about this
process for two reasons. First of all, I find that my
engineering colleagues around the table are showing a great
willingness to tackle real problems. By real problems I mean
getting into the "nitty gritties" of the mechanics of the
endothelial cell; to deal with non-linear processes in arteries
which include chemical phenomena, as well as strictly mechanical
phenomena; to look at fluid flow situations which we know we
cannot understand in detail and not let that deter us and deflect
us into problems that are irrevelant. By the same token I
think the physiologists have an appreciation for the type of
engineering approach to deal with conceptual models of the types
that we have proposed, or in fact they are proposing, is also,
I believe, a very healthy sign. I speak specifically of
Dr. Smith's suggestions regarding hypoxia; it is this type of
sophistication with respect to analyzing physiologic data that,
first of all, makes me encouraged for work with physiology
counterparts and, secondly, suggests that the interaction
is going to be a very fruitful one.

BIBLIOGRAPHY

1.   Bratzler, R.L., Chisolm, G.M., Colton, C.K., Smith, K.A.,
        Zilversmith, D.B., Lees, R.S.: The distribution of
        labeled albumin across the rabbit thoracic aorta
        in vivo. Circ. Res., 40:182, 1977.

2.   Bratzler, R.L., Chisolm, G.M., Colton, C.K., Smith, K.A.,
        and Lees, R.S.: The distribution of labeled low-
        density lipoproteins across the rabbit thoracic
        aorta in vivo. Atherosclerosis. In press.

3.   Bratzler, R.L., Chisolm, G.M., Colton, C.K., Smith, K.A.:
        Theoretical models for transport of low-density
        lipoproteins in the arterial wall. Atherosclerosis:
        Metabolic, Morphologic and Clinical Aspects.
        G.W. Manning and M. Daria Haust, Eds., Plenum Press,
        943-951, 1977.

4.   Gimbroni, M.A., Jr.: Culture of Vascular Endothelium and
        Atherosclerosis.In: Int'l Cell Biology, (B.R. Brinkley
        and K.R. Porter, Eds.) Rockefeller U. Press,
        649-658, 1977.

5.   Cornforth, J.W., Hunter, G.D., Popjack, G.: The biosynthesis
        of cholesterol from acetate. Arch. of Biochem. &
        Biophys. 42: 2, 1953.

6. Weinbaum, S., and Caro, C.G.: Macromolecule transport model
    for arterial wall and endothelium based on ultra-
    structural specialization observed in electron micro-
    scopic studies. J. Fluid. Mech. 74, 611-643, 1976.

7. Keatinge, W.R.: Mechanical response of arteries to stimula-
    tion of sympathetic nerves. J. Physiol. (London)
    185: 701-705, 1966.

8. Fry, D.L.: Atherogenesis: Initiating Factors, CIBA
    Symposium, New Series, No. 12., Associated Scientifc
    Publishers, Amsterdam, 1973.

9. Siflinger, A., Parker, K. and Caro, C.G.: Uptake of ^{125}I-
    albumin by the endophelial surface of the isolated
    dog common carotid artery: effect of certain physical
    factors and metabolic inhibitors. Cardio. Res.
    9:478-489, 1975.

10. Guyton, A.C., Granger, H.J., Taylor, A.E.: Interstitial
    fluid pressure. Physio. Rev., Vol. 51, 527-563,
    1971. and
    Wiederheilm, C.A., Dynamics of transcapilary fluid. J. Gen
    Physio., Vol 52, 29-63, 1968.

11. Gerrity, R.G. and Cliff, W.J.: The aortic tunic intima
    in young and aging rats. Exp. Mol. Pathol.,
    16:382-402, 1973.

12. Simionescu, N., Simionescu, M. and Palade, G.E.:
    Permeability of muscle capillaries to small hemepeptides
    Evidence for the existence of patent transendothelial
    channels. J. Cell. Biol. 64: 586-607, 1975.

13. Schwartz, C.J. and Gerrity, R.G.: Arterial endothelial
    structure and function with particular reference to
    permeability. Atherosc. Rev. (A.M. Grotto, Ed.)
    Raven Press, N.Y., 1978.

14. Bell, F.: Adamson, I.L., and Schwartz, C.J.: Aortic
    endothelial permeability of albumin: Focal and
    regional patterns of uptake and transmural distribu-
    tion of ^{131}I-albumin in the young pig. Exp. Molec.
    Path., 20, 57-68, 1974.

15. Gerrity, R.G., Richardson, M., Somer, J.B., Bell, F.P.,
        Schwartz, C.J.: Endothelial cell morphology in
        areas of in vivo Evans blue uptake in the aorta of
        young pigs. II. Ultrastructure of the intima in
        areas of differing permeability to proteins.
        Am. J. Pathol., 89: 313-334, 1977.

16. Ross, R.: Platelet mitogenic factor. The Smooth Muscle
        of the Artery. Wolf, S., Werthessen, N. (Eds.) 1975.

17. Caro, C.G.: Transport of material between blood and
        wall in arteries. Atherogenesis: Initiating Factors.
        Ciba Foundation Symposium 12 (New Series) pp. 127-
        164, Associated Scientific Publishers, Amsterdam,
        1973.

18. Caro, C.G., and Nerem, R.M.: Transport of C14-4-cholesterol
        between serum and wall in the perfused dog common
        carotid artery. Circ. Res. 32:187-205, 1973.

Chapter 7   HEMODYNAMIC CONTRIBUTION TO ATHEROSCLEROSIS

DR. MEYER: I will demonstrate some structural features
of the arteries which are probably related to hemodynamic
factors and appear to be important for the localization and
further development of lesions.

The curved segment of the internal carotid artery
which, located at the base of the skull, is known as the
carotid siphon, is of particular
Carotid Siphon   interest. This segment consists
of four arterial curves which
immediately follow each other (Fig. 7-1A and 1B). Thus, the
blood flow is diverted in this short segment several times. The
deflection of the blood flow probably results in different
functional load upon the opposite, i.e. concave and convex
walls of the curves, and, consequently determines distinct
structural differences between the opposite arterial sectors,
which are already present at birth. In newborn children,
intimal cushions consisting of numerous fine elastic fibers
are seen at the inner walls of the curves, whereas at the
opposite convex wall only a single primary internal elastic
membrane is present (Fig. 7-2). With growth, the intimal
cushions become more prominent (Fig. 7-3 and 7-4). and in
young adults they are often as thick as the underlying
(subjacent) media. They are rather poor in elastic elements
and mainly consist of loose collagenous networks and ground
substance. At the opposite, i.e. outer (convex) wall of the
curves and in adjacent sectors numerous new elastic sheets
appear internal to the internal elastic membrane and form a
prominent (hyperplastic) subendothelial (intimal) elastic
layer (Fig. 7-3 and 7-4).

The different structural components appearing at the
opposite arterial sectors show a different affinity for
calcium and lipids. Strong
Affinity for Calcium   subendothelial elastic networks
and Lipids   of the outer, i.e. convex and
lateral walls of the curves early
become a predominant substrate of calification.

In the upper (fourth), sharpest curvature of the siphon,
calcific deposits have been regularly demonstrated grossly
in all children aged 1 - 16 years (1,2,3,4). They regularly
appear above the orifice of the ophthalmic artery and often

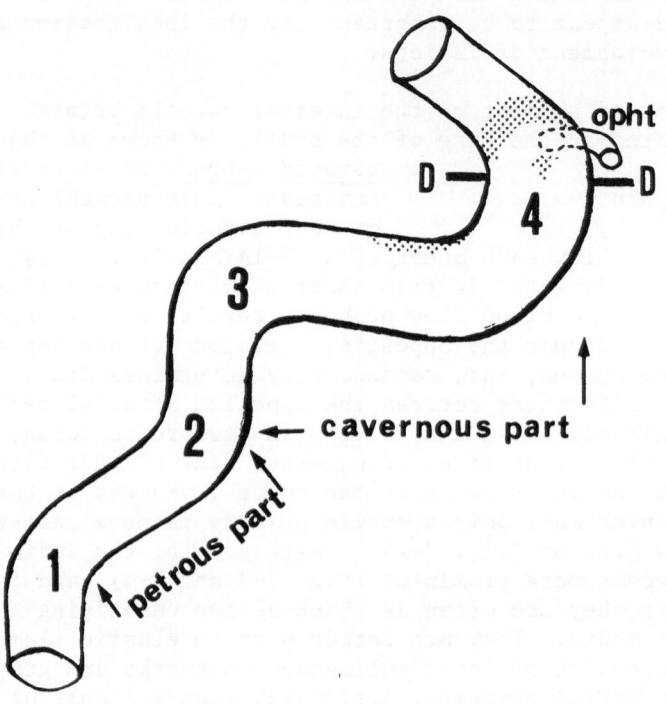

Fig. 7-1A: Schematic diagram of the right carotid siphon
showing sites of predilection for early calcification (dotted
area) and indicating the petrous and cavernous portions of
the internal carotid artery. The numbers refer to the
curvatures of the siphon. D-D = dura mater. Opht - origin of
the ophthalmic artery. (From Meyer and Lind, 1972).

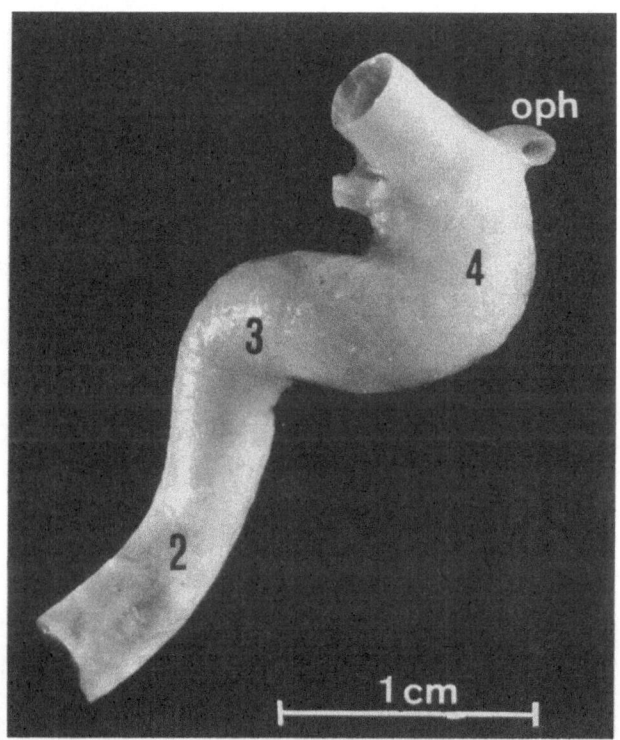

Fig. 7-1B: Carotid siphon of a four-year-old boy which has
been dissected free after fixation in formalin at a filling
pressure of about 90 mm Hg. The numbers refer to the
curvatures. (The first curvature was cut off and is not
seen in the figure). oph - cross- sectioned ophthalmic artery.
The small adherent part of the adjacent dura mater (D) indicates
the level of its perforation by the siphon. (From Meyer,
in preparation).

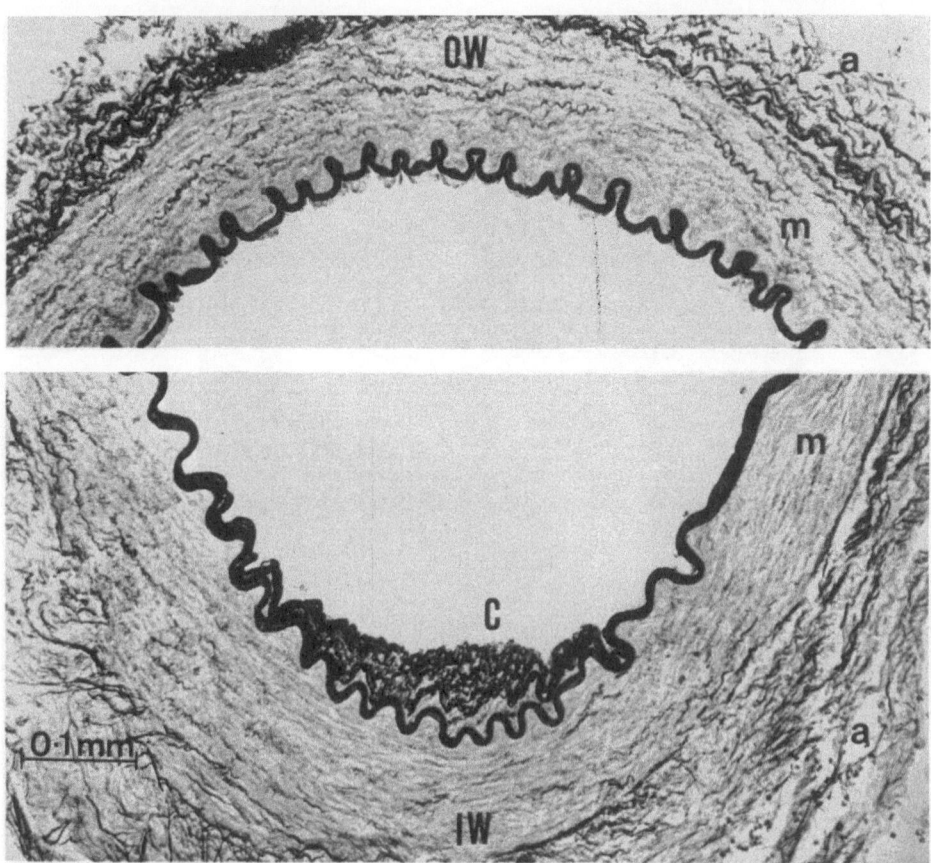

Fig. 7-2: Small intimal cushion (C, below) mainly consisting
of fine elastic fibers is seen at the inner (concave) wall (IW)
of the fourth curvature of the carotid siphon from a newborn
child. At the opposite sector (above), e.e., at the outer wall
(OW) of the curvature only a wavy internal elastic membrane is
seen below the endothelial lining. m - media; a - adventitia.
Case 46 K/76. Cryostat section. Weigert's resorcin fuchsin.
(From Meyer, in preparation).

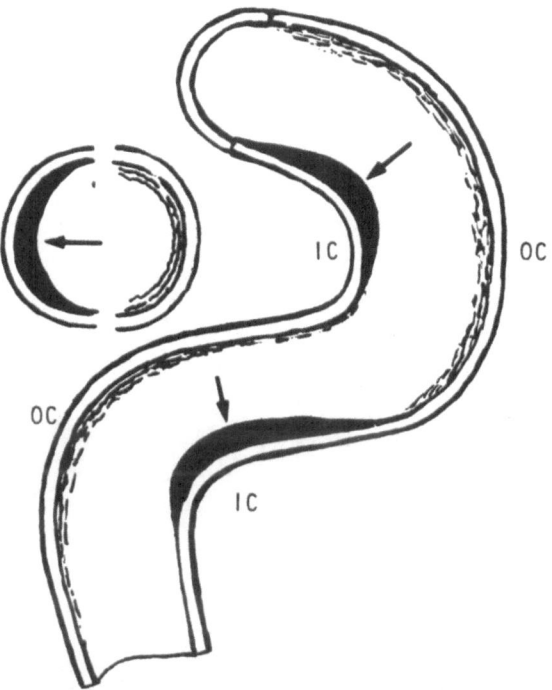

Fig. 7-3: Diagram showing a longitudinal section of the right carotid siphon which illustrates the location of intimal cushion and elastic tissue elements. In childhood, the subendothelial elastic layer is well developed along the outer walls (OC) of the curvatures, whereas prominent intimal cushions (arrows), consisting mainly of loose connective tissue and sparse elastic elements are present along the inner walls (IC) of the curvatures. Inset shows a cross-section of the vessel at the site of the arrows.

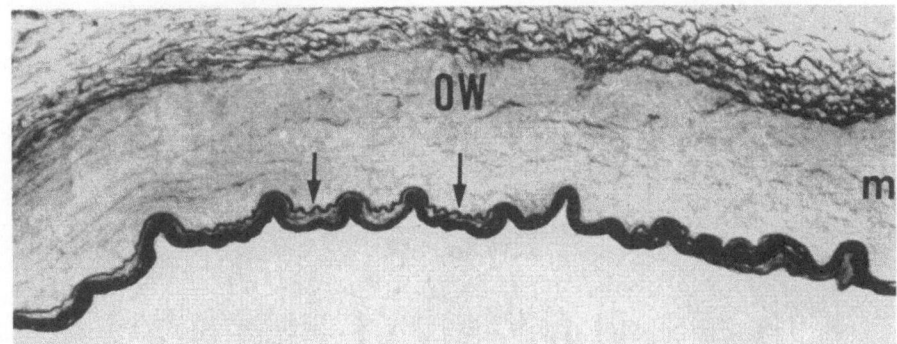

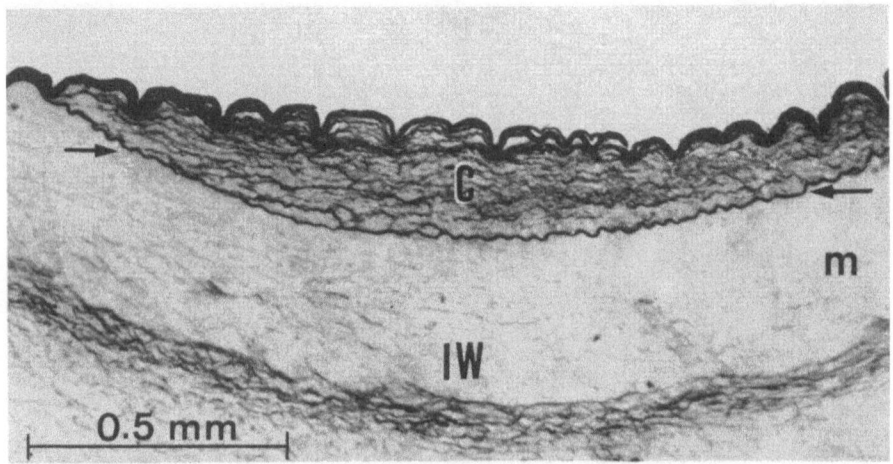

Fig. 7-4: Structural differences of the opposite sections of a
carotid siphon from a 13-year-old boy. At the inner (concave)
wall (IW) of the fourth curvature (below), a prominent intimal
cushion (C) rich in elastic fibers is seen internal to the fine
primary internal membrane (arrows). At the opposite outer
(convex) wall (OW), a thick hyperplastic secondary elastic
layer is present internal to the discrete primary internal elastic
membrane (arrows) showing a fine wavy pattern. m - media,
Cryostat section. Weigert's resorcin fuchsin. Case 58 K/76.
(From Meyer, in preparation).

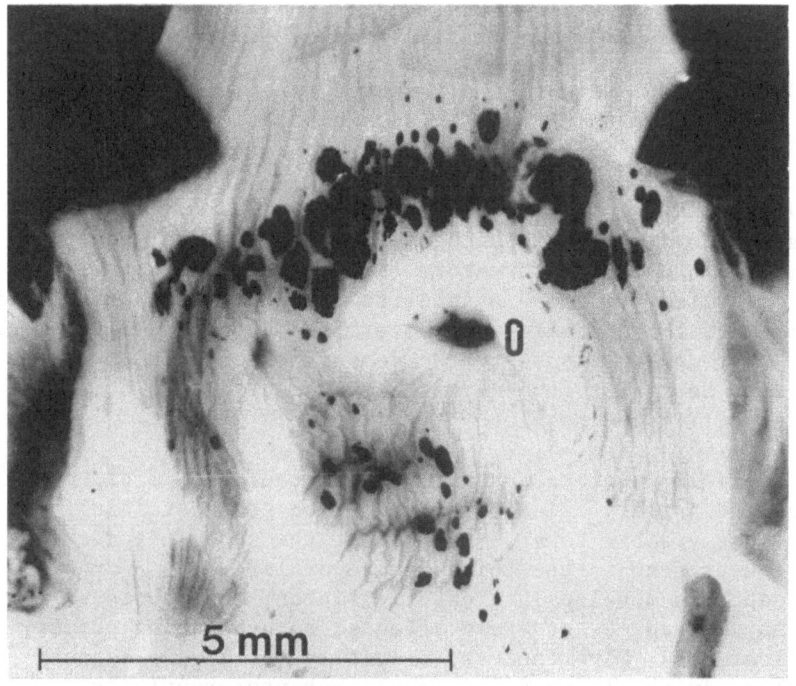

Fig. 7-5: Numerous, partly confluent early calcifications (black)
form a circularly arranged band above the orifice of the ophthalmic
artery (O). Scattered incrustations are also seen below the
orifice. Carotid siphon of a three-year-old girl who died after
accident. (Case 341/70). Von Kossa reaction. (Unpublished).

extend around a larger part of the arterial circumference at
this level (Fig. 7-5). Later the calcifications also appear
in the subjacent, i.e. more proximal portion of the siphon.
In young adults they often encircle the intimal cushion which
regularly develops at the inner (concave) wall of the fourth
(upper) curvature. The cushion itself remains free of calcific deposits for a long time (Fig. 7-6).

   DR. TAYLOR: How old is this person, Dr. Meyer?

   DR. MEYER: This siphon is from a 17-year-old man.

   DR. TAYLOR: Seventeen. I wanted to bring that out.
It is exciting to think that this calcification occurs at
such a young age.

   DR. MEYER: In the fourth decade of life, larger confluent
incrustations are also seen regularly in the dorsal wall
proximal to the fourth curvature (Fig. 7-6). Since this
wall is located at some distance from the bone, its predilection
to calcification can hardly be determined by physical parameters
of the surrounding tissues. The deposition of calcium
appears to be rather favored by hemodynamic factors arising
with deflection of the blood stream in this segment.

   The lipid deposits appear later in the carotid siphon
than do the primary calcifications. With gross staining
they become visible towards the end of the second decade and
are often present in the third decade of life (5). Thus, the
lipid deposits develop in a carotid siphon, some parts of
which may already be severely affected by preceeding primary
calcifications. Nevertheless, initially the lipids do not
accumulate in the incrustated areas, but preferentially
appear in the intimal cushions of the inner (concave) wall
of the curves. In young adults the different localization
of calcific and lipid deposits is distinctly seen (Fig. 7-7).

   DR. TAYLOR: How old?

   DR. MEYER: This siphon is from a 35-year-old man.

   At this age, calcification is often limited to the area
adjacent and proximal to the intimal cushion. Here, strong,
                              hyperplastic elastic sheets
Intimal Cushion   become the predominant substrate
                              of incrustation. In contrast,
elastic sheets extending further towards the intimal cushion may
be free of calcifications, but show a diffuse, pronounced lipid
infiltration, which is also seen in the intimal cushion
itself (Fig. 7-8).

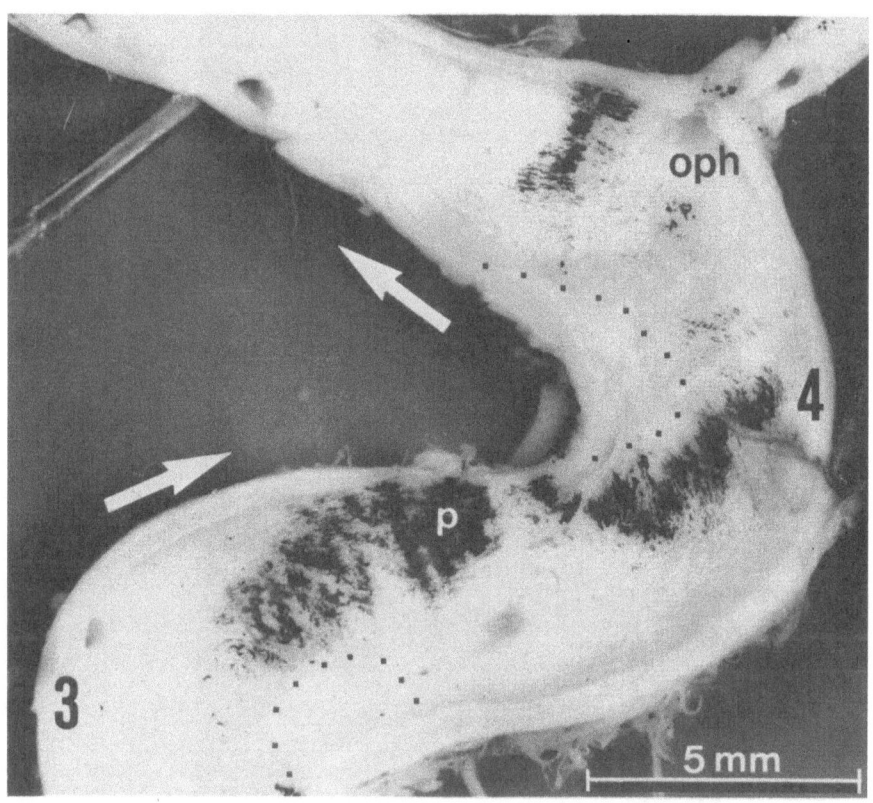

Fig. 7-6: Upper part of the medial half of the right carotid
siphon from a 17-year-old male who died in a traffic accident.
After von Kossa reaction, confluent axially arranged calcific
deposits (black) are seen above the orifice of the ophthalmic
artery (oph). The peak of the concave inner wall of the fourth
curvature (4) is free of calcifications, but tightly packed
confluent linear incrustations are seen below and in front of a
slightly raised intimal cushion (dotted line in the center of
the figure). A small intimal cushion was seen at the peak of the
third curvature (3) but it is not well seen here. Below the
peak of the fourth curvature, there is a large calcific plaque
(p) which is partly covered by grayish intimal connective tissue.
Fine calcific deposits are seen below the plaque. Gross staining
for lipid shows only a faint reddish tinge, i.e. early lipid
infiltration is present in the area of both intimal cushions
located at the peaks of the inner walls of the third and fourth
curvatures. Arrows indicate the direction of blood flow.
Case 43/72.

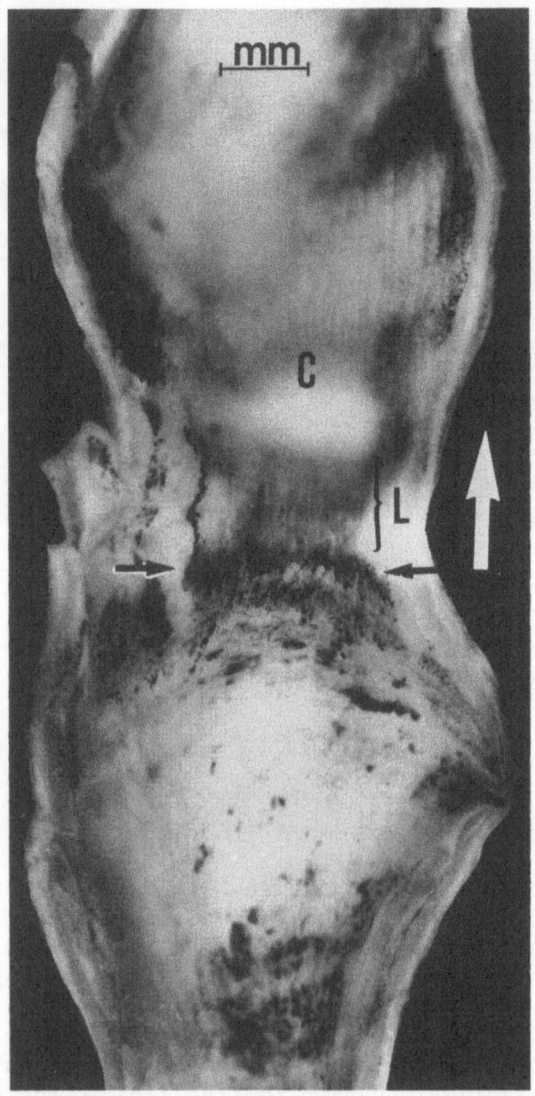

Fig. 7-7: The inner wall of the third curvature is seen from
above in the longitudinally opened siphon from a 35-year-old man.
(Cause of death: traffic accident). Von Kossa reaction and
gross lipid staining with Fettrot 7B. Just below the height
of the curvature, the luminal layer is densely interspersed with
fine (black) partly confluent calcifications (between arrows)
which extend circularly over a large part of the circumference.
In front of the incrustations, a lipid infiltrated area (L,
grayish), red-stained in the specimen, is seen. The lipid
infiltration extends up to the intimal cushion (C, white). White
arrow indicates the direction of blood flow. (See also Fig. 7-8).
(Unpublished).

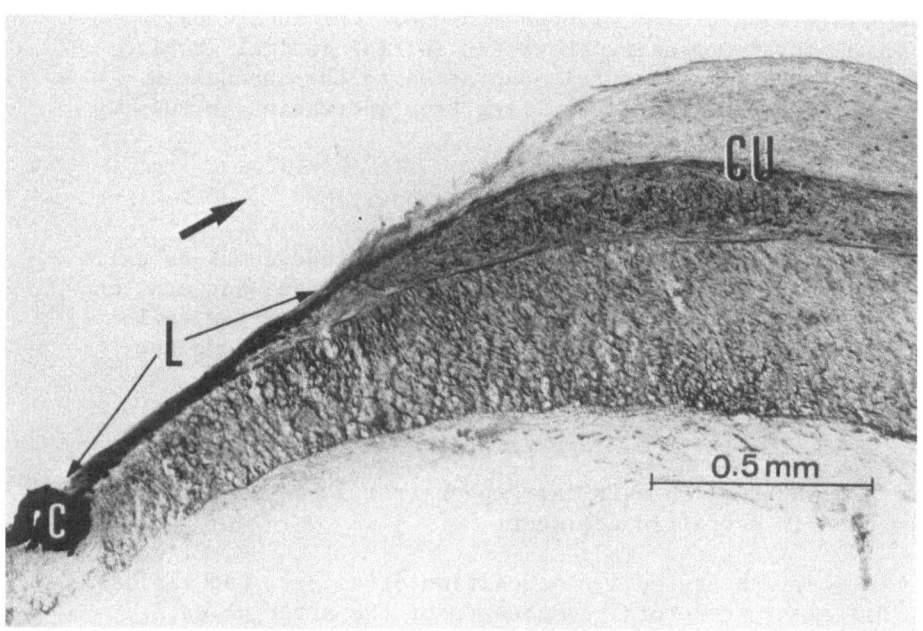

Fig. 7-8: Longitudinal cryostat section of the inner (concave) wall of the third curvature demonstrated grossly in Fig. 7-7. Roundish grain-like calcific deposit (C) penetrating the media is seen to the left. In the right part of the segment the media (m) is superimposed by an intimal cushion (CU) consisting of two well delineated layers. In the layer adjacent to the media fine, grain-like calcific deposits (black) are seen. Between the calcific deposit and the cushion the hyperplastic elastic intimal sheets are infiltrated with lipids (L) and stained deeply red in the section. They appear grayish in the photograph. The arrow indicates the direction of blood flow. (Unpublished).

DR. SCHWARTZ: You seem to have two components in the cushion.

DR. MEYER: Yes, this intimal cushion consists of two components, i.e. of two layers which are superimposed upon each other and delineated by a limiting elastic lamella. This structural feature is probably related to the widening and distortion of the siphon with age. The additional luminal layer appearing above the initial intimal cushion may represent a structural adaptation to the changes in blood streaming (flow) resulting from increasing tortuosity of the siphon in adults.

DR. WOLF: Is it a cellular composition?

DR. MEYER: The intimal cushions include numerous cells embedded in rather loosely arranged collagenous networks and ground substance. In contrast, there are only a few cells between the hyperplastic elastic sheets which become the substrate of calcification.

DR. TAYLOR: How old was he?

DR. MEYER: This is the siphon from a 35-year-old man who died in a traffic accident.

Later, the selective deposition of calcium and lipids in different structural components of the arterial wall becomes less prominant. The lipids, for instance, appear, additionally, in the thickened intima which develops over the incrustated elastic sheets. Moreover, the layer of the hyperplastic elastic intimal sheets may simultaneously be interspersed with fine grain-like calcific deposits and be diffusely infiltrated with lipids. Pronounced involvement of the carotid siphon by overlapping primary calcifications, lipid infiltration and atherosclerotic lesions occurs even at a relatively young age (Fig. 7-9). With the progression of lesions the assessment of factors which determine their localization becomes increasingly difficult.

This siphon is from a 32-year-old man who died of myocardial infarction.

The significance of the adjacent hard tissues, i.e., of the bone and the dura for the development of lesions arising in the carotid
Counter Pressure of Bone   siphon have not yet been precisely assessed. The tube of the siphon is mostly surrounded by venous sinus, which probably acts as a hydraulic suspension and damps the recoil arising with

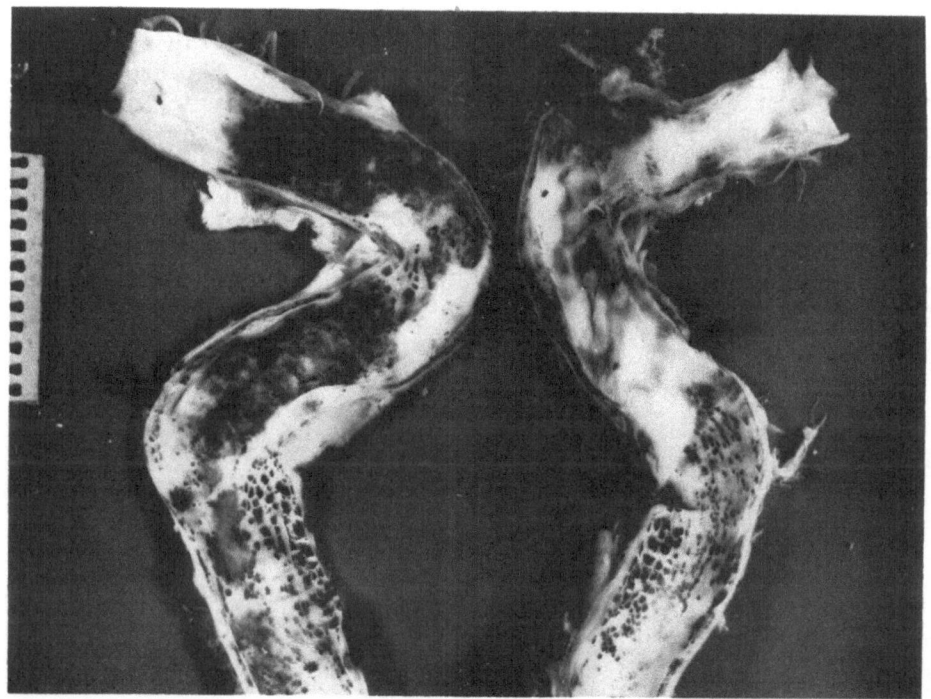

Fig. 7-9: Extensive primary calcifications (black) are seen in
the medial (left) and the lateral (right) halves of the longitudinally opened carotid siphon from a 32-year-old man who died
of myocardial infarction. In many areas calcifications are
covered by advanced atherosclerotic plaques (white). (The areas
of prominent lipid infiltration, which were red-stained in the
specimen, are not distinctly visible in the photograph). Millimeter scale left. Von Kossa reaction and Fettrot 7 B. Case 847/73.
(From Meyer, 1975A).

transmission of the pulse wave. In this way, the siphon is probably sufficiently protected against the counter-pressure of the adjacent tissues. However, with age and progressive dilatation of the arterial tube, the distance between the widening artery and the surrounding bones may become shorter and the "counter-pressure" of the bone more effective.

Remarkably, pronounced calcifications seldom appear in the petrous portion of the siphon which is embedded in an osseous channel. In contrast, only some parts of the upper cavernous portion of the siphon are located in the vicinity of the osseous tissue. Therefore, the greater invovlement of this segment by calcifications and atherosclerotic lesions appears to be related to its more tortuous pattern and additional hemodynamic factors arising in curved arterial segments. I should like to demonstrate three remarkable patterns of early lipid infiltration in the cervical part of the carotid artery, which appear to be closely related to the preformed structural characteristics of the involved areas (Fig. 7-6).

In the trunk of the common carotid artery the lipids initially appear below the orifice of the external carotid
Lipid Infiltration in   artery, extend proximally
Cervical Part of Carotid   along the antero-medial wall
Artery   during the second decade and
                                                form a longitudinal, triangular
                                                stripe (deposit) regularly
seen in young adults (Fig. 7-10 and 7-11). The characteristic shape of the lipid infiltrated area persists even in later ages.

Microscopic examination reveals conspicuous structural differences between the opposite, i.e. predisposed and resistant arterial sectors. At the predisposed antero-medial wall, a well delineated musculo-elastic intimal layer appears internal to the internal elastic membrane in the first decade of life, i.e. before the lipid infiltration becomes visible, grossly or microscopically. Toward the end of the first decade, a compact sheet of tightly packed strong, longitudinally arranged elastic fibers develops along the luminal aspect of the musculo-elastic layer and becomes superimposed by a thin luminal layer of a loose connective tissue which is rich in ground substance (Fig. 7-12 arrows). Both layers develop a moderate thickening of the intima at the predisposed arterial wall, whereas the intima of the opposite, resistant arterial wall remains thin in children and young adults.

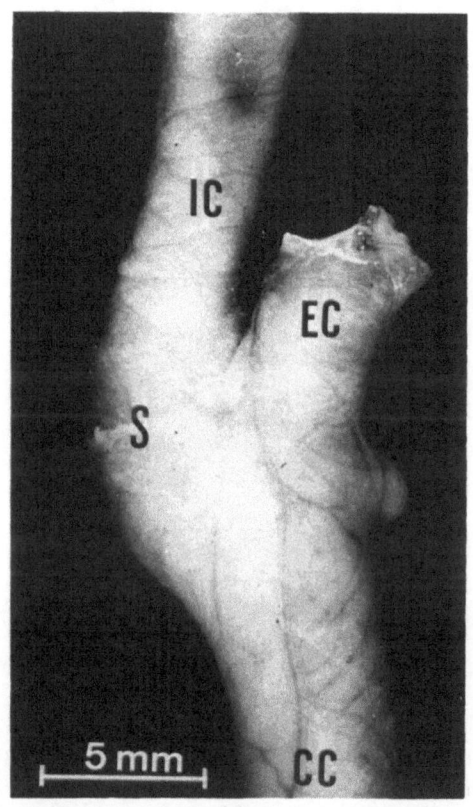

Fig. 7-10: Carotid bifurcation of an 18-month-old child dissected after fixation under pressure of 60 cm water formalin solution. CC – common carotid artery, IC – internal carotid artery, EC– external carotid artery. The protruding sinus area (S) is clearly seen.

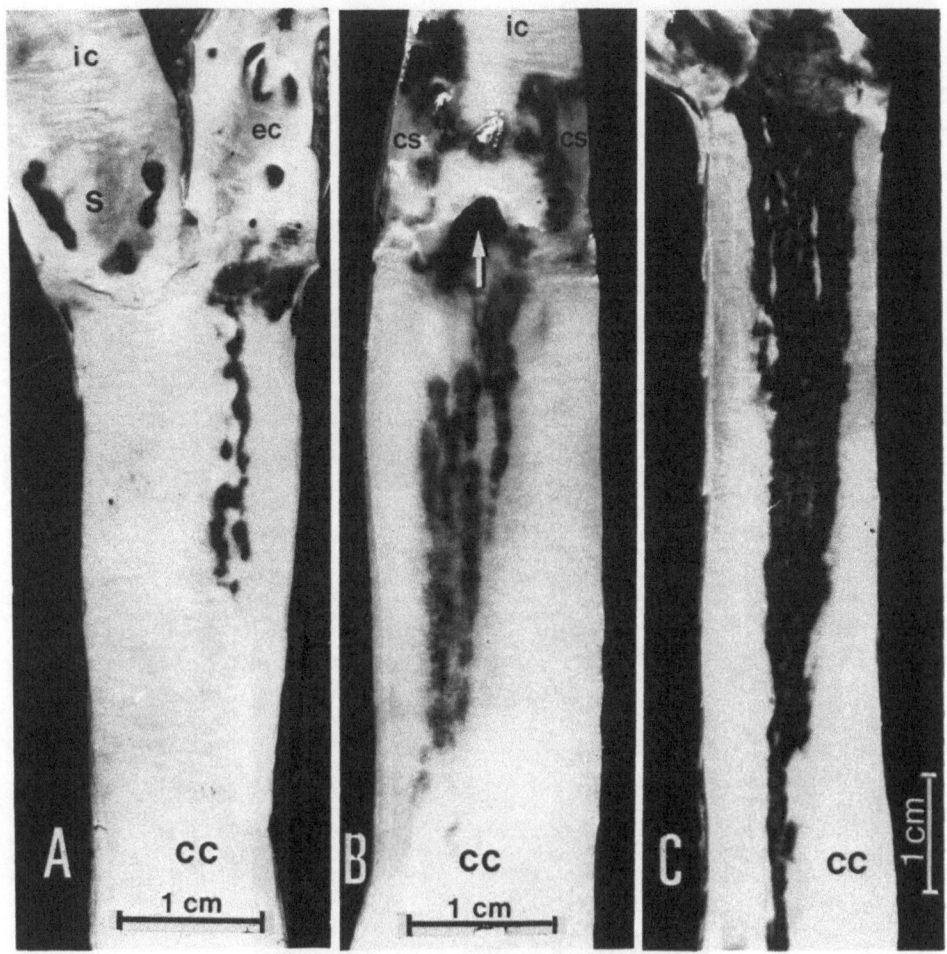

Fig. 7-11: Various stages in the development of gross patterns of
lipid depositis in the common carotid artery.
A. Lipid deposits (black) initially appear below the orifice of
the external carotid artery (EC) and extend proximally along the
length of the vessel. Lipid deposits are also seen in the
peripheral parts of the sinus (S). 20-year-old man. (Case 1243/73).
B. Deposits then become confluent along the antero-medial wall of
the common carotid artery (arrow) and extend around the central
part of the sinus. In this specimen the central sinus area (CS)
has been opened longitudinally and divided into two parts which
extend to the borders of the vessel. Note also the lipid-free
carina of the carotid bifurcation (arrow). 34-year-old man
(Case 227/73).
C. With more advanced lesions, lipid infiltrates the antero-
medial wall and the lesion assumes a characteristic triangular
form 31-year-old man (Case 127/72). Fettrot VII B.(From Meyer
and Noll, 1974).

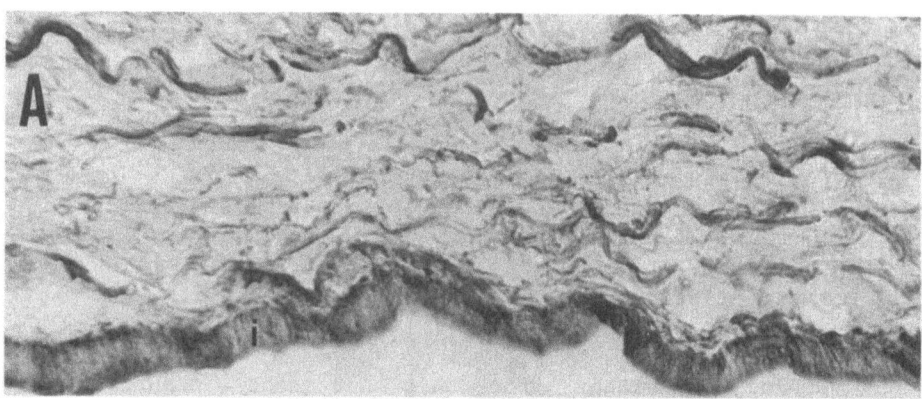

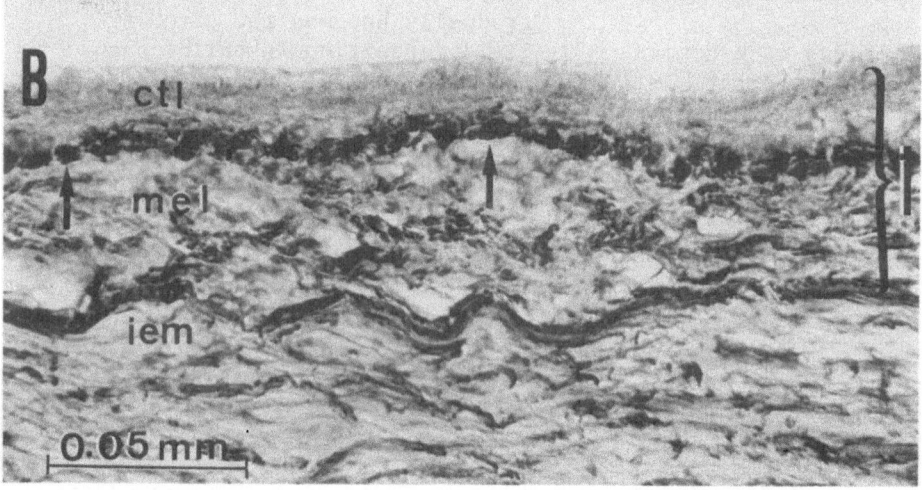

Fig. 7-12: Structural differences between the dorso-lateral (A) and antero-medial (B) walls are well seen on a cross section of an arterial ring taken from the middle of the common carotid artery from a 20-year-old man. Cause of death: traffic accident. In dorso-lateral wall (A), the intima (i) is thin. It consists mainly of a subendothelial layer formed by tightly packed elastic fibers. No internal elastic membrane is seen. In the antero-medial wall (B), the intima (i) is thickened and has a well-developed musculo-elastic layer (mel) between the internal elastic membrane (iem) and the compact sheet of strong longitudinal elastic fibers (arrows). Cross section of these fibers are seen below the thin connective tissue layer (ctl) of the intima. No lipids are present at this level. Cryostat frozen section. Weigert's resorcin-fuchsin. Case 1145/71. (From Meyer and Noll, 1974) (6).

DR. CARO: On the opposite side of the wall, is there a lack of cells?

DR. MEYER: The intima is thin at the resistant arterial wall and accordingly it includes fewer cells than the opposite predisposed wall.

The lipids seem first to appear selectively in the sheet of the strong longitudinal elastic fibers which develop along the luminal aspect of the musculo-elastic luminal layer (Fig. 7-13). Later the lipids also appear in the cells of the musculo-elastic layer, i.e. between the sheet of longitudinal elastic fibers and the internal elastic membrane.

In general, the extent of the thickened and differentiated intima seems to correspond to the triangular area which gradually becomes the site of lipid deposition in children and in young adults. Remarkably, the granular medial calcification, independent of intimal lipid deposits, sometimes also appears in the antero-medial wall of the carotid trunk and extends over approximately the same triangular area as do the lipid deposits (4). The appearance of both intimal and medial lesions in the same portion of the arterial tube suggests that a common hemodynamic factor may be responsible for their development.

Possibility of a Common Hemodynamic Factor. Antero-medial Wall of Carotid Trunk

The second remarkable area is the carotid sinus, i.e. the slightly protruding proximal portion of the internal carotid artery just above its origin from the carotid trunk (Fig. 7-14a). In children, the lipid deposits predominantly appear in the peripheral parts of the protruding sinus area (Fig. 7-14a). Later dot-like or linear lesions often conglomerate into a ring-like, slightly raised deposit, which may partly or completely encircle the central sinus area (Fig. 7-14b). Later, i.e., in the third decade of life, the entire sinus area often becomes almost completely covered by a thickened lipid-containing intima (Fig 7-14C and 7-14D).

Carotid Sinus

As in the carotid trunk, the early development of lipid deposits in the carotid sinus appears to be closely related to an early thickening and differentiation of the intima during postnatal growth (Fig. 7-15).

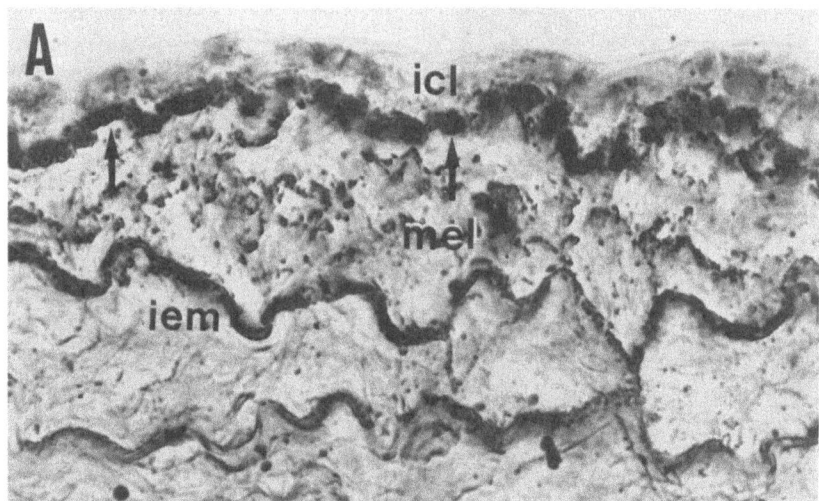

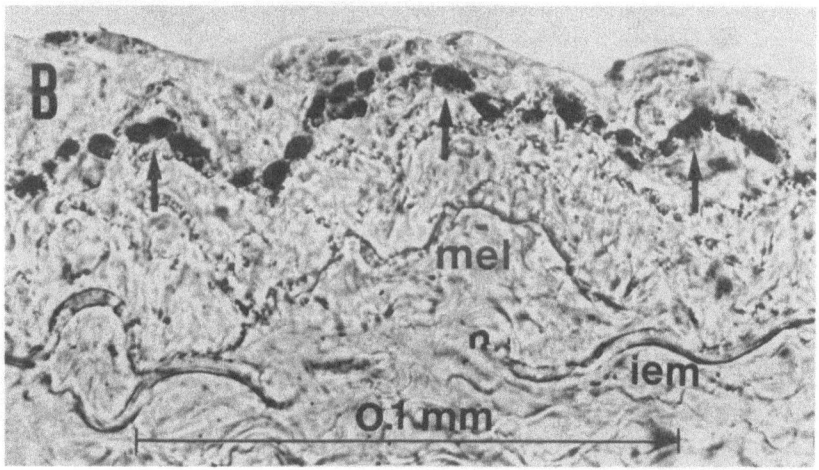

Fig. 7-13: Cross sections of the intimal luminal layer of the
common carotid artery showing selective deposition of lipids in
the sheet of strong elastic bundles. A. With Weigert's
resorcin-fuchsin stain, cross sections of strong elastic bundles
(arrows) are distinctly seen between a thin intimal connective
tissue layer (icl) and the intimal musculo-elastic layer (mel).
iem - internal elastic membrane. B. With Fettrot, the lipid
infiltrated, red-stained cross sections of the strong elastic
bundles (arrows) appear black. Note the fragments of the
internal elastic membrane (iem). 10-year-old boy (case 51/74).
Cause of death: traffic accident. (From Meyer and Noll, 1974).

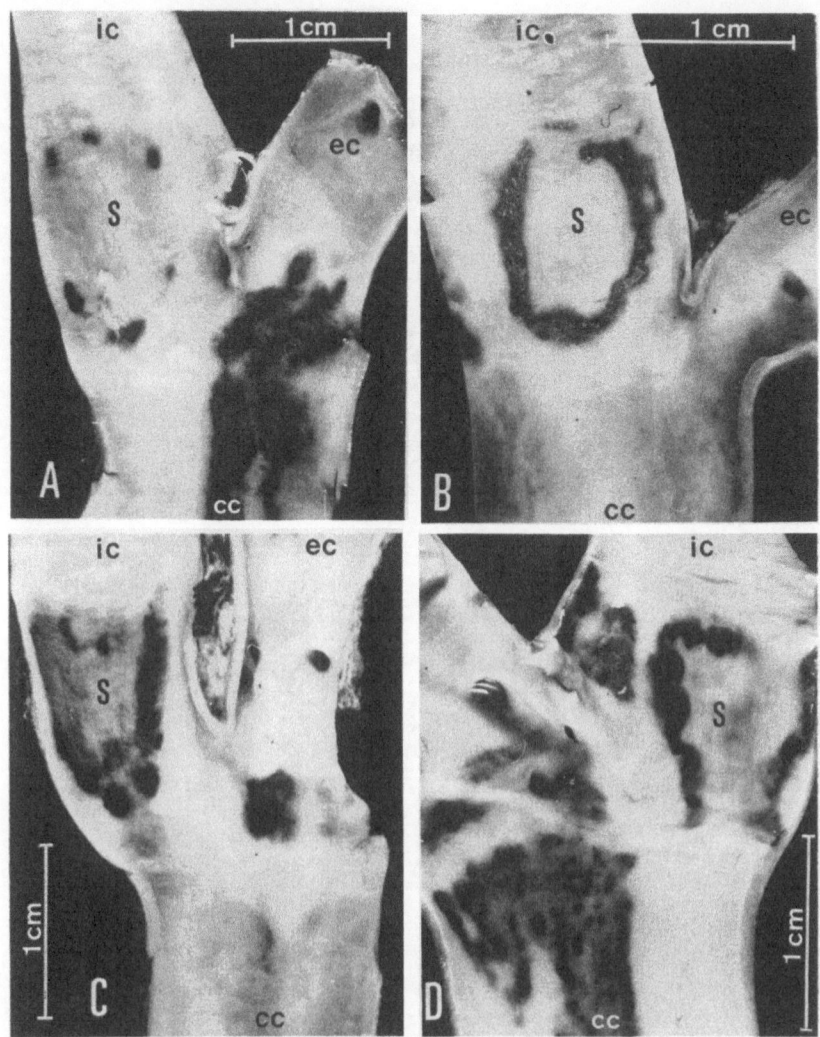

Fig. 7-14: Gross patterns of early lipid deposits in the carotid
sinus. A. Note scattered punctate lipid deposits (black) around
the periphery of the carotid sinus (S). 13-year-old boy.
(Case RM 183/74). B. A ring-like lipid deposit encircles the
central protruding sinus area. 10-year-old boy. (Case 51/74).
C. Extensive lipid deposits are present in the peripheral parts
of the sinus. A pale diffuse staining ("blush") is seen in the
central sinus area and along the antero-medial wall of the
common carotid (cc). 19-year-old women. (Case 1335/74).
D. Lipid deposits in the periphery of the sinus from a 30-year-
old man. Cause of death in all cases: traffic accidents.
Fettrot 7B. S-carotid sinus; ic - internal carotid artery; ec-
external carotid artery, cc - common carotid artery. (From Meyer
and Noll, 1974).

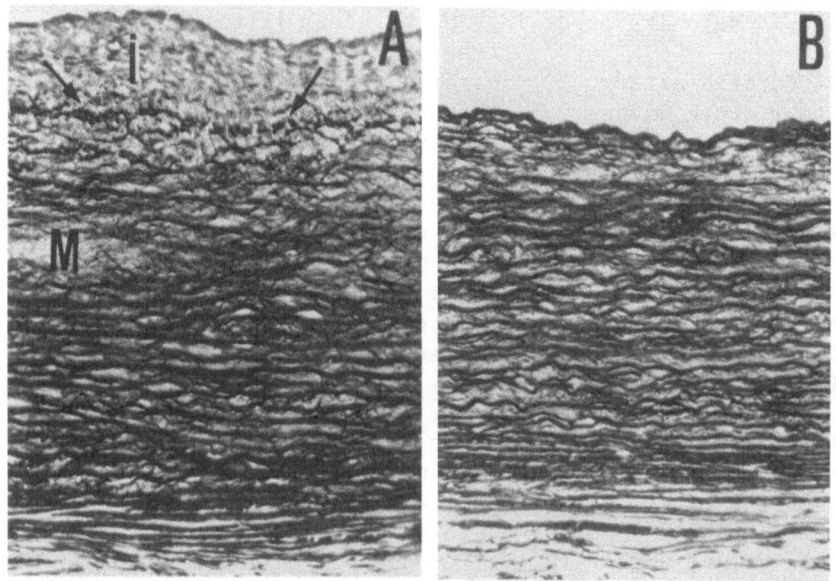

Fig. 7-15: Cross section of the protruding lipid-free area
within the ring-like lipid deposit in the carotid sinus (A)
and of the arterial wall external to the lipid deposit at the
same level (B). A. In the sinus, the intima (i) is about one-
fourth the thickness of the media (M). Arrows point to the
sheet of longitudinal elastic fibers which extends along the
inner aspect of the musculo-elastic intimal layer. B. In the
segment immediately external to the sinus, no intimal thickening
is present. 10-year-old boy. Case 51/74. Weigert's resorcin-
fuchsin stain. (From Meyer and Noll, 1974).

No difference in the microscopic structure could be found
between the intima of the peripheral parts of the sinus and
the intima of the central area. The peripheral portion is
the site of early lipid deposits, whereas the central area
initially stays free. The preferential accumulation of lipids
in the periphery of the sinus may be due to the differences
in functional load and the different elasticity of the central
and peripheral portions of the sinus.

The third conspicuous gross feature is the sharp delineation
of the lipid deposits appearing in the sinus from the lipid-
free portion of the internal
Internal Carotid Artery   carotid artery located immediately
Immediately above Sinus   above the sinus. Even with a
                                pronounced involvement, the lipid
infiltration ends abruptly above the sinus. Then, the border
between the affected and lipid-free parts of the arterial
luminal surface often appears as a straight horizontal line
(Fig. 7-16). Microscopically, the upper borders of the
lipid deposits regularly correspond to the transitional area
between the elastic and muscular arterial segments, where
the media assumes the structural pattern of muscular arteries
(Fig. (7-17).

At the same level, the thickened intima of the sinus
becomes progressively thinner. Thus, the lipid deposits are
limited to the sinus which belongs to the elastic arterial
segment and which is, moreover, covered by thickened intima.
The lipids do not appear in the immediately distal muscular
segment showing a thinner intima. It is still to be elucidated
whether the structural features of the media or the intima
or of both are responsible for different involvement of
these adjacent arterial segments. (See diagram Fig. 7-18).

The next three figures show the peculiar distribution
of lipid deposits in the cervical portion of the vertebral artery.
This portion is of special interest because it passes through
several successive ring-like osseous structures with soft
tissues in between (Figs. 7-19, 7-20, 7-21). This unique
topographic relationship suggested a way of determining
whether the localization of lipid deposits and atherosclerotic
lesions may be influenced by the physical characteristics of
the surrounding tissues, i.e. whether the arterial lesions
appear at the sites surrounded by bone or softer tissue (7).

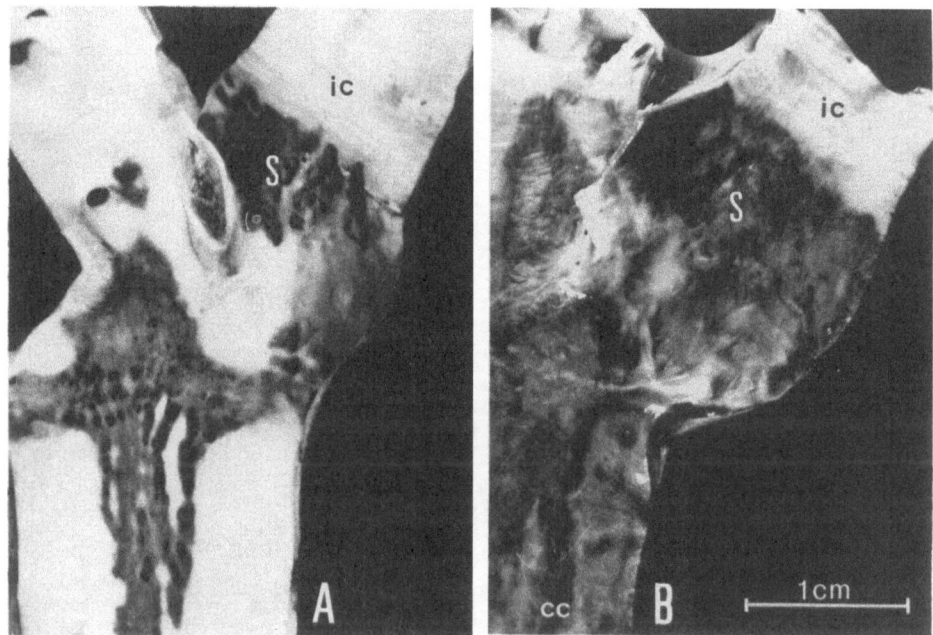

Fig. 7-16: Advanced lipid infiltration of the carotid sinus (S).
Note sharp delineation of the lipid-infiltrated area from the
lipid-free portion of the internal carotid artery (ic); common
carotid artery (cc). A: carotid artery from a 22-year-old
woman (1140/71); B: carotid artery from a 46-year-old man
(1126/71).

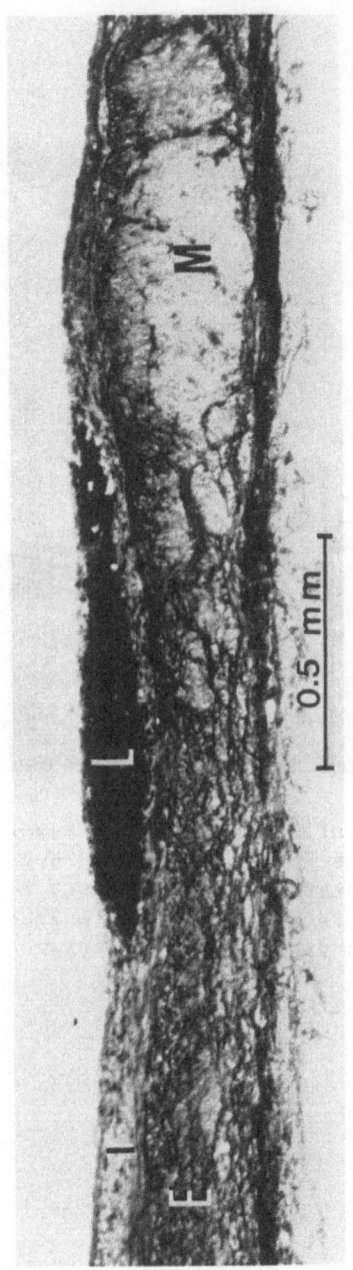

Fig. 7-17: Lipid deposits in the upper part of the sinus (L, black) are located in the transitional zone between the proximal elastic (D) and distal muscular (M) segments and do not extend into the muscular segment (even in old age groups). Note the pale (unstained) smooth musculature of the muscular arterial segment and the thickened intima (I(of the sinus. Resorcin-fuchsin and Fettrot stains. 27-year-old woman (Case 118/73). (From Meyer and Noll, 1974).

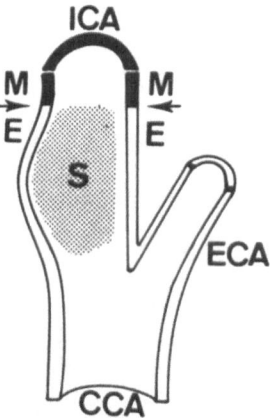

Fig. 7-18: Intimal thickening (dotted) in the carotid sinsu (S) stops abruptly at the demarcation between the elastic (E) and muscular (M) arterial segments (arrow). CC - common carotid artery, IC - internal carotid artery, EC - external carotid artery.

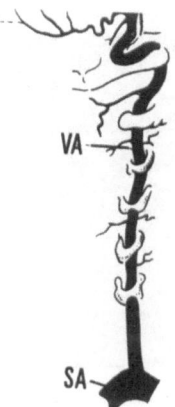

Fig. 7-19: Schematic presentation of the course of the vertebral artery (VA) through the costovertebral foramina. SA subclavian artery. (From W.W. Meyer, 1964).

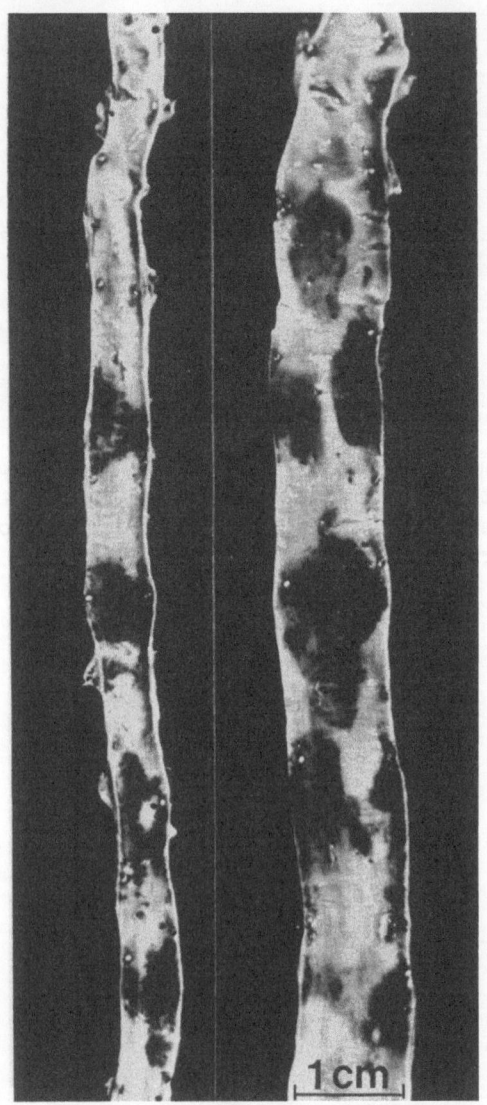

Fig. 7-20: Rhythmical arrangement of lipid deposits in the vertebral artery from a 54-year-old woman. The red stained deposits appear black in the photograph. The right vertebral artery was hypoplastic (left). Scarlet red staining. (From W.W. Meyer and Naujokat, 1964).

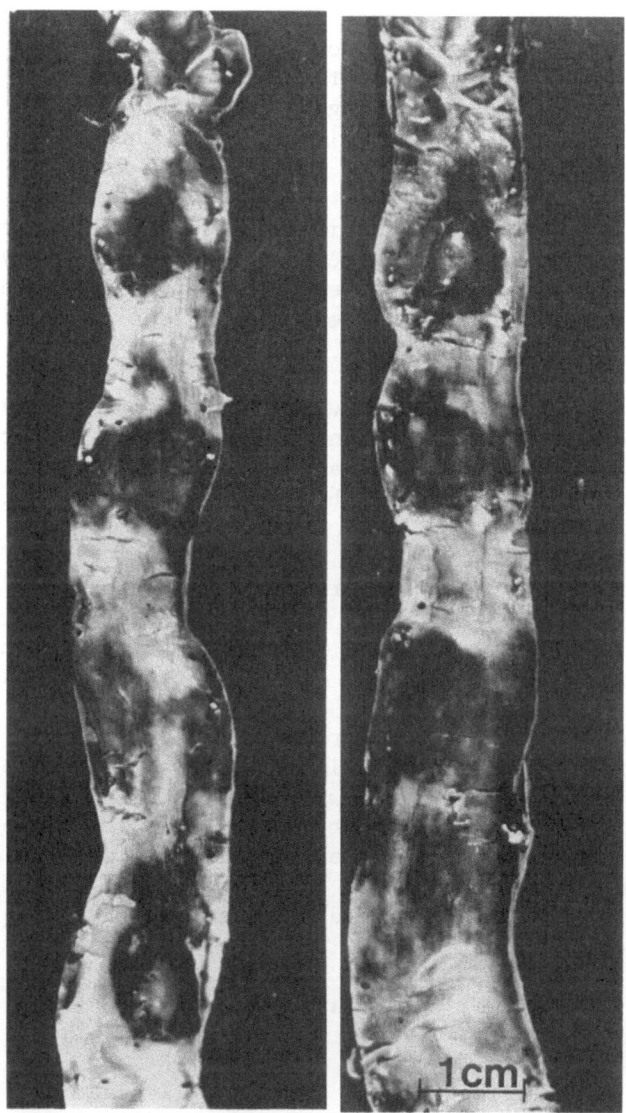

Fig. 7-21: Rhythmical arrangement of lipid deposits and atherosclerotic lesions in the vertebral artery from a 78-year-old man.
The lesions (black) predominantly appear in the ectatic segments
localized between the costotransversal foramina (Scarlet red
staining). (From W.W. Meyer and Naujokat, 1964).

But let us first look at the topographic situation. In the costo-transversal foramina of the cervical vertebrae, the artery is surrounded by bone. However, the arterial wall does not directly touch the osseous ring. A well developed venous plexus surrounds the arterial tube and may probably reduce the recoil of the pulse wave considerably. The spinal nerve and spinal ganglion are located immediately behind the artery. They obliquely cross the arterial tube and are immediately adjacent to its dorsal wall.

The lipid deposits initially appear at the dorsal arterial wall adjacent to the spinal ganglion. They later extend above the spinal nerves, i.e. into the segment of the artery which is located between the osseous rings, i.e., costotransversal foramina.

In some cases, this results in a regular sequential arrangement of fatty streaking. Even with a further prgression of lesions, a sequential arrangement may be distinctly visible as demonstrated in the vertebral artery of the 78-year-old man (Fig. 7-21).

Age changes of the arterial tube, for instance the ectasia, probably favors the sequential arrangement of lipids. Arterial segments

Age Changes   located between the osseous rings become more ectatic with age compared to segments surrounded by bone. This results in change in caliber along the intravertebral segment of the artery. On the other hand, with ectasia the distance between the arterial wall and the surrounding bone in the costovertebral foramina decreases and the recoil of the pulse wave may become more effective. Both factors could be significant for the localization of lipid deposits and their sequential arrangement.

DR. WERTHESSEN: Where are the nerves that measure the oxygen?

DR. MEYER: The wall of the sinus is penetrated by numerous nerves, and in some areas the media appears interrupted by small bundles of nerves. It could not be excluded that this structural peculiarity favors lipid deposition in the intima of the sinus.

There is, in fact, a proliferation of the intimal cells preceeding the lipid deposition at young age.

This is true of the carotid sinus as well as of the predisposed area of the carotid trunk. The proliferation of the intimal cells and formation of a differentiated, thickened intima may be interpreted as a structural adaptation to the increasing hemodynamic load.

DR. WERTHESSEN: I was just interested in whether or not the nerve endings which measure the blood, are in the lipid area.

DR. MEYER: This is a very interesting problem, but as far as I know there is no exact information on the question.

DR. TAYLOR: As far as I know, no one has studied carotid sinus reflexes in arteriosclerotic carotid sinuses.

DR. CHIEN: It is not clear to me whether the red stained lipid infiltration area can be free and behind the cervical spine? Are these areas surrounded by bone or next to the nerve?

DR. MEYER: The lipid deposits appear first at the dorsal wall of the vertebral artery adjacent to the spinal ganglion.

DR. LEE: In regard to your calcium deposits, which are very interesting, have you looked at any other vessels other than the carotid arteries? Children have such calcium deposits. Do you know the vitamin D content of human milk or is vitamin D supplementation the culprit?

DR. MEYER: The predilection of the common and internal iliac arteries for calcifications may be due to the higher blood volume flow to which these arteries are exposed during fetal development as a part of the placental circuit. They show an accelerated growth, and wear and tear changes may occur in these arteries already before birth. In Germany, calcifications of the iliac arteries and of the carotid siphon have been demonstrated grossly in all children aged one year or older. An overdosage of Vitamin D may occur in Germany and could be a pathogenetic factor.

DR. LEE: We have studied Vitamin D and Fred Kommeror studied Vitamin D, and concluded that it induces widespread arterial calcification.

DR. CARO: I would like to congratulate Dr. Meyer on
those marvelous pictures. I have seldom seen anything so
fine. I wondered if you or anyone has made any studies of
the vertebral arteries under normal pressure. Does the
artery bulge in between the areas where it is suported?

DR. MEYER: In the older individuals the segments
located between the osseous rings appear ectatic. No measurements
of the internal diameters have been made.

DR. CHIEN: I think the decisive factor responsible for
lesions of the siphon is its coiled shape. The siphon, at
least in childhood, is surrounded by a venous plexus.

DR. MEYER: Yes, the siphon seems to be well protected
against the osseous tissue by venous plexus at least in
younger individuals. However, with age, ectasia of the
siphon occurs. Then, the distance between the arterial wall
and the surrounding osseous tissues may become significantly
shorter and the recoil may become a factor influencing the
development of lesions. (2,4,8,9).

DR. TAYLOR: It makes that terrible siphonic turn too,
Dr. Meyer. I don't think bone is as good a cushion as liver,
spleen, kidney, or brain tissues. These are superb soft
external arterial cushions.

DR. CARO: Dr. Meyer tells us that there is ectasia of
the vertebrals. Now if I can go back to Dr. Dewey's presentation,
I think that we have two findings that have a lot in common.
We are seeing lipid deposition occurring in two regions of
ectasia. In one of these the deposition may stop where the
flow reattaches, or at least accelerates and Dr. Meyer
showed us that the lesion stopped where I would guess that
the flow channel narrows again.

DR. SCHWARTZ: A brief question. I was impressed with
Dr. Meyer's beautiful demonstration of the close affinity of
elastic tissue for lipid. The question I ask of the engineers
is simply this: Can they conceive of any mechanism where
abnormal fluid mechanical stresses would in some way modify
the structure and composition of elastin, and thus change
its binding capacity for lipoproteins and lipid?

DR. COLTON: Has a detailed examination been made of the
conformation of those macromolecules? Is the conformation
dependent upon anatomical position or extent of deformation
of the tissue? Perhaps the sites for interaction with lipids
are exposed to a greater extent in some regions than in others.

DR. SCHWARTZ: We still have to ask that set of questions.

DR. SMITH: Elastin is a very non-polar protein and it
appears that the non-polar aminoacids are grouped together
to form hydrophobic regions; Keller and Mandl isolated large,
non-polar polypeptides from hydrolysates of elastin (10).
Elastin is resistant to acid and to alkali in aqueous media, but
is rapidy hydrolysed in the presence of organic solvents.
Robert (11) has suggested that organic solvents and lipids may
react with hydrophobic regions, rupturing the hydrophobic interactions and leading to a partial "unfolding" of the molecule,
which then becomes more susceptible to hydrolytic or protease
attachment. He also suggests that "stretched" elastin may be
more permeable to lipid; this may be largely speculative,
but the idea that stretching facilitates lipid infiltration,
which in turn facilitates proteolysis, fits very well with
the histological picture.

DR. MEYER: I would like to ask the engineers whether
the different structure of the concave and convex walls of
the carotid siphon could be explained in terms of hemodynamics.
I discussed this question with a colleaque privately and
learned that centrifugal forces are probably negligible in
the curved arterial segments and cannot be responsible for
pronounced hyperplasia of the intimal elastic sheets at the
outer walls of curves. What other physical forces may be
involved which could explain the structural differences in
curved arterial segments?

DR. DEWEY: In a vessel with an extremely sharp radius
of curvature there is a difference between the stress in the
wall at a given point of pressure on the inside versus the
outside. It may be that this difference in stress particularly
in the carotid bifurcation alters the curve.

DR. COLTON: I would like to reiterate the point raised
by Dr. Schwartz that the binding capacity of the various
macromolecules in the arterial wall, such as collagen, elastin
or the glycosaminoglycans may be dependent on the stress to
which they are exposed and the resulting deformation they
undergo.

Change in the applied stress could open sites which might
be closed at a lower degree of stress, consequently the
effect of local variations in stress might be to change the
capacity of the wall to hold the lipid that passes through
it, and not necessarily to alter the endothelial permeability
to lipoproteins.

DR. NEREM: There is no direct evidence for the involvement
of fluid mechanics in the initiation of atherosclerotic lesions.
Someone may wish to take exception with such a denial of
direct evidence but in fact it is indirect evidence upon
which we "hang our hats," base our NIH grants, and write our
papers for the variety of meetings where we go around and
talk to each other.

Fortunately, there is at least some indirect evidence,
and what I will comment on briefly is what I consider the
                              primary indirect evidence,
Pattern of Disease   i.e., the pattern of disease.
                              Fig. 7-22 is the classical drawing
out of Spain's 1966 article in Scientific American (12)
illustrating that basically there is a pattern to the disease,
I think we all accept this as fact even though we may not
agree on the pattern.   However, it appears that it is the
abdominal region of the aorta, the carotids, and the coronaries
which are the positions in the vasculature having the highest
predilection for developing atherosclerosis.   If we look at
the coronary system in detail, and even if one accepts that
there may be involvement of most of the extramural coronary
vessels, there still are regions which seem to have a higher
predilection than others.   These are primarily regions of
branching, and in some cases of sharp curvature, and these
are certainly regions of interest from a fluid mechanic
viewpoint.

Unfortunately, we do not have enough detail on the
pattern of the disease.   For example, I am not sure that
anyone at this point can really state whether at a bifurcation
initiation of the disease occurs on the flow divider or on
the outer wall.   Now this may be something that we will want
to talk about further.   Certainly, there were some very
interesting results presented by Dr. Meyer that would suggest
a certain type of region as being the favorite.   Now I am
extremely reluctant to use terms like 'low shear' and 'high
shear' because those of us who have been in this area of
research for a long time realize that low shear or high
shear may have absolutely nothing to do with it.

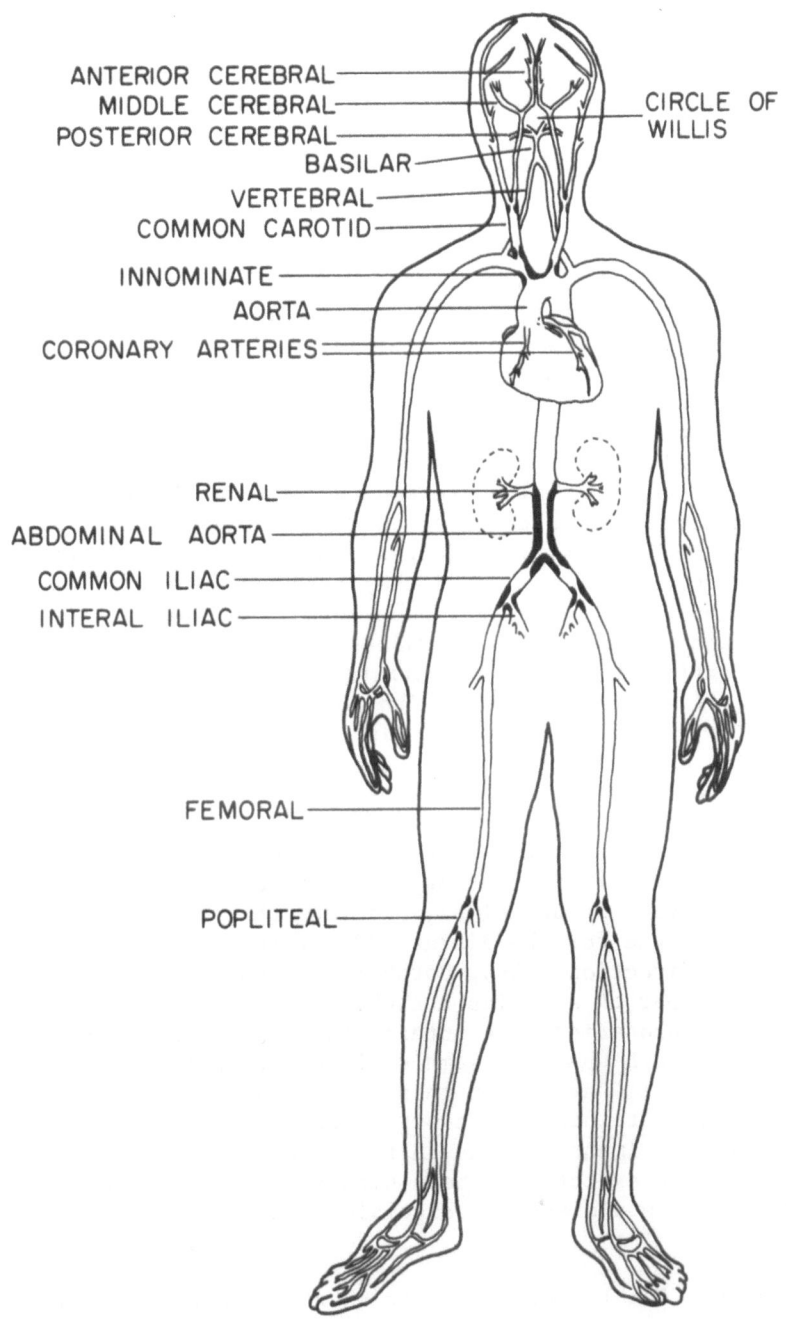

Fig. 7-22: Illustration of vascular sites having greatest predilection for the development of atherosclerosis (from Spain, 1966).

But at least there are regions which one can characterize in
this fashion as long as one realizes that the underlying
reasons may be totally different and not shear dependent.
In this context, some of Dr. Meyer's data certainly suggest
that the preferential regions are ones where maximum stresses
would not be expected to occur and where, if anything, the
opposite is true, i.e., they are suspected of being low
shear regions.

    Recently there have been at least two groups that I
know of who have been trying to determine in some detail
and quantitatively where lesions initiate. One of these
efforts is at NIH. Dr. Fry is not here today, and I am not
sure how far along this effort is; however, an effort is
being made to quantitate data on the distribution of fatty
streaks and lesions in the aorta from subjects that I believe
were obtained from the Baltimore County morgue. The other
approach involves cholesterol-fed animal experiments and is
the work at the University of Western Ontario by Fred Cornhill
(13) and Margo Roach (14). Here they have used a rabbit as
a model. They have looked at branch vessels eminating from
the aorta, and using a polar coordinate system, they have
mapped the pattern. This is illustrated in Fig. 7-23. The
lesions here represent staining with Sudan III so they are
sudanaphillic lesions. The solid line here is the outline
of the celiac artery orifice and the dashed line is the
outline of the staining as measured for that particular
case. Combining all these results, one obtains a pattern in
terms of a polar coordinate system--it is nothing more than
a quantitative way of pinpointing the orifical pattern--for
particular location in an animal, and from this there is a
definite preference for the distal side of the orifice in
terms of flow direction. Drs. Cornhill and Roach have
looked at a number of arteries branching off the aorta
including the coronaries, the intercostals, and the renal
arteries. Although there is some difference, it is the
distal side that is favored in this particular experiment.
Note, however, that this is not normal human atheroma. This
is a feeding experiment and the distal side in terms of
stresses would be expected to be a high shear stress side
although again I would add the disclaimer that I earlier
voiced.

    DR. CARO: Can I ask, were they short or long duration
experiments?

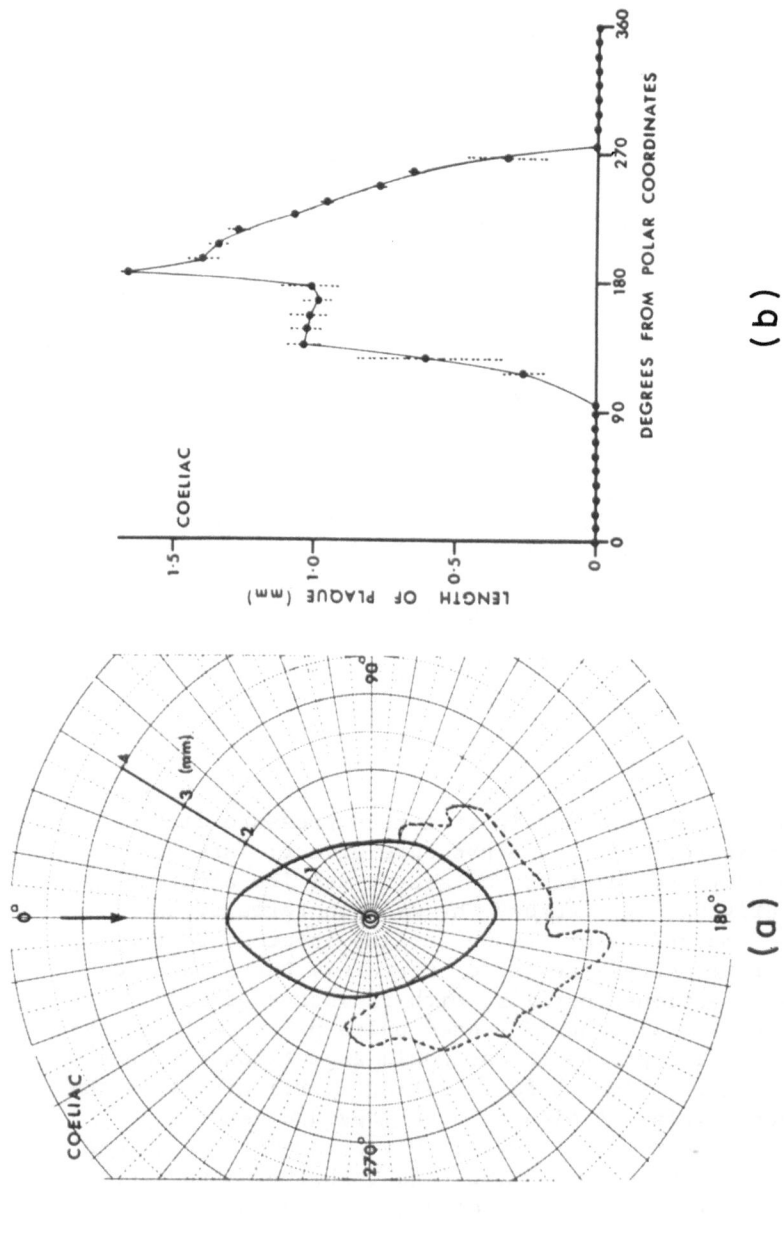

Fig. 7-23: (a) Polar coordinate representation of aortic lesion (dashed line) around the coeliac orifice (solid line); (b) rectangular coordinate drawing from (a) with the dotted lines showing the SEM of 5 measurements. Note that the lesion is entirely distal (from Cornhill and Roach, 1974).

DR. NEREM: I think these are eight-week experiments.
The rabbits were on egg yolk with rabbit pellet diets.   I
mention this because I think we need more detailed information
of this type and because I believe that this pattern of the
disease is the chief, if not the only, indirect evidence for
fluid mechanics--hemodynamics--being a primary or any kind of
a signficant factor in the disease process.   I thus would urge
people, who are in a position to obtain this kind of data, to
help us in developing this type of quantitative approach and in
developing data bases which look very carefully at differences
between animals and between spontaneous versus induced atheroma
so that ultimately we may be able to answer this question in a
very definitive way.   This is one series of questions that we
should be able to answer if we are able to organize our efforts.

In talking about fluid forces being involved, we should
recognize that we are talking about either the pressure or the
frictional force on the wall, i.e., the wall shear stress, the
frictional force or shear stress very much influenced and
determined by the detailed flow characteristics that are
associated with the particular vascular flow situation, the
local geometry and wall elastic properties and so forth.   Before
going on to talk about the coronary system, I would like to say
just a word about these forces.   First, if we talk about
pressure, the main reason for our interests is that hypertension
is the one risk factor which seems to have some relevance to
hemodynamics being involved.   However, we are in a rather poor
state in terms of understanding what that pressure influence is,
i.e., what the role of hypertension is in terms of risk factor
information.   For example, is it a mean pressure diastolic/
systolic pressure, or a pulse pressure effect?   Are we
talking about vessel distension, are we talking about an
increased driving force across the wall in terms of the
transport of materials or are we talking about distortion of
the vascular geometry--the latter certainly has some appeal
to it.   As I mentioned earlier, with an increased mean
pressure there is also an increased pulse pressure, and with
an increased pulse pressure, one would expect considerable
alteration in the flow characteristics, particularly in the
shear stress levels.   A higher pulse pressure generally
would mean a higher peak velocity, but also a change in the
velocity wave form so as to give rise to higher shear stresses.
Thus, what exactly is the role of pressure in this whole
problem?

In considering the role of shear stress, Dr. Dewey gave
us some background as to where we think we are in terms of
understanding the general magnitude of these stresses.

However, I would like to make a few additional points with the next few figures. Fig. 7-24 presents some calculations by Pedley (15) of aortic wall shear stress. These are based on the measured ascending aorta velocity waveform which is presented. Although you can measure velocity profiles with such instruments as hot-film anemometers and pulsed ultrasonic doppler units, to determine a wall shear stress from a velocity profile is a highly risky business. One approach is to take the basic waveform and use that as the input to a theoretical calculation. There are a number of ways to go about this and such calculations only represent reasonable estimates. Pedley, in taking the wave form here which was measured by Nerem, Seed, and Wood (16) at Imperial College, arrived at these estimates for shear rate.

There are a couple of things to note; first, the peak shear rates independent of whether you are talking about forward flow or reverse flow, reach a level of 4000 inverse seconds. In terms of shear stress, that would be something over 100 dynes per square centimeter. The interesting thing is that there is at least as large a stress during the period of reverse flow as there is during peak systole. This is because as the flow reverses very steep velocity gradients at the wall result so that the reverse flow may have very high stresses associated with it. A second important point is that the peak shear stresses associated with such pulsatile flows are in order of magnitude larger than the mean stress associated with the basic mean flow through the vessel. Thus, when we are trying to understand the pattern of a disease and the hemodynamic involvement, I think one has to be looking at more than just mean flow characteristics.

At NIH, Dr. Robert Lutz and his colleagues (17) have been carrying out some experiments in a plastic model of the aorta, i.e., an actual cast of the aorta of a dog and some of the major branches. The measurements presented in Fig. 7-25 were carried out with an electrochemical technique and for steady flow. Without going into a lot of detail, on the flow divider--Lutz measured a peak shear rate of 700 inverse seconds which would be about 30 dynes per square centimeter. This is the peak stress in the region of the flow divider and this for a steady flow. If one allows for a pulsatile flow through that same type of geometry, one could again expect that the stress associated with the pulsatile flow might be as much as an order of magnitude greater than what Lutz measured.

Measurements of Shear Stress by a Plastic Model of Dog's Aorta

DOG

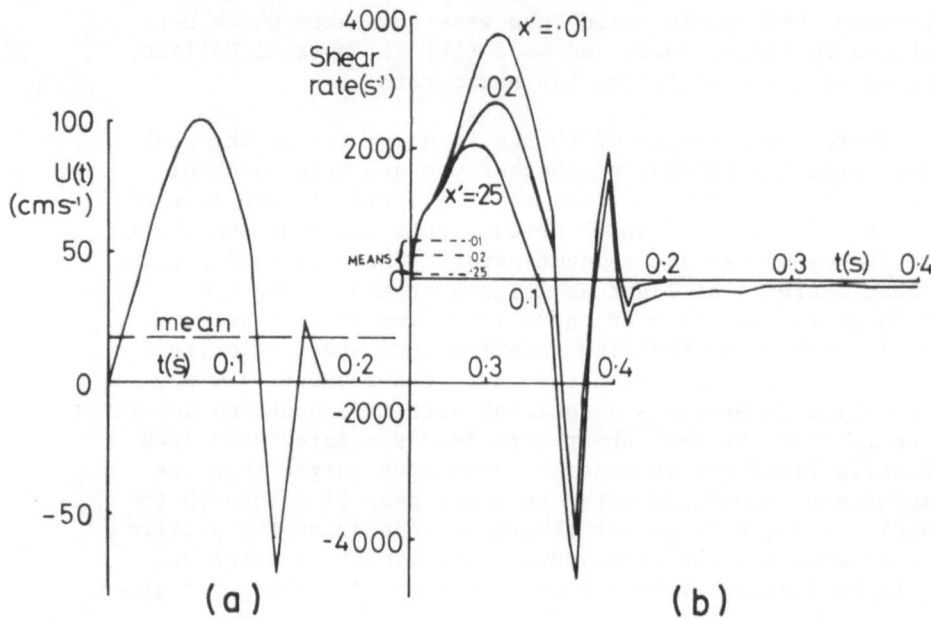

Fig. 7-24: Calculation of aortic wall shear rates using velocity waveform in (a) time history of wall shear rate shown in (b) for different values of x', the ratio of the distance from the aortic valves to the distance flow travels in one pulse (from Pedley, 1974).

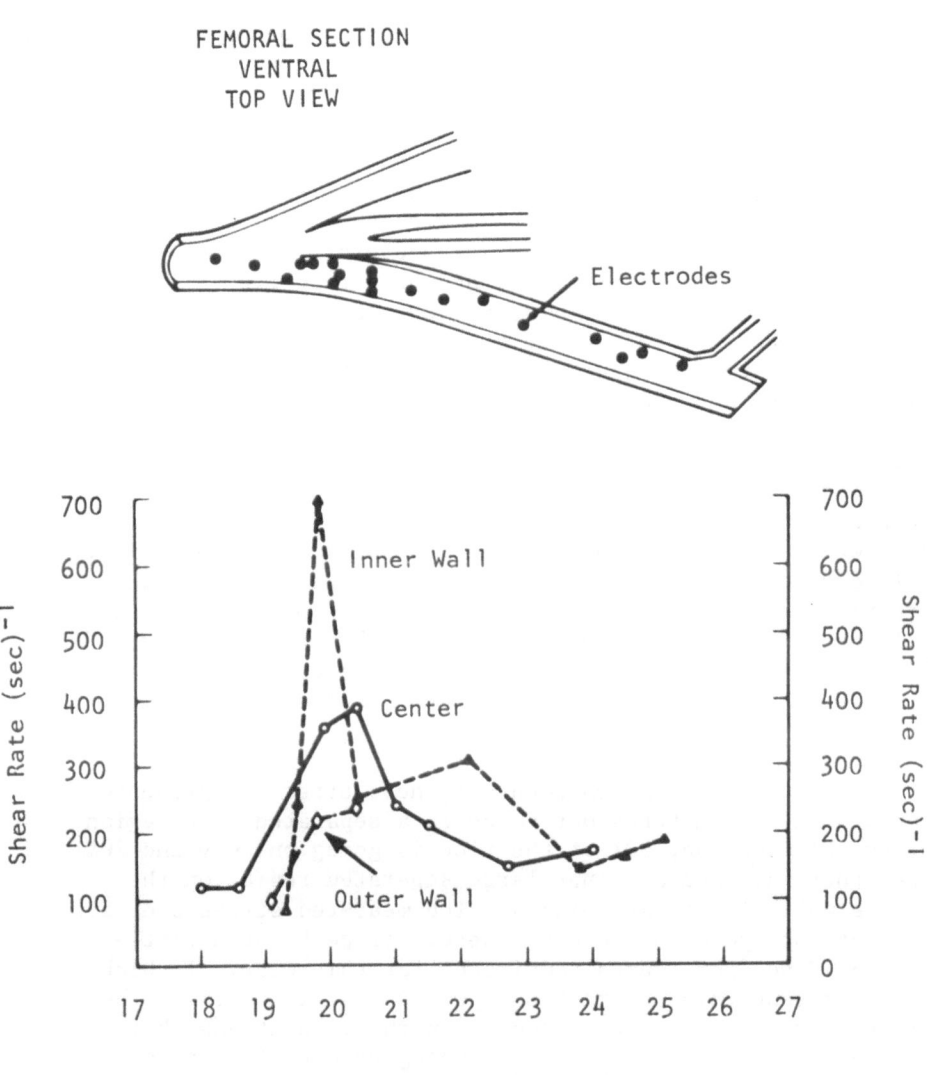

Fig. 7-25: Shear stress distribution pattern on ventral side of model femoral artery section. Electrode positions are indicated in the schematic drawing of the artery at the top of the figure. Electrodes were placed on the inner wall, midline, and outer wall of the femoral branch (from Lutz et al, 1974).

Thus, instead of 30 dynes per square centimeter we are
talking more on the order of several hundred dynes per
square centimeter as a maximum shear stress. From either of
these two situations, one thus can conclude that a shear
stress on the order of 100 to 200 dynes per square centimeter
is not unrealistic in terms of the arterial system.

    One other perspective on this shear stress problem is
given by the experiments presented in Fig. 7-26 and 7-27.
These were carried out in Aachen, Germany by Dr. Niranjan
Talkuder (18) when he was there as a doctoral student.   The
model is that of a bifurcation, and pulsatile flow experiments
were carried out with Reynolds numbers on the order of a
couple of hundred, not unlike that in the coronary system.
Dr. Talukder went to great lengths to look at the effect of
flow division and some of these results are illustrated in
Fig. 7-26. Dr. Dewey in his presentation certainly pointed
out the importance of this, and this brings us back to some
of the comments in this meeting from researchers working on
regulatory mechanisms.   These regulatory mechanisms are the
ones which will determine how the flow divides which ultimately
will decide what the actual stresses are that exist in the
arterial system and what the detailed flow characteristics
will be.   It is very easy for someone like myself to say,
"Don't tell me about the system; I am interested in local
details," but in fact those local details are determined by
system characteristics.

    In Fig. 7-27 a measurement of shear stress is presented
for a point which turns out to be in a separated flow region.
At the bifurcation, 30% of the flow is going one way and 70%
the other way, and a rather large separated region on the
inside wall results at point A.   The measured stress over a
time of one cycle is presented here. It peaks at a little
over 30 dynes per square centimeter for this case. I think
the important thing is that the peak stress is again on the
order of a factor of ten larger than the mean stress that
one would calculate for the flow going through that branch.
The mean stress, t_{Am} by the way, is very close to what you
would calculate for a parabolic Poiseuille profile, but t_{AP}
the rms stress level is a factor of 2-4 higher and the peak
stress is a factor of ten larger--even though you are in a
recirculating separated flow region, a region which one
might be tempted to characterize as being a dead water or
stagnant region.

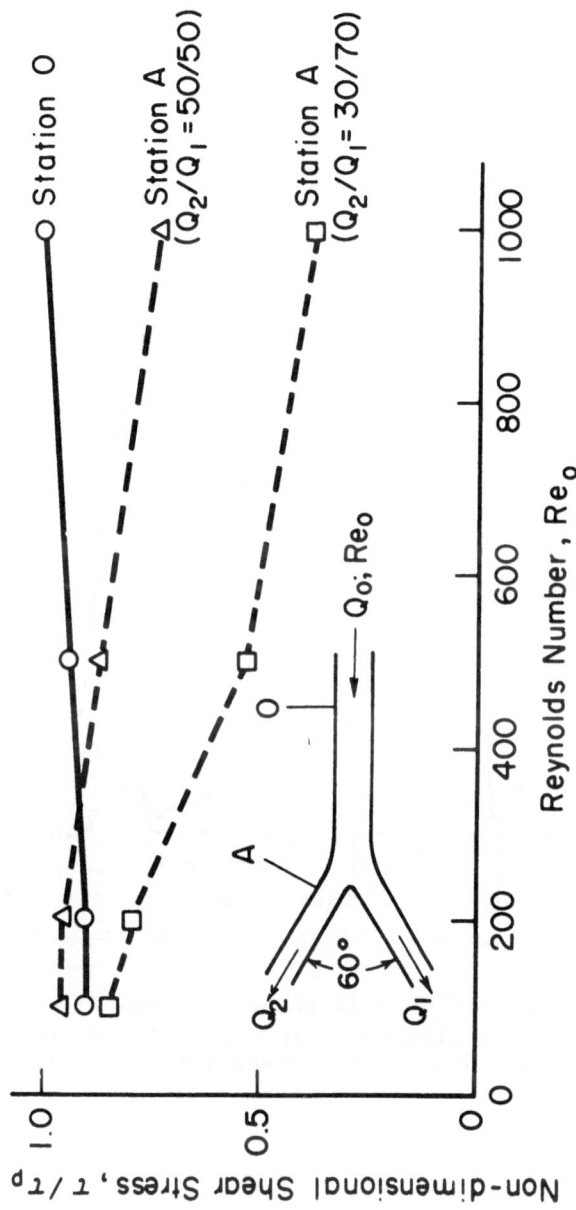

Fig. 7-26: Steady flow shear stresses normalized by corresponding Poiseuille flow values measured as a function of Reynolds number in a model bifurcation. (Talukder, 1974).

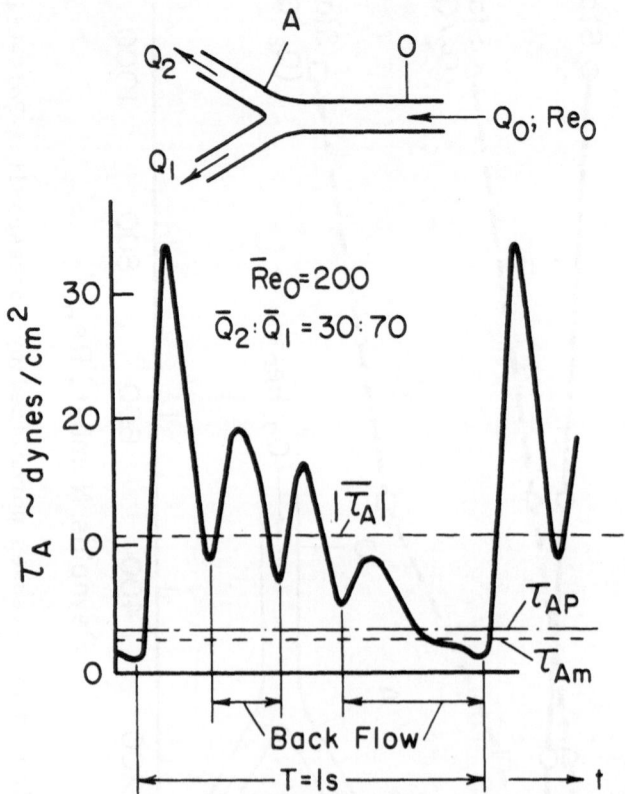

Fig. 7-27: Pulsatile flow wall shear stresses as measured at position A in a model bifurcation; $|\bar{\tau}_A|$ is root mean square value, τ_{AM} is mean value, and τ_{AP} is Poiseuille shear stress value (Talukder, 1974).

Secondary flows--this corkscrewing type of motion is certainly
very much associated with the asymmetries that we see through
vessel curvature and branching. Flow separation--in our
measurements we have not been able to detect flow separation,
but that is probably only an indication of the crude level
at which we are operating. I really think that flow separation
is possible, particularly on the outside walls. The pulsatile
nature of the flow--although we don't see turbulence in the
coronary system, we do observe oscillations which are of an
extremely interesting nature.

     Just to talk a minute about the velocity asymmetries in
the coronary system, (Fig. 7-28 and 7-29) present our hot-
film measurements of the point
velocity at various positions in
the extramural coronary vessels
of the horse and with our probe
moving across the lumen of the vessel from the outside wall to
the inside wall. Fig. 7-28 shows a diagram of the left
common coronary bifurcation into the LAD and the left circumflex
in the horse. X marks the spot where we positioned the
probe. The vessels are curving over the heart, so that the
plane you are looking at is really a plane that is curving.
Thus, as we come in with our probe, we are moving from the
outside wall, in terms of the plane of curvature, toward the
inside wall. This corresponds to going from your right to
your left in terms of these profiles. These are for various
times through the cardiac cycle -- one-fourth of the way,
one-half of the way, three-fourths and full stop through the
cardiac cycle. As you can see, there are only a very limited
number of data points. The vessel is maybe eight millimeters
in diameter, and the probe is on the order of a millimeter
in diameter. Thus, we are only able to get maybe half a
dozen points across the lumen of the vessel. And yet consistently
in the left common coronary, we get an asymmetry which is
essentially favoring the outside wall, i.e., the flow is
pushed toward the outside wall.

     This is totally opposite to what one sees in the aortic
arch, where the flow is if anything pushed toward the inside
wall. However, the aortic arch is a totally different fluid
dynamic situation. Viscous effects are minimal there, being
confined to thin boundary layer regions. In the coronary
system, the flow is much more fully developed and for a
fully viscous flow in a curved pipe you would expect the
peak velocity to be pushed toward the outside wall. So
this type of profile is obtained from the left common coronary
artery and is consistent with what we know about viscous
flow in a pipe.

Velocity Asymmetries in
Coronary System

HORSE

It is in fact anything but that, particularly in a pulsatile
flow situation, and one gets considerable variation in
stress and considerable peaking, certainly during what would
be here representative of the systolic portion of the cycle.
This is presented only to provide some perspective on this
whole problem of how the shear stresses are acting in the
arterial system.

Obviously we need to obtain much better information on
what the stress levels are in the vascular system. Of
course, when we talk about pressure--and again I am interested
in pressure because hypertension is a risk factor which I
can't ignore in trying to put basic fluid mechanics and
transport studies together with the etiology of the disease--
but when we talk about pressure, it may not really be a
fluid mechanic or a hemodynamic effect at all. It conceivably
could be a hemostatic effect, in terms of the kind of stress
loading that Dr. Kenyon talked about. However, whatever it
is, we need better information on these stress levels and
this is something on which we should be able to make considerable
progress.

I would like to say a word about coronary flow characteristics.
Some of the characteristics of interest are asymmetry in
velocity profiles, secondary flows,
flow separation and the oscillatory
or pulsatile nature of the flow.
The view point I am coming from
is that you start out by saying I understand fully developed
laminar or Poiseuille flow and the parabolic profile--a
classical type of flow situation--and then say that one
never sees this in the larger vessels of interest to a group
like this. The lists above are the kinds of phenomena which
Dr. Dewey talked about and which really alter the flow from
the nice well behaved situation and make it interesting. I
just want to comment briefly on some of these relative to
the coronary system. Velocity profiles, the ones we have
measured are admittedly crude, but at least give us some
ideas of the type of skewing present in the coronary system.
Turbulence--I suppose we could spend a day talking about
turbulence in the arterial system, although I have seen in
the aorta velocity waveforms that look very much like turbulence,
I have never seen anything that looked like turbulence in
the coronary system. Distal to a highly stenosed region,
one presumably could have a turbulent jet, but in terms of
the normal vasculature--the normal coronary system--I don't
believe turbulence will be found.

Coronary Flow
Characteristics

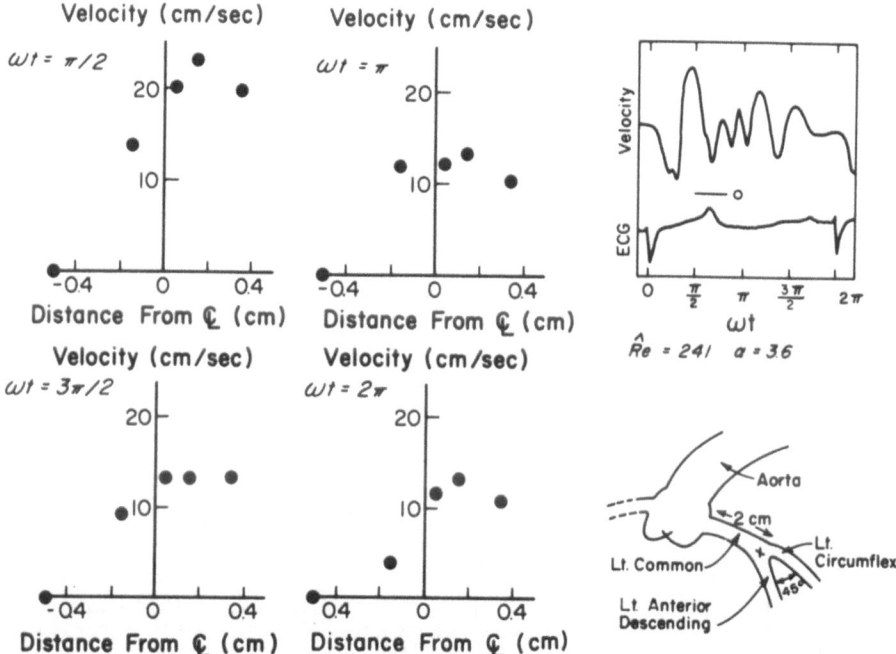

Fig. 7-28: Centerline velocity waveform, ECG, and velocity profiles for the indicated times and location of measurement in the left common coronary artery of an anesthetized horse. Measurements were performed in the plane of curvature of the artery.

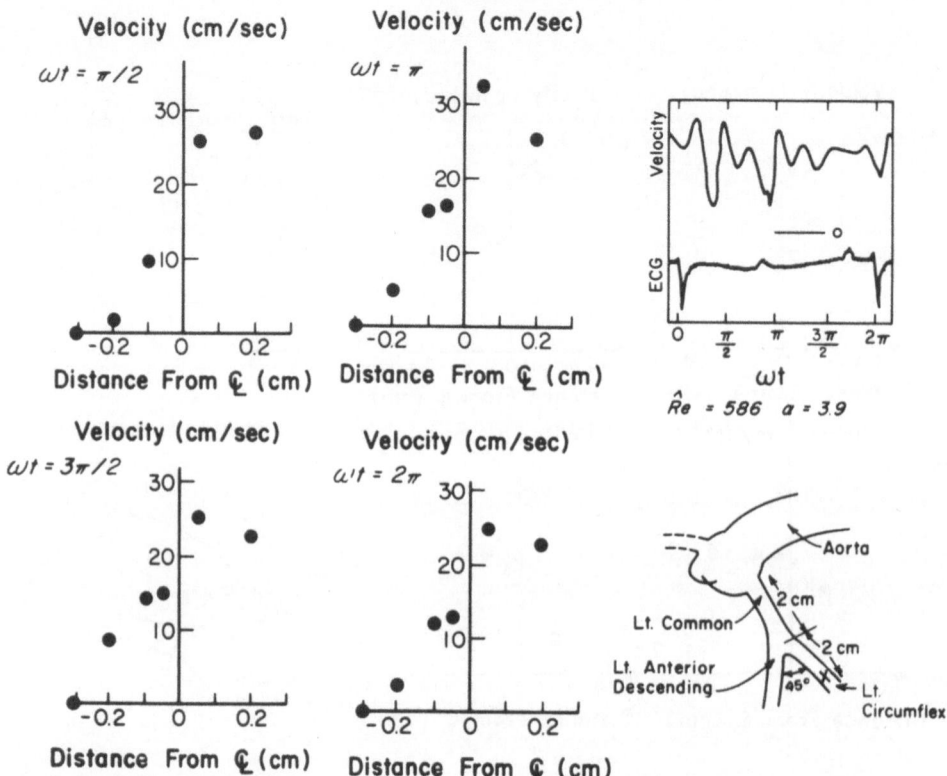

Fig. 7-29: Centerline velocity waveforms, ECG, and velocity profiles for the indicated times and location of measurement in the circumflex coronary artery of an anesthetized horse. Measurements were performed perpendicular to the plane of the bifurcation.

It also suggests that the highest shearing stress should be at the outside wall and not the inside wall, again in contradiction to what we think is the case for the aortic arch.

Now this is proximal to the bifurcation point. If you move distal to the bifurcation point, the picture does not change that much. As seen in Fig. 7-29 here again we have the bifurcation into the LAD and the left circumflex. Our probe is not now positioned perpendicular to the plane of bifurcation but coming in as much as possible at an angle so we can observe the effects of the flow being divided at the bifurcation. Ideally you would want to position the probe in the plane of the bifurcation, but we are only able to come in at about a 45 degree angle. The velocity profiles we have obtained do not suggest higher velocities being toward the flow divider side, but rather suggest that the higher velocities are away from the flow divider. Remember, we are not in the plane of bifurcation. We are not orthognal to that plane, but moving at about 45 degrees.

Furthermore, although you have the flow divider which would be expected to produce high velocities near that inside wall, at the same time you have a curving plane of bifurcation which is producing its own secondary flow effect. The net result is that the peak stress point quite possibly has been moved away from the flow divider to a slightly different position. There has been a rotation due to the combination of these two secondary flows of curvature effects.

I mentioned the fact that we see an interesting oscillation in the coronary system. Fig. 7-30 presents measurements in the left common coronary artery

Oscillation in the
Coronary System

of the horse, both with a hot-film placed at the center line of the vessel as well as with an electro-magnetic flow meter cuff. You can observe low frequency large amplitude oscillations which are present both on the hot-film and on the flow meter waveforms. We also see these oscillations in pressure waveforms, although the amplitude is somewhat suppressed there. However, if you take the pressure waveforms and try to compute a pressure gradient, then again one sees rather large amplitude oscillations which, of course, would have to be present in as much as the flow is pressure driven. As we move the probe across the lumen of the vessel, we see no change in the phase of these oscillations. Thus, the entire flow seems to be sloshing with this five to ten Hertze frequency.

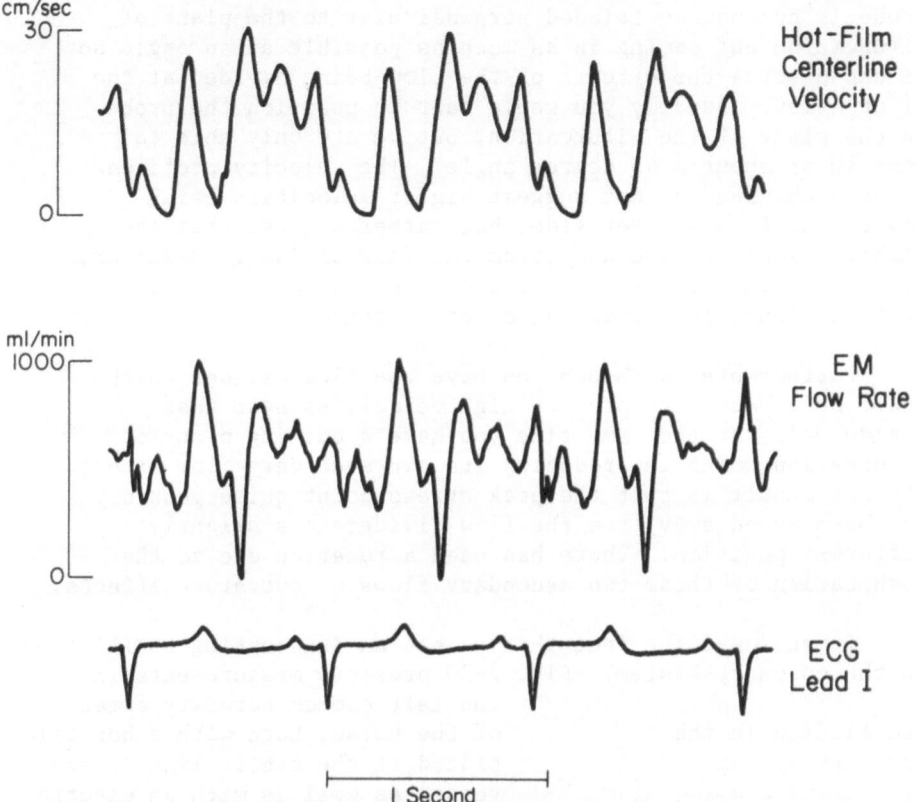

Fig. 7-30: Simultaneously measured centerline velocity waveform and electromagnetic flow meter waveform together with ECG for left anterior descending coronary artery in an anesthetized horse.

We believe that this is a reflection type phenomenon, some
type of resonance phenomenon, and to test this, we have
devloped a computer model which includes a number of nonlinear characteristics of the system, e.g. the wave speed
dependence on pressure and some of the elastic characteristics
of the wall. Fig. 7-31 shows a comparison between this
standard computer model and a flow measurement from a horse,   HORSE
the former using pressure measurements from the horse as
input to the computer program. The solid line is the experimental
data -- note again the oscillations, and the dashed line is
the computed waveform. Agreement is certainly not especially
good. However, we hope to be able to modify the program
systematically and parametrically to do better. One of the
things I need to point out is that with this computer program,
which in the diastolic region actually does a reasonable job
of predicting the oscillation characteristics, we can essentially
do a parametric investigation on the effect of size on this
typed phenomenon. What we find is that as one goes to
smaller and smaller animals, the frequency of the oscillations
increases slightly and the amplitude of the oscillations
decreases considerably. There is some evidence that oscillations
like these are present in dogs. Dali Patel at NIH has seen   DOG
oscillations in some animals. Heinz Pieper in our Physiology
Department at Ohio State, has seen oscillations in a number
of animals. Some of Gregg's classical waveforms also show
oscillations of this type. In the horse we see these oscillations
almost all of the time, while in smaller animals the amplitude
is less, as we predict with our computer model and the
observations are not as consistent. I think when you get
down to smaller animals as opposed to the horse, the presence
of such oscillations is very sensitive to the exact wave
speed associated with the coronary vessel or system.

DR. COX: Do you see these same kinds of oscillations
in the anterior descending coronary artery or only in the
left circumflex?

DR. NEREM: You see them also in the LAD and in the
circumflex.

DR. COX: What about the right artery?

DR. NEREM: We have not been over on the right side.

DR. COX: We see them always in the left circumflex
coronary, but very rarely in the anterior descending coronary.

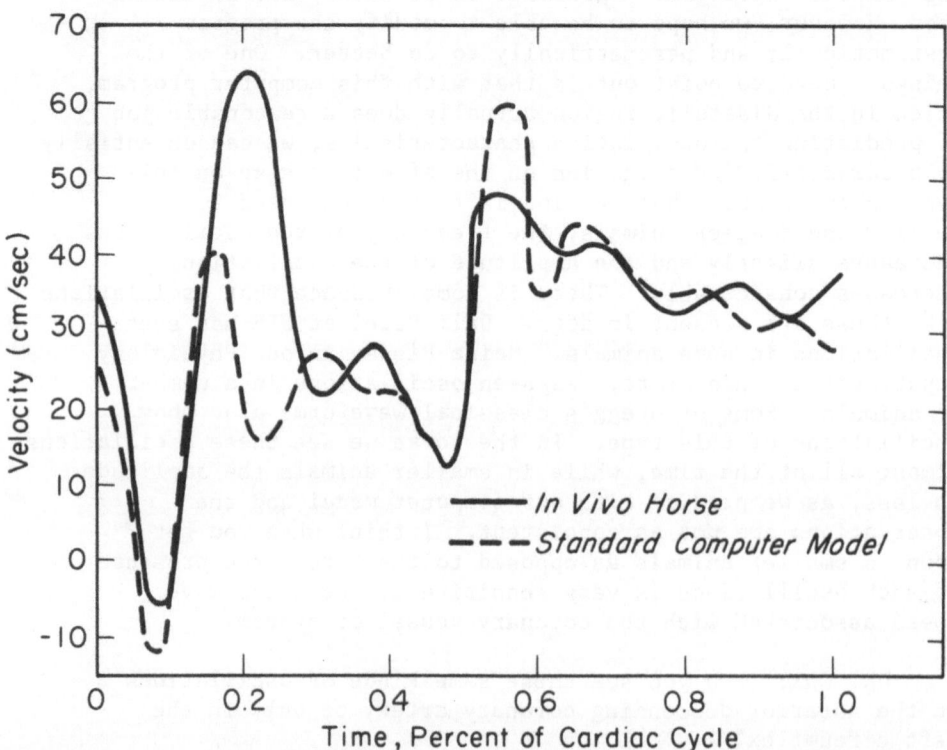

Fig. 7-31: Comparison of standard computer model calculation and
in vivo flow velocity measurement from a horse at a position 15 cm
distal to the left coronary ostium.

I am just wondering to what extent these oscillations may be related to compression by the cardiac muscle since there is a very large difference in the distribution of flow in the circumflex versus the anterior descending artery.

DR. NEREM: Our model allows for flow into branch vessels and we have parametrically varied that effect. It does not seem to have a major influence on the predicted oscillation characteristics. That is all I can say in response to your question.

DR. MANSFIELD: In man the right coronary is usually, not always—but usually, the dominant vessel as far as flow reception is concerned. The flows you are talking about on the left side are mainly diastolic flows. In the right coronary vessels there is relatively low pressure, and systolic. So where you find your oscillations will depend on the size of the vessel, the line of flow and whether they are systolic or diastolic.

DR. STONE: May I add to that. One difficulty with what you just said, which is true, is that the flow distribution from the right to the left side would be under the same physical principles as the left load. The flow penetration to the myocardium through that right artery will still be a diastolic component.

DR. MANSFIELD: The number in man is much smaller, it is only about 20% versus 80% of the flow in man going through the right coronary.

DR. STONE: I understand that, but what I am saying is that the flow distributed from the right coronary artery to the left ventricle to the posterior septal wall and the posterior ventricular wall, will be exposed to the same physical force as anything coming through the left side, so the flow penetration from right to left will still be diastolic.

DR. NEREM: Even though we do have turbulence, there are waveforms in the coronary system which can be very complicated and the flow that goes with them can be equally complicated. We have not investigated at all yet how certain pharmacologic interventions would affect such oscillatory activity. That is an area that Lowell Stone and I have talked about and think it would be well worth pursuing. If in fact as Dr. Dewey says the coronaries are where the action is in terms of ultimate pay-off, there is a lot of work for fluid mechanics researchers to do in terms of understanding better what is going on in that coronary vasculature.

Let us approach how fluid mechanics might interact with the endothelium. Fig. 7-32 is just one illustration of the atherogenic process and I do not want us to feel constrained by this particular series of events, but just to raise what I think is a very important question and one in which I know Dr. Werthessen

Two Types of Roles for
Hemodynamics or Fluid
Dynamics in Disease
Process

is interested. As you follow through with some disease process, starting with a normal intact endothelium and proceeding, we essentially can talk about two different types of roles for hemodynamics or fluid mechanics. One is in terms of primary endothelial damage. This could be a very traumatic insult to the system or it might be a different type of primary damage in the sense that, when we are talking about a disease that has a 40 year time course, primary damage presumably can be very subtle. However, at least one possibility is some way to have hemodynamic factors involved in the primary damage. The other possibility is that somehow hemodynamics gets involved in the wall's ability to respond to whatever insult has been provided it, e.g. that could be through some sort of platelet adhesion process such as I will talk about in a minute. But I do want to raise the question -- knowing we are not in a position to answer it today -- that hemodynamics, in general, even if it does play a role, and as I mentioned earlier the evidence is indirect, still could be either primary in nature or it could be a response type or mediating role. Now, let us talk briefly about some potential mechanisms through which hemodynamics could enter into the process.

We have all been talking about yield stresses, about a magic number of 400 dynes per square centimeter; in addition, Dr. Mansfield had some very interesting results from his studies on the influence of flow on the endothelium. One view is that in some way the flow irreversibly alters endothelial cells, that there is a primary physical insult to the endothelium that comes from the flow. The stress levels I mentioned earlier don't make this totally impossible. However, I would have to admit that my own feeling is that, for the kind of disease process about which we are talking, I would not vote for that one.

Beyond actual physical trauma, there is the whole area of mass transport.

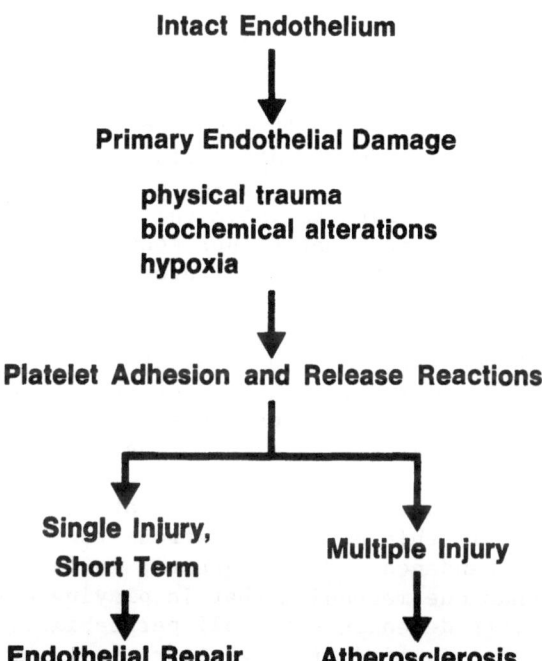

Fig. 7-32: Illustration of possible steps in atherogenic process.

There are a lot of materials moving in and out of the wall
and certainly fluid mechanics
Wall Permeability a can, in some way, play a role
Function of Wall Shear in accelerating or decelerating
Stress certain transport processes.
Now much of the emphasis has been
on the transport of cholesterol and lipoproteins. This
is true of the in vitro work, in which Dr. Caro and myself
(19) and also Dr. Carew (20) have been involved -- also some
of the work of Dr. Schwartz. We do not know the roles these
molecules play in the disease process, but it is still of
interest to study the transport problem. One of the things
that has been determined is that there is a dependence of
the transendothelial transport rate on the shear stress
applied to the endothelium. If you take all the available
data and try to correlate it into a single picture, you
obtain a pattern such as illustrated in Fig. 7-33 where the
wall permeability, a characteristic velocity for the wall
transport process in centimeters per second, is presented as
a function of wall shear stress. There are two points I
want to bring out here.

First, if you take the low shear stress data, i.e. the
work by Dr. Caro and myself and some of the later work,
there is a very weak shear stress dependence. If you talk
about the higher shear stress levels, the first piece of
work in this area was Dr. Carew's Ph.D. dissertation. We
have subsequently done some experiments at high shear stress
levels (21) and in this high shear stress region, there is a
much steeper dependence. This suggests, in fact, that there
may be more than one mechanism that is playing a role in
this shear stress dependence of wall permeability. So we
need to bear that in mind, that whether these shear dependent
transport processes are intrinsic to the disease process is
really open for question at this point.

Now the other point I want to make is that the transition
from one type of shear stress dependence to another type of
shear stress dependence occurs
Pulsatile Shifts from around 50 dynes per square
Low to High Shear Stress centimeter. Based on my values
for the level of shear stress
in the vascular system, it would appear that the mean shear
stress corresponds to the low shear stress dependence region.
However, as the flow pulses, at least in the aorta and
certain regions of the coronary system, the shear stress
moves up into the high shear stress dependence region.

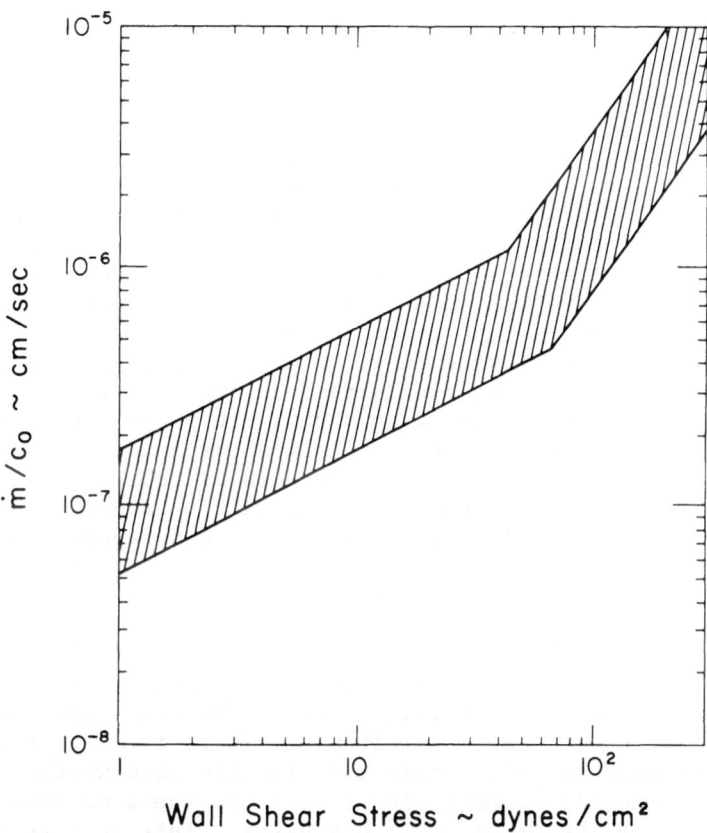

Fig. 7-33: Illustration of shear stress dependence of wall permeability (m/C_O) to blood–arterial wall macromolecule transport; m, wall transport rate, and C_O, blood concentration.

So you are moving back and forth from a low shear stress to
a high shear stress dependence, and if there are two different
mechanisms involved here, then you are moving from one type
of shear stress influence to another type of shear stress
influence and back again as the flow pulses. Some of the
experiments we have carried out -- as well as those by
others in this area too -- suggest that the arterial wall is
in fact very sensitive to flow pulsations. To quickly
sketch an experiment that we completed approximately nine
months ago (22), we were interested in the transport of
serum cholesterol into the arterial wall for pulsatile flow
conditions. This was an in vitro experiment using excised
carotid arteries. ^{14}C cholesterol was introduced into the
serum and we used that tagged molecule to measure the transendothelial transport rate -- not looking at wall concentration
gradients, as Dr. Colton quite correctly has suggested we
should start doing, but just looking at a total wall uptake.
It is purely an oscillating flow. There is no mean flow at
all. In that oscillating flow situation, we find that the
rate of wall uptake of this tagged cholesterol molecule is
dependent on both the frequency of pulsation and the amplitude
of pulsation. In fact, however, the data all correlate with
peak shear stress, i.e., one can collapse the frequency
dependence and the amplitude dependence into a dependence on
peak shear stress --actually peak shear rate -- which gives
results which are quite consistent with the steady flow
experiments summarized earlier. Now as you can see in Fig. 7-34
there is considerable scatter in the data, and yet there is
still an unmistakable trend that the wall permeability is a
function of the wall shear rate. As may be seen, this is
true both for cholesterol and albumin. There is a definite
shear dependence of wall uptake even in this case where
there is absolutely no mean flow at all and where we have
oscillations on the order of 1 to 4 Hertz. This is a relatively
low frequency, but on the same order as some of those oscillations
I showed earlier in the coronary system.

So much for transport phenomena; now let us talk about
some other possible mechanisms through which hemodynamics
might play a role.

Actually the next one I'll mention is a transport
process also. I don't know whether Dr. Dewey and I can agree
on this one, or may be we
would agree and that agreement
would be in disagreement with the
investigators who are working
specifically in this field.

Hypoxia--Diffusion
of Oxygen through
Blood to the Wall

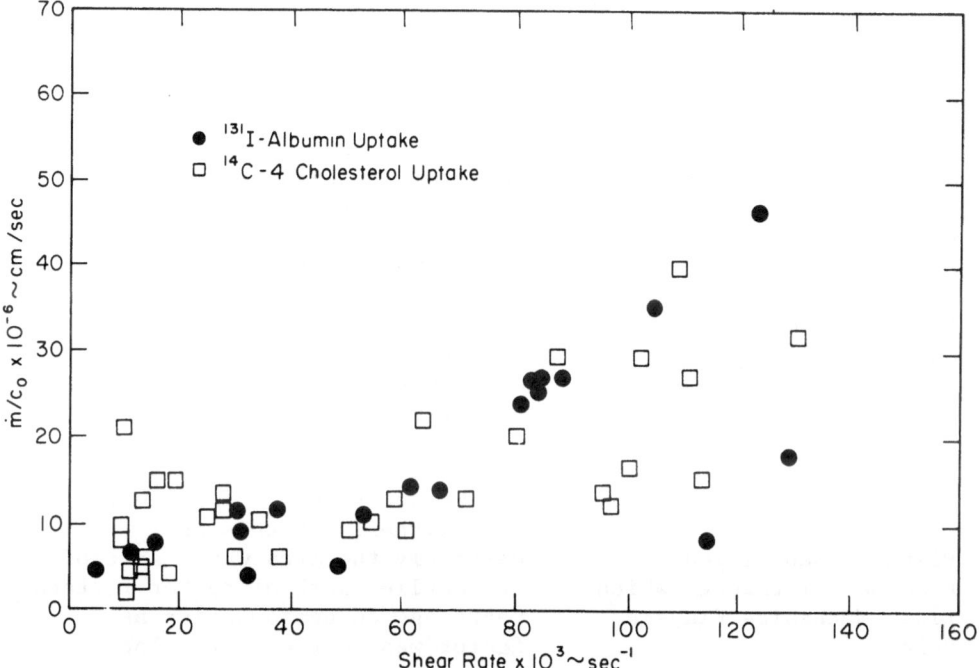

Fig. 7-34: Wall permeability (m/C$_O$) for the transport of
^{14}C-4-cholesterol and ^{131}I-albumin in serum perfused carotid
arteries as a function of peak wall shear rates; m, wall
transport rate, and C$_o$, serum concentration (from Mack, 1975).

However, there is a sizeable effort out at U.S.C., as part of
their atheroscleorsis project, to look at hypoxia, particularly
in terms of hemodynamics playing a role. In other words, it
is their contention that the rate limiting step in the
transport of oxygen to tissue is not the movement of oxygen
through the tissue, but the diffusion of oxygen through
blood to the wall. Back (23) has made estimates of the
resistance on the plasma side of the interface versus the
wall side of the interface, and has come up with a ratio on
the order of a factor of two. I think it is a very preliminary
estimate, and I will say that the few oxygen tension measurements
through the wall with which they have been able to compare
their calculations are in agreement. I do not think we can,
at least on the evidence we now have, discount the possibility
of fluid mechanics influencing oxygen transport and playing
a role in hypoxia such as Dr. Smith suggested. Here I am
suggesting, however, that in addition to looking at how far
a location in the wall is removed from the endothelium, we
also need to look at transport characteristics in the plasma,
particularly where there are separated flow regions. Although
some separated flow regions would be very highly disturbed
and one would expect very good mixing, I am not sure that
this is true of all separated flow regions, for example the
outside wall in the region of a bifurcation. So, I think
hypoxia is a possible mechanism through which fluid mechanics
could exert an influence and which cannot be discounted.

Platelet deposition is another mechanism through which
fluid mechanics can play a role. We don't know a lot about
this either, but this is
certainly the area where some of
the earlier work of ten or fifteen
years ago on hemodynamics as a
factor was carried out. The
hypothesis is that flow somehow
influences the deposition and adhesion of platelets to the
wall and that when the wall has been insulted, it is not a
question of where the insult occurs, but where hemodynamics
will preferentially allow platelets to interact with the
wall and which thus determines the pattern of the disease.
Many of you know of the work of Perry Blackshear's group at
the University of Minnesota, and based on an admittedly
specific model as to how platelets get to the wall, they
predict that platelets will deposit on the wall based on a
parameter which involves the wall shear rate (24). This
parameter involves the shear rate in the denominator.

**Platelet Deposition:
A Mechanism through which
Fluid Mechanics Plays a
Role**

Thus, low shear regions correspond to a large value of this parameter, and on this basis they hypothesize that low shear regions are the ones where you will find the disease developing because that is where platelets will preferentially deposit and interact.

DR. CARO: There is a requirement for a very substantial filtering.

DR. NEREM: Yes, it includes filtering of fluid through the wall. That is correct. There is one other possibility that I will mention. Markle and Hollis at Penn State (25) have been doing some work in which they have been looking at shear stress and its influence on albumin uptake. They also have been looking at the effect of shear stress on aortic wall histamine synthesis and they find a relationship that we are totally in the dark about at this point that suggests a different way for fluid mechanics to play a role. One could hypothesize, purely for the sake of argument, that one way wall permeability gets changed with wall shear stress is that the shear stress induces aortic histamine synthesis which alters the wall permeability. In other words, it is this biochemical step which is influencing wall permeability. I am not here to either support or detract from any such an hypothesis, but only to suggest that there are a lot of things that we don't know anything about in terms of a hemodynamic influence and that is a definite possibility. This also raises questions about other kinds of influences on the biochemistry of the artery that might be present. How does the wall respond to stresses that are imposed on it? Is it just a mechanical response or is there something else? Some of Dr. Smith's comments -- certainly in terms of collagen synthesis -- would suggest that the wall does respond in a chemical or metabolic way. So the question, or at least another question, is through which of these mechanisms, or through whichever other mechanisms we have not identified yet, does hemodynamics play a role in the disease process?

Aortic Histamine Synthesis Alters Wall Permeability

I now come back to the following question: In terms of the coronary system, where does atherosclerosis first develop? For example, in a region of a bifurcation, is it on the flow divider? If so, is that because of high shear stresses that are denuding the endothelium?

Where does Atherosclerosis First Develop?

Is it because of increased synthesis of histamine? Or, in
fact, does it start first on the outside of the wall? If it
is on the outside wall, it makes a big difference as to
whether this outside wall is slightly upstream or slightly
downstream. This is because there is possibly a separated
flow region and this has certain implications in terms of
the various types of mechanisms I have talked about. If it
is slightly downstream and in fact is in the region where
this separated flow is now re-attaching, then this is where
high shear stresses would be expected to occur. So there
are some basic questions about the pattern of the disease
that do relate to a mechanistic point of view.

The same question can be raised about regions of sharp
curvature in the coronary system. Of course in comparing
the coronary system with the aortic arch it must be remembered
that we expect in the left common coronary artery, based on
HORSE our horse experiments, that the higher shear stress will be
on the outside wall, and yet in the aortic arch we expect
the higher shear stress to be on the inside wall.

But where in fact does atherogenesis initiate and, of
course, what mechanisms then seem viable? And then finally
I bring us back to the earlier illustration of the pattern
of the disease. What are we talking about when we attempt to
explain this pattern? People like myself would like to
believe that we are talking about local flow details; however,
as I mentioned earlier those local flow details could very
well be determined by regulatory mechanisms. If we consider
the major left side coronary branch, how much of the flow
goes the circumflex route versus the LAD route? The answer
depends very much on peripheral resistance and how that flow
is going to divide. Of course, maybe it is not a hemodynamic
problem; maybe it is a hemostatic problem and it is just the
basic pressure loading on the system with stress concentration
in regions of certain types of geometry and where certain
types of tethering are important. I guess all I can do is
add to the list of questions and hopefully stimulate some
discussion.

DR. WERTHESSEN: In your Fig. 7-34 you showed the
predisposition of various areas of the vessel to become
                                        atherosclerotic. Haimovici did
Haimovici's Translocation   the classic experiment of
Experiment   switching sections of the dogs'
                                        aorta around (26). Then he put
the dog on atherogenic diet.

The visceral section which is predisposed in the normal animal, remained predisposed even when in the chest. I have a hunch that with the improved technology available today, you could do some really beautiful experiments.

It is also true that there is a drastic difference in the biochemical aptitude, if I can use that term, along the length of the aorta. For example, in both swine and bovine aortas, there is a 10% difference in concentration of cholesterol between the aorta and the bifurcation. There is also a wide range of change along the aorta in its biosynthetic capacities. Those differences could provide fluid dynamicists today with today's surgical technology, the means to do some critical experiments. You can take out a patch and put it somewhere else and see how it misbehaves or rearranges its metabolism to fit its altered location.

DR. SMITH: I am interested in Dr. Werthessen's description of Haimovici's translocation experiment, because working constantly with human aorta one is enormously impressed by the different type of lesion that is developing in the lower abdominal aorta compared with the thoracic and upper abdominal aorta. It is certainly a more fatty lesion, it is very different in character, so I think that this translocation experiment is extremely interesting and I do think that you are right and that this could very usefully be studied further. Now this raises a whole lot of problems.

One of the things we looked at some years ago was the relative concentrations of intact LDL in different segments of the aorta. These had very clear distribution. If we took the upper abdominal as 100% the thoracic segment was somewhere around 150% and the abdominal segment about 95%. So, in fact, the retention of lipoprotein was lowest in the abdominal segment and highest in the thoracic segment (27). One tends on the whole to get large fibrous plaques in the thoracic segment and these very insidious fatty type plaques in the lower segment.

Translocation Experiment Raises Many Problems

Another question. All this beautiful work on vesicular transport and yet nobody, as far as I can see, knows what the condition of the endothelium in the middle aged human is. Do we, in fact, actually have a beautiful endothelium as has been shown in the experimental animals?

Or, by middle age have we got an endothelium that is pretty
fatty so that there is passage of lipoprotein between cells
as well as vesicular transport? I don't know how this
question can be answered but it seems to me that it is
extremely relevant when one is thinking of the endothelial
barrier. And going back again to the transposed aorta it
seems to me that it is extraordinarily difficult to isolate
the structure from atherosclerosis. I suppose that these
were adult dogs that Haimovici was using; if you did this to
a newborn puppy and let the animal grow up with this patch
and after it was fully grown fed it cholesterol, I wonder
what you would get then? This brings me around to Dr.
Meyer's work. Dr. Nerem and I tried to do a joint exercise
to see if we could decide where the lesions developed at the
bifurcation. So far the results have been so complicated
that we have not been able to arrive at an answer.

DR. CARO: What bifurcation was this?

DR. SMITH: The iliac bifurcation. The wall is different
around the iliacs, and you have thin patches and thick
patches. Are these really innate structural differences or
are they early atheroma? How do they influence atheroma
development? This is extremely relevant at branching
points where the whole architecture of the underlying vessel
is changed. I find it extremely difficult to know whether
an intimal cushion is atherosclerosis or architecture.
Quite apart from the fluid dynamics, we do not even know
what the actual structure itself is doing?

DR. MANSFIELD: A couple of points about the translocation
experiments. It is a very interesting way of going at it.
You have significantly altered the segment that you are
talking about and when you have denervated it because you
have removed it from its initial nervous connection, you
have also removed at least the common pathways in the vasa
vasorum in that area when you are translocating, for example,
from the abdominal aorta to the thoracic aorta. So I think
you have to be very careful in terms of your interpretation
of what you find. It is not at all infrequent as you may
see, for example, clinically to take an artery from one area
and move it to another. For example, the hypogastric artery
moved up and used as a bypass for the renal artery, the flow
going to each of these then becomes different and it is a
denervated segment and it does tend to get quite atherosclerotic
and dilated with time, but it does not tend to obliterate
its lumen, although it may increase its size three and four
fold.

Why this should occur under certain circumstances we really
cannot explain. But part of it is probably due to the fact
that we have changed the base line and we have denervated a
segment. These are important considerations when we are
doing that type of experiment.

DR. WERTHESSEN: Do these transplants ever become
innervated? Have you been able to check? The reason I
asked is that we have data that indicates that denervating
the artery alters lipid metabolism (28).

DR. MANSFIELD: I would not be surprised. Reinnervation
has not been thoroughly studied. You can demonstrate,
however, that the vessels can respond locally to drugs.

DR. MALLIANI: We should indicate that atherogenesis is
likely to be the result of very many different processes,
different in the various species and in the various types of
patients. In others words, a kind of common end point for
different pathways. In addition, it is obvious that in the
course of decades of life the multiple factors may variously
act at different times.

DR. BJORKERUD: Dr. Smith suggested possible presence of
injured endothelium and/or changed endothelium in the artery
segments of human arteries obtained at surgery and kept
alive in tissue culture medium for a short time. We stained
the specimens by a technique which is rather similar to the
one used in the tissue cultures to indicate decreased viability,
the so-called dye exclusion technique. We tried a lot of
stains for this purpose and found the stereo isomer Trypan
Blue, Evans blue to be most suitable. Fig. 7-35, shows a
segment from a human femoral artery cut open; the blue spots
are endothelial cells that cannot exclude the stain, i.e.
they are, to some extent, injured. Interestingly, there are
fewer injured cells around the orifice of a branch which is
difficult to reconcile, I think, with current hemodynamic
concepts. The explanation could be that the branches constitute
a source of new endothelium for areas in the major vessel
subject to severe strain.   Another thing which is interesting
and should be emphasized is that more visible (i.e. stainable)
lipid is present in areas with intact endothelium. However,
this is histochemically stained lipid. As measured with
chemical methods there is much more lipid in areas with
injured endothelium. I think one should keep this paradox
in mind when interpreting histological slides, because
strong lipid staining does not necessarily mean there is
more lipid there.

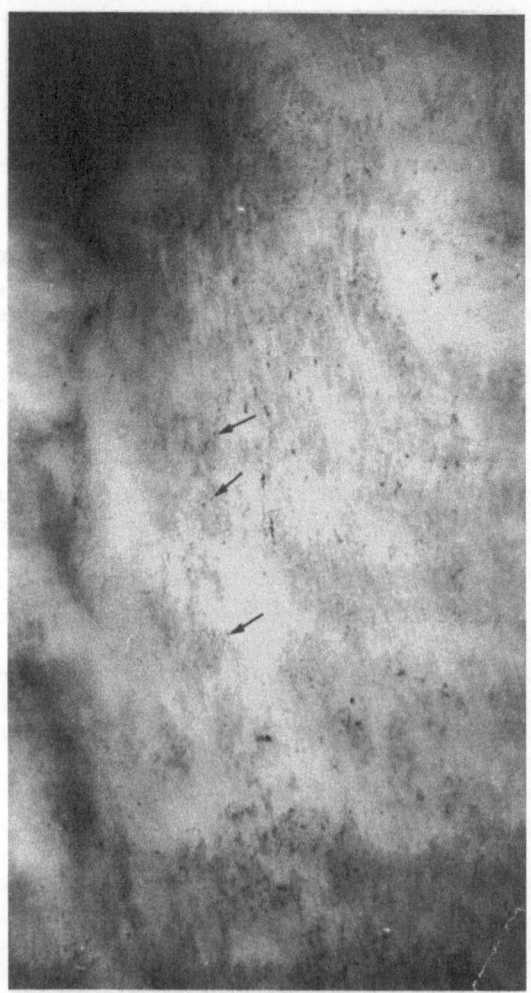

Fig. 7-35: View of inner surface of an area of a segment of
the femoral artery from a 36-year-old man. The leg was removed
for clinical reasons and the artery subjected to dye exclusion
test with uncomplexed Evans blue immediately after excision.
The black spots (arrows) are nuclei of injured endothelial
cells which take up the stain. Uninjured endothelium does not
stain and appears white. In the upper left corner is the
opening of a small branch. Ca. 40 X.

I want to make a comment on what Dr. Nerem said. Is endothelial injury really something of importance or is it a secondary rather unimportant factor as compared to classical atherogenic factors such as hypercholesterolemia? If endothelial integrity changes from the most integrated endothelium to the most disintegrated endothelium which we find in the normal non-manipulated rabbit, we find an increase of lipoprotein transfer -- as evaluated from transfer of labelled cholesterol ester, of about 4 times. If we denude endothelium, i.e. we create a situation with minimal endothelial integrity. The transfer is about 30 times higher. These figures should be compared with the ca. 10 times increase of lipoprotein transfer which occurs when altering the serum cholesterol level in the rabbit from ca. 50 mg% to 400 mg% (29). This might indicate that the state of the endothelium as influenced by mechanical factors may be as important as lipoprotein abnormalities in atherogenesis.

Mechanical Factors may be as Important as Lipoprotein Abnormalities in Atherogenesis

DR. COLTON: What was the label of cholesterol you used?

DR. BJORKERUD: It was tritiated cholesterol.

DR. COLTON: How was that incorporated into the lipoprotein?

DR. BJORKERUD: We labeled the lipoproteins with the technique described by Whereat and Staple (30). This technique has been shown not to denature the lipoproteins.

DR. COLTON: Did you determine the extent to which you had labeled cholesterol ester and free cholesterol?

DR. BJORKERUD: Yes. The radioactivity was rather evenly distributed between the d- and the combined B- and pre -B fractions at all time intervals tested during 24 hours after the injection.

DR. CARO: It would seem entirely analogous to what Dr. Fry and we find, something like a six to ten fold increase in flux when the vessel is denuded of endothelial cells. On the other hand, I do not think this helps to answer the question of what happens in an experiment of twenty years duration.

DR. TAYLOR: I will review two phenomena of arteriosclerosis and arterial repair which, in the main, defy teleological explanations.

1. The immunity of healed intimal arterial scars to fatty
atherosclerotic deposits baffles me; these intimal scars
                            must have first healed in
Immunity of Healed   animals with normally low serum
Arterial Scars to   lipid levels. My co-workers and
Atherosclerosis   I, did such a study in 1963 (31);
                            this study was done in monkeys.
Review of the literature, in depth, revealed that a similar
phenomenon had been observed in rabbits in 1929 (32).
Interestingly after damaged arterial scars had been permitted
to heal for 3 months and animals were then made hypercholesterolemic, those portions of arteries with no healed scars were
highly susceptible to atherosclerosis whereas the scars that
had healed while serum lipid levels were normal were immune
to lipid deposits (atherosclerosis).

2. In 1960 Economou et al., (33) produced aortic injury in
dogs by employing several methods. Two methods resulted in
                                    central and/or external medial
Restoration of Functional   damage with no injury to the inner
Vascular Tissue   media, internal elastic membrane,
                                    subendothelial space and endothelium
  Fig. 7-36 injection of Urokon (70% acetizoate) into central
media, and Fig. 7-37 excision of the outer 1/2 to 2/3 of
the aortic media. In both of these types of aortic injury
there was no reparative reaction and aneurysms present at
the time of surgery, still persisted 30 weeks later, Fig. 7-38.
Two different forms of injury resulted in damage to the
subendothelium and inner media Fig. 7-39 transmural freezing
of the entire aortic wall, (33) and Fig. 7-40 - surgical
removal (employing a cork borer) of the endothelium, subendothelium
and internal elastic membrane and inner media. Within 6
weeks the aneurysms produced by transmural freezing Fig. 7-39
or excision of the inner media, subendotehlium and endothelium
Fig. 7-40 were completely healed by the proliferation of new
vascular tissue. In a third study we removed about 1/2 of
the outer media then tramsmurally killed all medial cells
of 1/2 of the aneurysmal lesion by hypothermal injury Fig. 7-41
and diagrammatically shown in Fig. 7-39 and illustrated in
the photomicrograph Fig. 7-42   Only the transmurally frozen
half of the lesion had a reparative intimal scar and half
its aneurysmal dilatation had been corrected Figs. 7-41 & 42.
Our group concluded that in order for completely restorative
arterial repair to occur the subendothelial space and internal
elastic membrane must be stimulated by injury; we feel that
there are multipotential cells in the subendothelial space
which respond to injury by rapid proliferation and formation
of new elastic, collagen and smooth muscle cells to restore
an adequate quantity of functional vascular tissue.

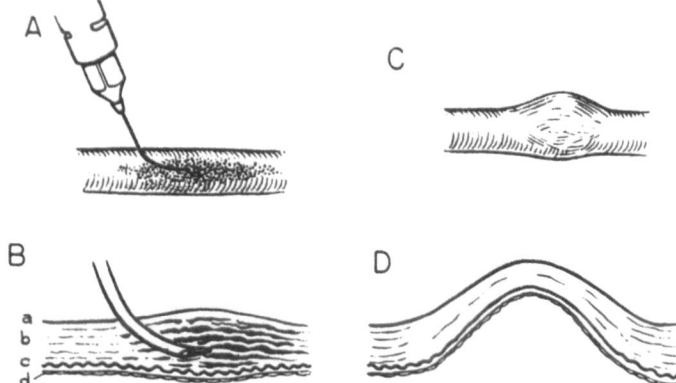

Fig. 7-36: Diagrammatic illustration of method of intramural injection of 70 per cent acetrizoate. A. A 45 degree curve in the needle makes it easier to maintain the orifice of the needle in an intramural position. B. The contrast material dissects laterally and separates the elastic lamellae. a. Adventitia; b. media; c. internal elastic membrane; d. endothelium. C. Aneurysmal dilatation observed as early as 3 weeks after intramural injection of the contrast material. D. Microscopically there is destruction of the central portion of the media. There is no apparent injury to the internal elastic membrane and sub-endothelial layer. No subendothelial reparative scar was noted as long as 30 weeks after intramural injection of Urokon (acetrizoate).

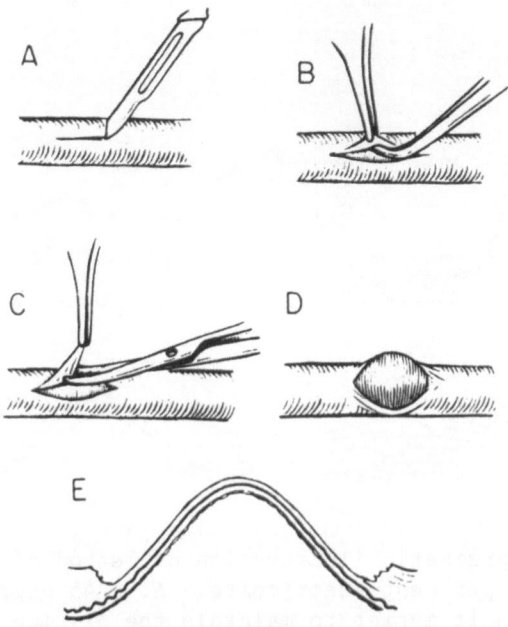

Fig. 7-37: Diagrammatic presentation of formation of aneurysm
by stripping of outer 70 per cent of the media. A. With gentle
strokes of the scalpel the desired depth of dissection is
reached. B and C, at the depth of the incision the media could
be peeled along a cleavage plane. An elipse of the dissected
media is exised, allowing full development of the aneurysm.
D. With removal of more than 70 per cent of the media, acute
rupture of the resultant aneurysm occurred. E. Aneurysmal
formation showing stretching of internal elastic membrane.
Even though 70 per cent of the media had been removed without
injury to the subjendothelial space and internal elastic
membrane, there was not reparative response.

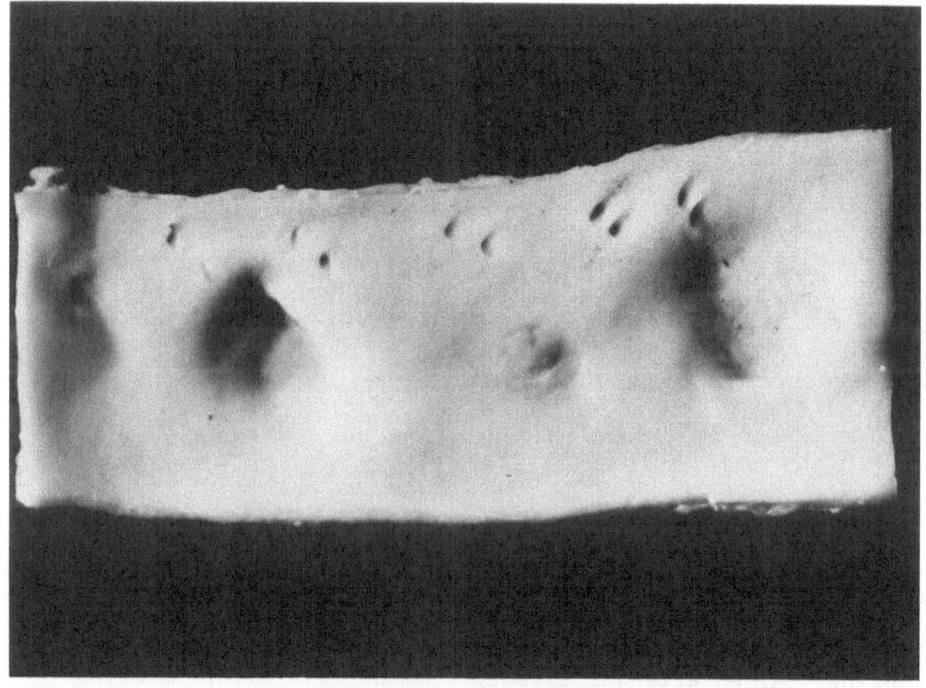

Fig. 7-38: Persistent aortic aneurysms in dogs abdominal
aorta 30 weeks after surgical removal of 70 per cent of outer
media and adventitia. Aorta has been opened longitudinally
and shows intimal surface.

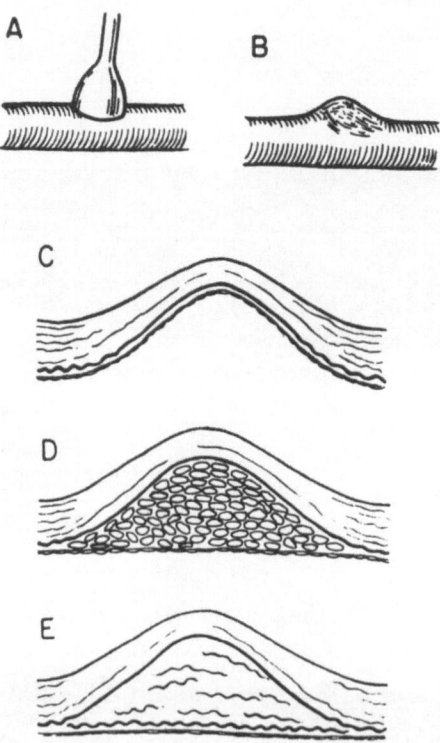

Fig. 7-39: Diagrammatic illustrations of effect of transmural
freezing, (A) on arterial tissue. Immediately after freezing
aneurysm develops at site of freezing (b) and persists for
several weeks. C. Illustrates straightening and disruption
of elastic lamellae and dissolution of killed cells in area
frozen. During the first 2 weeks there was not proliferation
of multipotential subendothelial cells (C); however, during
the third week these cells proliferated abundantly and
essentially filled the aneurysmal defect (D). The multipotential cells differentiated and formed an essentially new
vascular wall at about the sixth week (E), after 6 weeks mature
cells and new elastic and collagen fibers have restored the
artery to its original caliber and repaired the aneurysm.

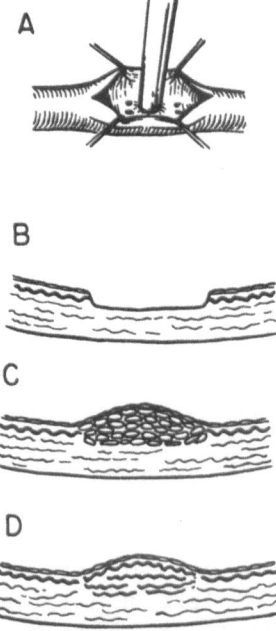

Fig. 7-40: Diagrammatic illustration of response of aorta to
stripping of endothelium and subjacent elastic lamella. A
shallow circular cut is made by gently rotating a 1/2 inch
diameter cork borer (A). Endothelium, subendothelium, and
internal elastic membrane are then dissected away leaving
shallow circular defect (B). As shown in C at about 3 weeks a
thick tuft of subendothelial cells and a thin layer of endothelial
cells cover the defect. At about 6 weeks the intimal scar
covering the small area of injury has differentiated into mature
vascular scar tissue with elastic and collagen fibers (D).

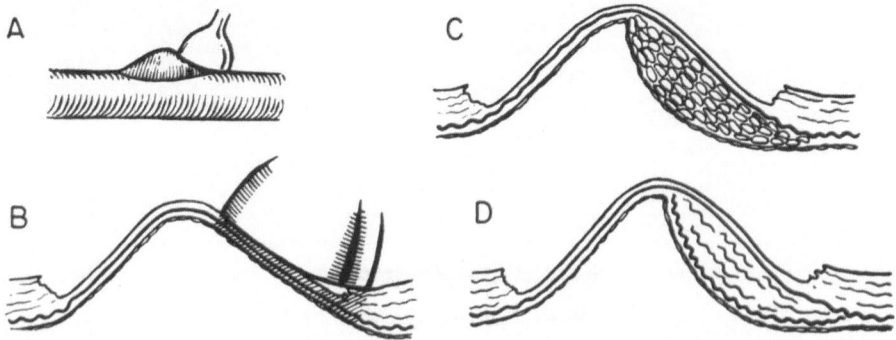

Fig. 7-41: A and B, transmural freezing of one-half of aneurysm
which had been produced by excision of 70 per cent of outer
media. The other half was left undisturbed. C. Whereas there
was no reparative process in the portion of the aneurysm which
was left undisturbed, there was brisk proliferation of subendothelial cells in the portion of the aneurysm that had been
transmurally frozen. D. The multipotential subendothelial cells
have differentiated and formed an essentially new arterial wall
in a thickened intima at the site of transmural freezing.

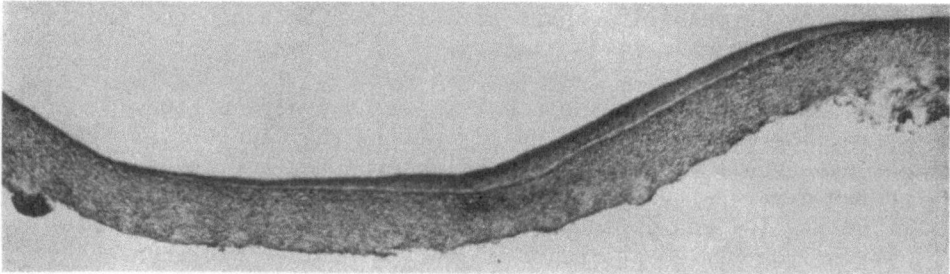

Fig. 7-42: Photomicrograph of Weigert's elastic tissue stain of
lesion produced by excision of outer media. Cut ends of outer
elastic lamellae are visible on the lower surface of the aorta
near each lateral margin of the photograph. After excision of
the outer media two-thirds of the aorta on the right was
trasmurally frozen; 2 months later this right-hand portion of
the aneurysm showed a thick intimal scar containing a rich
elastic network. The aneurysmal dilatation on this side of
the aneurysm was markedly corrected by this intimal scar.

DR. SCHWARTZ: Dr. Bjorkerud has shown something very
important, I think. The hypercholesterolemic effects on
                                    endothelium are probably
Hypercholesterolemic   terribly important; they occur
Effects on Endothelium   at very low levels before any
                                    significant hypercholesterolemia
has in fact occurred. We, like yourself, have demonstrated
very marked increases in the influx of protein into the arterial
PIG wall in hypercholesterolemia in the pig. Stefanovitch and Gore
RABBIT have done this in the rabbit with iodinated albumin (35).
The influence of very minor elevations in the serum cholesterol
level in a matter of days or weeks produced a spectrum of
changes in endothelial ultrastructure. I think this is a
point which is perhaps not appreciated, and it appears that
hypercholesterolemia is producing in the human an enhanced
level of permeability, part of which may be accounted for on
the basis of endothelial injury.

DR. LEE: In this connection we have done a study on
thymidine incorporation and mitosis in the endothelial cell
RABBIT of the rabbit after feeding cholesterol for one day and
three days. After three days of cholesterol feeding, the
labeling indices of endothelial cells doubled from 1/2 of
1% to 1 or 2%. This indicates that certain rapid changes
are taking place in the arterial wall including endothelial
cells. The increased mitosis and labeling indices indicated
that some endothelial cells are dying and being replaced at
a faster rate. As I mentioned earlier, after the dead
endothelial cells are washed away into the bloodstream and
before the denuded vascular surface is covered again,
noxious blood constituents would have an easier access to
subendothelial spaces through these denuded areas.

DR. SMITH: I want to comment on these very short term
effects; I have already referred to a paper by Day and
Proudlock (36) showing greatly increased cholesterol esterification
just three days after feeding cholesterol. In those three
RABBIT days, the rabbit's cholesterol went from something like 70
mg% to something over 400 mg%. And when you get this extraordinary
change in environment, I wonder whether one can relate it to
the sort of thing that might happen to you and me. I cannot
imagine any situation by which I could put my cholesterol up
seven fold in three days.

DR. LEE: I have to correct my earlier statement. I
said that we have carried out thymidine incorporation and
mitosis studies in rabbits.

This statement is not correct; the animal we used for those
studies was young swine and it was not rabbits. The serum   RABBIT
cholesterol level of control swine was around 90 mg% and it
increased to approximately 150 mg% after three days of   PIG
cholesterol feeding.

DR. SCHWARTZ: Do the ultrastructural changes also
occur without any marked increase in the circulating cholesterol?

DR. LEE: Right. In the early stages of atherosclerosis
in these swine, the pre-proliferative phase of atherosclerosis,
we have observed certain ultrastructural changes including
more frequent dead or dying cells and necrotic debris in the
media of the aorta. These findings suggest that some active
metabolic changes are taking place in the arterial wall even
in the very early stages.

DR. BJORKERUD: As related to what Dr. Schwartz said
about the relationship between endothelium integrity and r-
lipoproteins, HDL; we had a series of rabbits which were   RABBIT
kept at a constant serum cholesterol level for about a year.
We dosed the cholesterol individually as guided by the
individual serum cholesterol levels in each specific animal.
We had obtained levels which were rather constant which is
similar to the situation in the human being. Interestingly
enough, in the animals below about 350 mg% of cholesterol in
serum the integrity of the endothelium was largely unchanged.
Above a level of ca. 350 mg% the integrity of the endothelium
seemed to decrease.

DR. CARO: Margot Roach at Houston, at the Cardiovascular
Fluid Mechanics course last November, reported on some
volunteers who were starved, as I recall it, for several
days and then ate several eggs and bacon and it seems their
serum cholesterol rose from a hundred to many hundreds mg%.
I think she mentioned the number 800 mg/100 ml.

DR. DEWEY: There are at least two very disturbing
pieces of information that have come out of this conference
and that have been subliminally
plaguing me for several years. I
would like to pose this as a
question. What is the relationship
between animal experiments and
human conditions? Dr. Mansfield very subtly touched on the
differences in the endothelial cell, from site to site
within man or differences between one animal species and
another.

What is the Relationship
between Animal Experiments
and Human Conditions?

And I find this very disturbing, if we expect the endothelial
cell to be an important element in the whole process that we
are looking at.

The second disturbing fact is the difficulty which
exists in trying to infer natural disease-producing mechanisms

Inference of Natural
Disease-Producing
Mechanisms for Trials
in Animals

from intervention trials in
animals. If you take data from
experimental animals--coarctation
experiments for example--one sees
the flow dividers will be spared
in certain circumstances in test
animals such as dogs' can one then apply that knowledge to the
human circulation? So I pose this as an open question:
What should we do? Should we try to duplicate human physiology
or do experiments we feel relevant, in a very strict sense,
to the human condition? Or should we attempt to understand
animals and animal conditions where we have more access to
details of the biochemistry and the physiology and the
uptake for example, for the various labeled materials in the
arterial wall? It seems to me that this is a very real
problem.

DR. NEREM: I will respond in two ways, Dr. Dewey.
First, I think many of us have felt for a long time that

High Shear and Low Shear

talk about high shear and low
shear was almost irrelevant in
the sense that one had to speak
in the context of a particular position in the vascular system.
What is high shear one place, may be low shear some place else.
Because whatever way shear is entering into the process, it
makes a difference in terms of how it relates to the wall

Shear & Relation to
Biochemistry

biochemistry and that is critical,
the balance between the various
steps involved. One situation may
require a different level of
shear than another--assuming that shear is a factor. There
is a more general problem. I feel we need basic data independent
of whether they are related to the disease or not. I don't
know whether people working on vesicular transport are
really working on the right thing, but I think that is a
process that we need to study in order to understand this
whole area of the dynamics of arterial flow.

DR. WEINBAUM: What is your intuition at this time,
Dr. Schwartz, as to the relationship of your short term
studies to either the formation of fatty lesions, or to the
development of early lesions?

I think we could eventually understand your experiments, but it is the gap between short term experiments and the actual disease process that is the big mystery.

DR. SCHWARTZ: I quite frankly can't answer that. We have to be able to answer numerous biologically-oriented questions that relate to the different components of the process, including vesicular transport, mechanisms of endothelial injury, modifications to endothelial structure and so on. Intuitively one has the feeling that transport of certain macromolecules into the vessel wall may be very important, and that certain hemodynamic factors may modify transport rates and/or fixation of these molecules in the arterial wall. Even to cope with the problem of getting macromolecules in or out of a vessel is a significant issue and to extrapolate further to the details of atherogenesis is a tall order. We do know that certain areas with arterioles as delineated by the uptake of Evans Blue, have abnormal transport rates, and a wide variety of other differences. We also know from Dr. Fry's data that lesions occur preferentially at these sites. These sites differ metabolically, using a wide variety of labeled precursors, and in their response to insulin. Additionally, in early hypercholesterolemia there is an accelerated rate of accumulation of lipids in blue areas relative to white areas. While I believe that blue areas are pre-lesion sites, the sequence of events leading to the established atheromatous lesion is complex and not fully understood.

DR. CARO: We must appreciate that for material entering the artery wall there are a number of resistances arranged in series, and we lack the information at present to assess their significance. Thus, whether an area is 'blue' or 'white,' in relation to Evans Blue labeled albumin, may be of no significance in a transport process with a time scale of thirty or forty years. Nonetheless, I think we should continue to study the basic biology, for example endothelial cell pinocytosis, because it may have great relevance to some other process.

I would also like to ask what work you have done with low molecular weight materials because, apart from our own work with acetate which is reported in the CIBA Foundation Symposium (37), I know of no other with small molecule materials. We found a negligible shear stress dependence and that the transport was not controlled by the diffusion boundary layer.

DR. SCHWARTZ: Yes, but only using the Evans Blue areas for in vitro metabolic studies.

DR. WERTHESSEN: I would like to comment on an implication in Dr. Fry's earlier remarks. The risk factor in hypertension is, as I see the epidemiological data, an expression clinically of the underlying disease and not necessarily of the amount of atherosclerosis. I think this is a point we often forget.

DR. FRY: The principle increases in risk are an increased incidence of coronary occlusion and stroke. Your point is well taken. So far as I know, careful measurements of the amount of atherosclerosis in these two circulations as a function of chronically elevated blood pressure have not been made. Myocardial infarction correlates with the presence of coronary atherosclerosis and presumably with the extent or amount of coronary disease. However, the relationship of the extent of atherosclerosis in the cerebral vascular system to the incidence of either hypertension or stroke is less clear. Cerebral hemorrhage secondary to medial degeneration of the small intracerebral vessels apparently accounts for a large amount of the increased risk of stroke in hypertension. The relationship of this disease process to atherosclerosis is not obvious.

DR. SCHWARTZ: There is a fairly consistent relationship between the elevation of arterial pressure and the amount of atheroma in the coronary arteries. The relationship of hypertension to atheroma in the cerebral vessels is nowhere near so clear cut (38,39). One can obtain a correlation coefficient, but for the single individual it does not mean much.

DR. FRY: I did not mean to imply that fatty streaks always evolve into atheromatous plaques. I presented data from our studies in experimental atherosclerosis that showed that the sites at which atheromata occur frequently correspond to sites that were originally occupied by fatty streaks. This correlation is particularly convincing at the bifurcation of the left circumflex and anterior descending coronary arteries, on the ventral aspect of the lower abdominal aorta, and in the internal iliac arteries just above the deep femoral orifices.

DR. GREENE: One means of investigating the importance of the fluid mechanical parameter to atherogenesis is to change the nature of the fluid.

This methodology has not been discussed thus far at the
conference, but if fluid mechanics is important, then let us
alter the fluid's constitutive equation so as to change its
response to some of the short term phenomena such as turbulence,
separation, and reattachment. Any variation in physiological
or other effects in response to fluid manipulation would
offer a degree of confirmation to this hypothesis.

The methodology used in the present experiments has
been to change fluid behavior in a manner which primarily
affects the short time processes
Change of Fluid Behavior   occurring in the flowing
fluid. Addition of an elastic
component to the normal fluid response yields a fluid which
is termed viscoelastic. This response is quite separate and
distinct from the viscoelasticity we have talked about
concerning the arterial wall, or the erthyrocyte itself.
Thus, under appropriate conditions we are able to talk about
blood as a continuum with some component of induced elastic
response. Viscoelastic response is brought about primarily
by adding small amounts of water soluble polymers of very
high molecular weight. This causes the fluid to exhibit a
certain amount of drag or friction reduction under some
circumstances, but in all cases to follow a constitutive
equation that involves a certain amount of elasticity. From
a spring-dashpot model approach, we have added the response
of a Hookean spring to the fluid. One limiting criterion,
however, is that the amount of elasticity added to the blood
response is so very small, and the memory of the fluid is so
terribly faint, that one only notices this effect for very
short time processes which occur in the arterial system, in
vitro, or wherever. Fortunately, viscoelastic effects are
observed at low concentrations of soluble polymer addition,
so that any gross effects of adding a foreign material to
the fluid are minimized. Polymer levels in the neighborhood
of 50 to 75 parts per million on a weight basis are typical.

Several previous studies have dealt with the effects of
polymer addition on blood turbulence. In one study, the
mean frequency of disturbances distal to a contrived occlusion
in the descending aorta of dogs was measured with and without
polymer addition.

Results showed that with a small amount of the viscoelastic
agent added to the blood, the frequency of the turbulence
generated distally drops significantly, in the neighborhood
of 60 or 70%. If one relates the frequency of these disturbances
to the flux of momentum, the fluid shear stress at the wall
distal to the occlusion is diminished.

    A second study has involved the problem of blood hemolysis
in roller pumps. Perfusionists have been working for quite
                                    some time with the problem of
Hemolysis During Life   hemolysis during life support
Support   with extracorporeal pumps, and
                                    have found problems with
mechanical trauma to erythrocytes related to long term
support. Roller pumps manufactured by Pemco and Travenol
were tested to determine the effects of polymer addition on
the level of hemolysis in calf blood. Interestingly, it was
found that hemolysis levels decreased by 30-60% when certain
polymers were added prior to pumping.

    To understand this phenomenon we must review the design
of this pump along with the fluid mechanical problems it
poses. Fluid is pumped through a tube by squeezing it between
a roller and a wall. The rollers are adjustable so that
one can change the minimum clearance between the tube walls
and, as most perfusionists point out, one does not run at
quite complete occlusion of the tube walls. The reason for
this is that many red blood cells would be crushed between
the opposing walls of the tube. Instead one tends to run
these pumps so that there is a slight unoccluded area,
perhaps the thickness of a few sheets of paper, between the
opposing walls of the tube which nearly eliminates crushing
red blood cells in the process of perfusion. This presents
a very interesting fluid mechanics situation as shown in
Fig. 7- 43. Viewing flow from right to left, one has the
possibility during motion of the roller, of a rather giant
axial pressure gradient between forward and reverse sides of
this moving roller, allowing for considerable fluid motion
and a great deal of regurgitation of fluid from the high
pressure side to the low pressure side. It has been hypothesized
that high rates of fluid acceleration, large local shear
stresses, and high frequency flow disturbances in this
region are responsible for much of the observed hemolysis.

    To confirm this hypothesis, sucrose solutions with
effective viscosities about the same as blood and containing
small quantities of tiny wood particles were circulated
through the roller pumps. High speed cinematograph was
utilized, with the aid of a Fairchild, Model HS-401 Motion
Analysis Camera, to photograph the roller region at about
1500 frames/sec. Tracing the paths of the small particles
in the course of their motion from frame to frame allowed
estimation of regurgitation velocities as high as 10 meters/sec.
along with generally turbulent conditions.

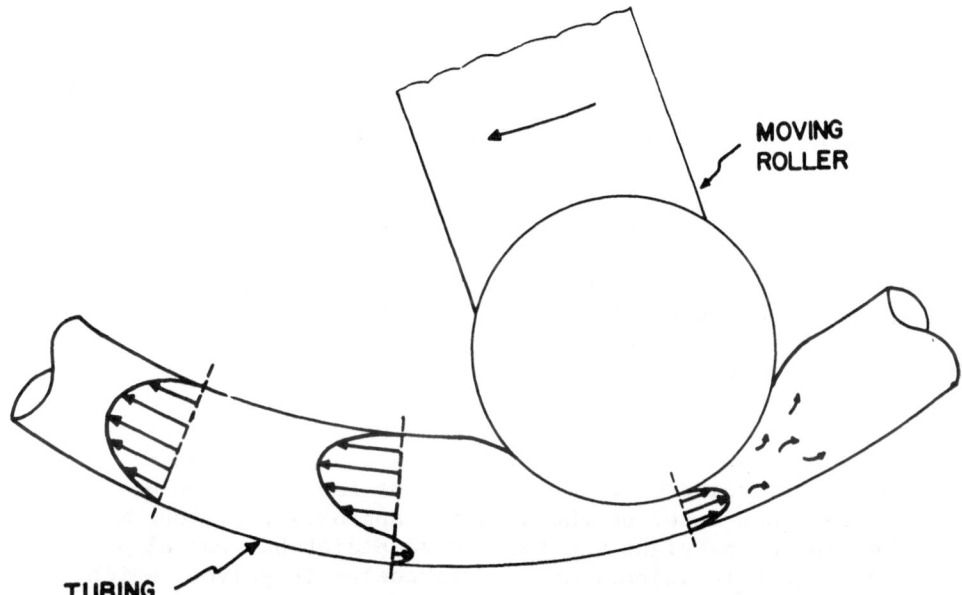

Fig. 7-43:   Roller Pump Schematic.

Hence, much of the hemolysis that occurs in roller pumps may
be caused by the extreme trauma of these red cells being
regurgitated under extreme conditions of turbulence; certainly
this would imply that high shear stresses must be exerted on
the wall of the erythrocyte. With the addition of polymer
to the sucrose system we have also looked at the possibility
of reducing a certain amount of that turbulence, reducing
the short-time response as a semi-elastic material for very
short-time processes. Results after polymer addition (100 PPM)
showed maximum regurgitation velocities of only 6 meters/sec.
but more importantly, eddies appeared considerably larger
and less chaotic than previously. A typical frame is shown
in Fig. 7-44.

RABBIT   We have also completed an in vivo experiement using
rabbits on high cholesterol diets. The experiment, carried
                                        out by Drs. Mostardi and Nokes
Fluid Mechanic Effects   at the University of Akron,
                                        involved a four month duration
test with a series of rabbits fed high cholesterol diets
such that their cholesterol levels ran upwards of a thousand
mg%. If fluid mechanics are important and short time processes
are important, as Dr. Nerem has questioned, then let us
again do something about changing the fluid response in vivo
for short time processes. This was done as before by maintaining
a circulating polymer level of about 60 PPM in the vascular
systems of half of the test animals. The animals were
sacrificed and examined at the conclusion of the experiment.
The pieces of tissue shown in Fig. 7-45 are descending
thoracic aorta from a matched pair of rabbits. The one on
the left has received the diet for approximately four months.
The one on the right was fed the same diet but was also
given periodic injections of a viscoelastic polymer which
altered the blood response to a very short term process,
meaning that many of the turbulent phenomena, disturbances,
separation, occurring at the highest frequencies were partially
suppressed. I cannot explain the process physiologically;
we have to date made no detailed studies of the tissue other
than these gross ones but certainly the fatty streaking, for
the no-polymer rabbit aorta on the left is in marked contrast
to the rabbit whose blood was doctored, so to speak, with a
small amount of viscoelastic polymer.

    DR. CARO: Is that a stained section?

    DR. GREENE: No, it is not. Next, Fig. 7-46 shows
comparative sections in the abdominal aorta of test rabbits;
the differences in plaque formation are not quite as apparent
here.

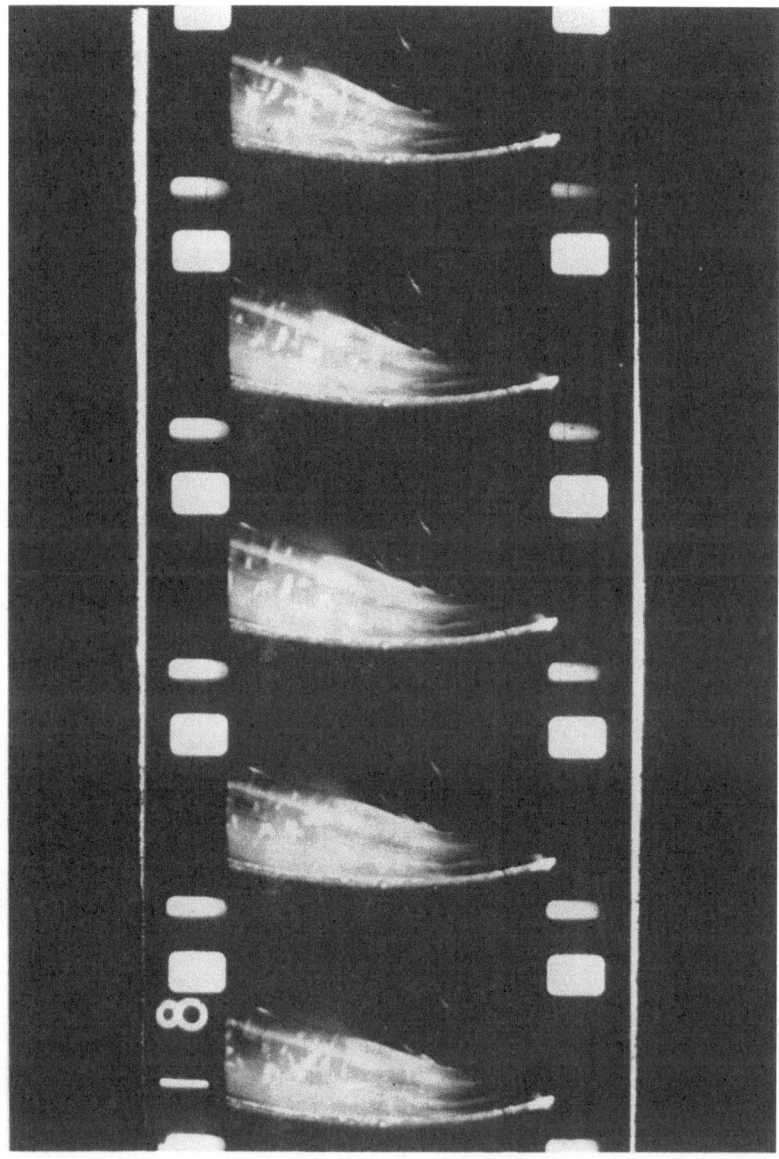

Fig. 7-44: Typical high speed cinematography of area behind moving roller showing wood particles in sucrose solutions.

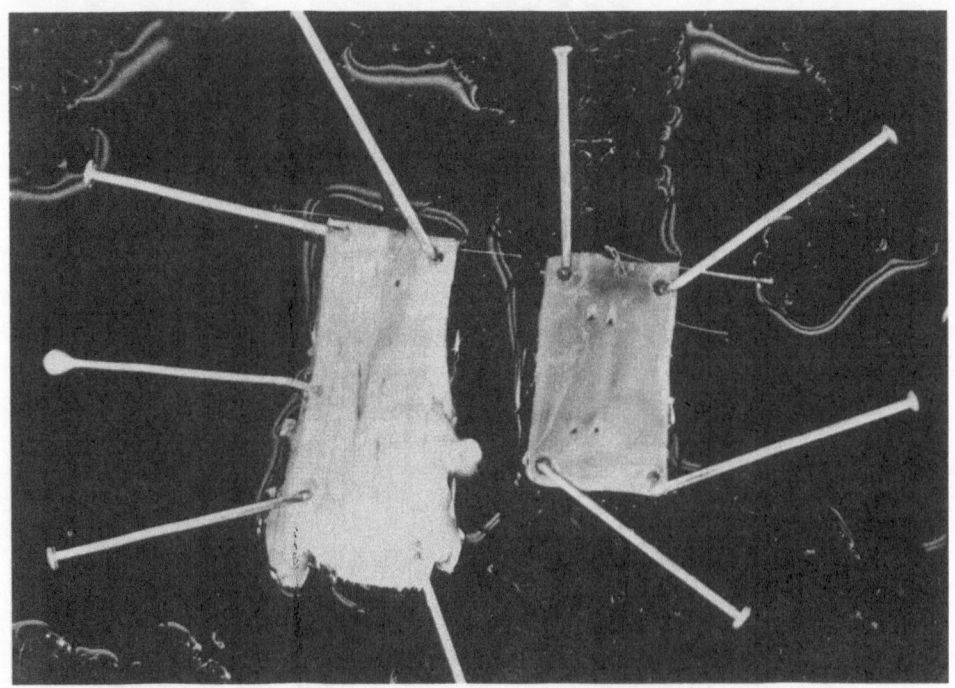

Fig. 7-45: Samples of descending thoracic aorta from no-polymer rabbit (left) versus polymer rabbit (right).

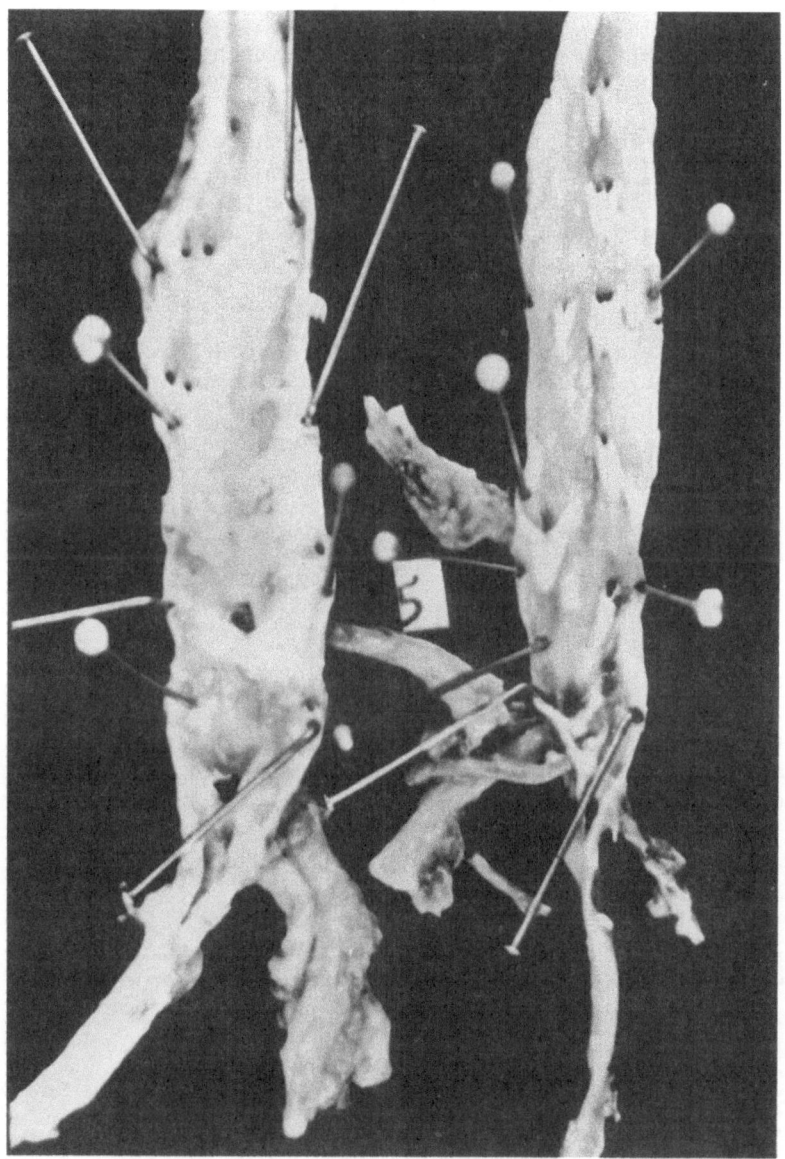

Fig. 7-46: Samples of abdominal aorta from no-polymer
rabbit (left) versus polymer rabbit (right).

It is the section again on the left which was taken from
the control rabbit on the high fat diet. The rabbit on the
right received the high fat diet as well as periodic injections
of the polymer solution. Again, on a percentage involvement
basis, there seems to be a significant difference between
the involvement of the rabbit aorta on the right versus the
involvement of the aorta on the left.

In summary, I want to point out that these studies have
all been designed to involve a new dimension in experiments
in blood flow. That dimension is to change the rheological
nature of the fluid, and, if fluid mechanics are important,
to see what effect this has on the course of a vascular
disease or a rheological event. There are many additional
studies which could be performed in this manner, for example,
some of the oscillating wall experiments that Dr. Nerem has
done would be very interestingly repeated with additions of
a small amount of polymer, so that the fluid was made viscoelastic.
We might see some significant changes in wall permeability
or uptake rate of albumin.

VOICE: Did you see any difference in growth rates
between those two?

DR. GREENE: I believe that while the external factors
such as growth and weight increase, as best as I can recall,
were reasonably similar, there may have been some slight
hemolytic effects with the polymer. Nevertheless, note that
I am not suggesting that we use polymer addition as a therapeutic
device at this time, I am primarily stressing the fluid
mechanical effects.

DR. WOLF: How frequently did you have to inject the
polymer over a four month period?

DR. GREENE: Roughly two and half times a week. We had
run some previous experiments with tritiated polymer and it
appears to have a half-life of about 36 hours in vivo.

DR. SMITH: Were the serum cholesterols the same?

DR. GREENE: Yes.

DR. COLTON: What polymer did you use?

DR. GREENE: This happened to be a polyacrylamide (Separan AP-30), a polymer made by Dow Chemical Co. It has a molecular weight of about two to three million. Of course it degrades with time, I suspect, both biologically and because of mechanical trauma in vivo.

DR. KENYON: How do you characterize the influence of the polymer on blood?

DR. GREENE: The apparent viscosities of the blood versus the blood with small amounts of polymer are nearly indistinguishable. There is a very slight increase in blood viscosity as one might suspect if one adds a small amount of polymer solution to the blood but only by a couple of per cent. The biggest chang. appears to be in the addition of the viscoelastic factor which can be characterized rheometrically by the first normal stress difference. I have no really good data from making total rheological measurements on blood yet; it depends strongly on what instruments you use. We have found in equivalent "viscosity" sucrose solutions, that adding sufficient polymer to induce a just normal stress difference of about five dynes per square centimeter generally gives significant differences in in vivo or in vitro effects for a given study.

DR. CHIEN: What was the shear rate at which you measured the blood viscosity?

DR. GREENE: It went from one reciprocal second or less to well over a thousand, but we tended to be interested primarily in the values obtained at higher shear rates since these are probably more appropriate in vivo for the larger arteries. Now whether this is the optimum shear rate, I don't know.

DR. CHIEN: The reason why I asked that is because the polymer induced aggregation and the increase in viscosity probably can be seen only at very low shear rates.

DR. GREENE: We have carried out some ESR measurements and microscopic observations on treated blood and we have found that even though many of these polymers are used for particle flocculation (and this scares one off immediately in terms of any kind of in vivo study) one finds that for circulating polymer concentrations of less than 150 parts per million these properties seem to be absent. So I don't think RBC aggregation is important here.

DR. DEWEY: One frightening feature that you have
pointed out to us in these results is the decrease in the
high frequency components of what apparently is turbulent
flow. At least disturbed flow. I would propose that perhaps
this might be the way of altering the fluid mechanic stress
at the wall, that could be potentially significant from the
experimental point of view. There have been a number of
studies. Dr. Schwartz has done some, for example, on coarctation
of the aorta. Dr. Fry and many people here have performed
experiments in which they have found significant changes in
the staining charactersitics of the endothelial cells distal
to a coarctation and one would correlate the regions of
damage and change with regions in which you would expect
very high wall pressure fluctuations and wall shear fluctuations.

There are relatively straightforward methods by which
one could obtain the power spectral density of the fluctuations
themselves. By that I mean that if you look at the spectral
content and the energy contained at the various frequencies,
one finds a rather characteristic type of turbulent spectrum
in these coarctation groups. It is easily characterized for
ordinary blood or for example in a Newtonian fluid. I would
expect on the basis of your results that the turbulent power
spectral density would change dramatically with the addition
of the polymer and if it is the high frequency content, and
as Dr. Weinbaum and others have suggested, which is as
important if not more important than the actual magnitude of
the shear, this might be a possible way on an experimental
basis to change this specific parameter without changing
other gross fluid properties. In this way one might be able
to see differences in staining or the uptake in which we are
able to vary one specific hemodynamic parameter without
influencing gross properties in flow.

DR. NEREM: I accept what you say, Dr. Dewey, in terms
of that particular type of situation; but I would be somewhat
surprised if those were present in the rabbit aorta under
similar conditions. However, in terms of your story, Dr. Greene,
are you sure that what you have done is to alter fluid
dynamics? Is it possible at this point that this polymer
has had a chemical effect on the endothelial cells?

DR. GREENE: I have no conclusive answer to that question
RAT at this time. In one set of early experiments with rats using
tritiated polymer, we did try to find out whether there was
any build up of polymer in or on various organs or the
arterial wall itself; we found no specific activity in those
regions.

DR. NEREM: I was thinking of the cells in some way changing shape or whatever.

DR. GREENE: I think what Dr. Weinbaum was discussing, the possible alteration of the motion of endothelial cells, would have some bearing on the result, but we have found no changes in shape of erythrocytes.

DR. WERTHESSEN: I do not know if you can do this but as an experimentalist may I suggest the use of a spontaneously developing lesion such as in the White Carneau pigeon?

DR. GREENE: We now have about 30 pigeons under study   PIGEON
and are currently working on this.

DR. WERTHESSEN: Good, good. Because if you can inhibit the development of lesions, then I think you have something.

DR. GREENE: That is precisely where we are proceeding.

DR. STONE: When you are increasing viscoelastic properties, does this tend to increase the viscosity?

DR. GREENE: Not significantly, that is a separate and distinct property. We are not making the fluid thicker although I mentioned that inadvertently one increased the viscosity slightly by polymer addition. We have run in vitro controls where we have significantly increased only the viscosity of the blood just by adding a viscous agent, but have not found corresponding reductions in say, hemolysis.

DR. STONE: Would this be similar to a hyperproteinemia?

DR. GREENE: What do you mean?

DR. STONE: Where you have increased protein content in the blood itself.

DR. GREENE: Does that affect the apparent viscosity of blood?

DR. STONE: Yes.

DR. GREENE: Molecular weight, what would it be?

DR. CARO: Fibrinogen, principally.

DR. GREENE: We have found no significant viscoelastic effects for molecules under a couple of million.

DR. STONE: They build them now in the M.A.A. Radio Isotope field, these are relatively large macroalbumin particles, you can get them quite long.

DR. GREENE: A much more appropriate set of experiments would be to try to build something that one could be sure would be fairly compatible...

DR. CHIEN: The largest dextran has a molecular weight of approximately two million.

DR. GREENE: I have not seen any data on that.

DR. CHIEN: This is the blue dextran manufactured by the Pharmacia Laboratories in Sweden.

DR. STONE: What is the actual count of Siren D, the hydrogenated size of those two million molecular weight particles?

DR. GREENE: It varies quite a bit depending on what fluid you put it in and the stresses present during flow.

DR. SMITH: Have you looked at the interaction between this material and any of the plasma constituents? I was thinking that if LDL in fact stuck itself on to this material it could make such a large molecule that it would not filter.

DR. GREENE: We have not considered that possibility.

DR. WERTHESSEN: You have an excuse for getting an ultracentrifuge.

VOICE: Does it change the behavior of the platelets, first question. Second question: Did you investigate the serum lipoprotein profile in the control and experimental animals with regard to, for instance, the presence of HDL?

DR. GREENE: I would guess that the answer to all of those is no, we have not investigated such factors, which is the reason why I call these extremely preliminary experimental findings.

DR. CHIEN: I am glad that Dr. Greene brought up the problem of blood properties in relation to the problem of atherogenesis.

Just to continue this vein of discussion, Fig. 7-47 is taken from the work of Goldsmith (40). What it shows is that the velocity profile is altered, if you have cells suspended in the media. And this parabolic profile is shown by the dotted line when you turn your fluid so that you have 38% red blood cells made into ghosts by removing the hemoglobin after osmotic lysis. The reason for doing that is to allow the visualization of the few cells that remain with the ghosts. Then you can map the velocity profile which shows blunting in the center and a steepening of the gradient near the wall. When a very high cell concentration (92% cells) is used, the degree of blunting in the middle is even more severe and the steepening of the gradient near the wall becomes more prominent. This will change the shear rate near the wall and hence also the shear stress at the wall. Of course, the velocity profile is also dependent on the flow velocity, the deformability of the cells, and a number of other factors. So the conversion of the mean velocity into shear stress at the wall is a rather complicated problem in the presence of cells (Fig. 7-48). In the presence of cells another thing that happens is that there will be collision between the cells and this again is taken from the work of Dr. Goldsmith (40). He tracked the path of individual red cells with time as the cells flow through a cylindrical tube. The abscissa shows the radial location in the tube plotted as a fraction of the tube radius. His observations indicate that the path of the cells is not a straight one, i.e. it is erratic. In the presence of neighboring cells, cell-to-cell collisions cause sideway motions of these red cells (8 micron in diameter) in the tube. When latex particles with the diameter of one or two microns are used to simulate platelets, it is observed that the path is even more erratic. The particles move across the tube over a very wide radial distance with time. Therefore, for the smaller particles such as platelets, collisions with red cells cause a very large excursion in their paths. What this means is that there is a larger chance for the interaction of the particles with the wall. This is true for the red cells to some degree and even more so for the smaller particles.

Figure 7-49 is again taken from Goldsmith's work (40) on the flow pattern beyond a partial obstruction created in a tube by gluing a latex sphere to the side of the tube. The behavior of particles such as red cells or latex particles flowing past such a spherical obstruction can be observed microscopically. An enlargement shows the detailed picture as the cells streaked by at rather high velocity past the obstruction, but once

Relation of Blood Properties to Atherogenesis

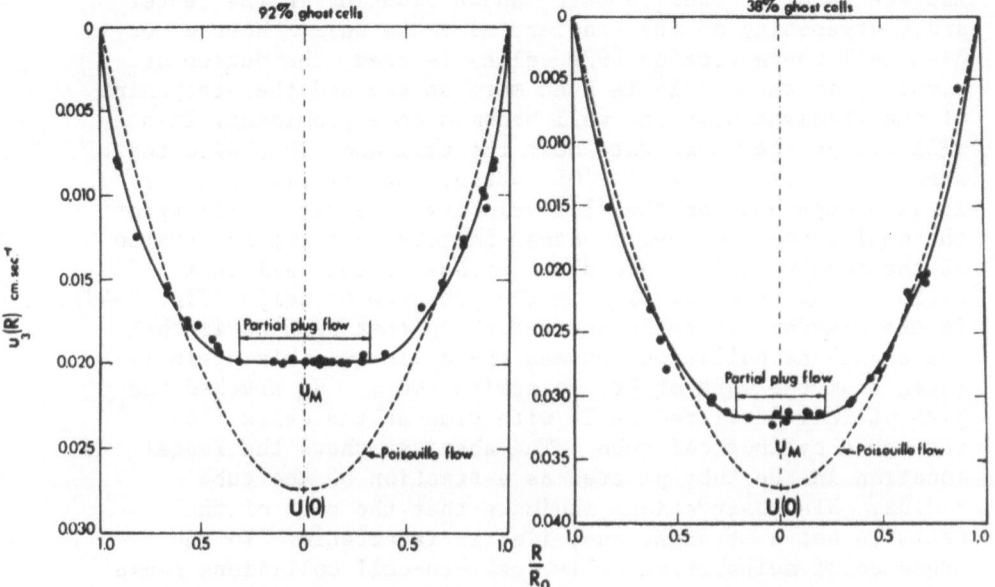

Fig. 7-47: Velocity distribution obtained with tracer human red cells in ghost cell suspensions at two cell concentrations: left, 92%, right 38%. The velocity along the longitudinal direction of the tube, $U_3(R)$, is plotted as a function of the radial position in the tube, R, normalized for the tube radius, R_0. $R_0 = 42$ μ. Courtesy of Dr. H. L. Goldsmith.

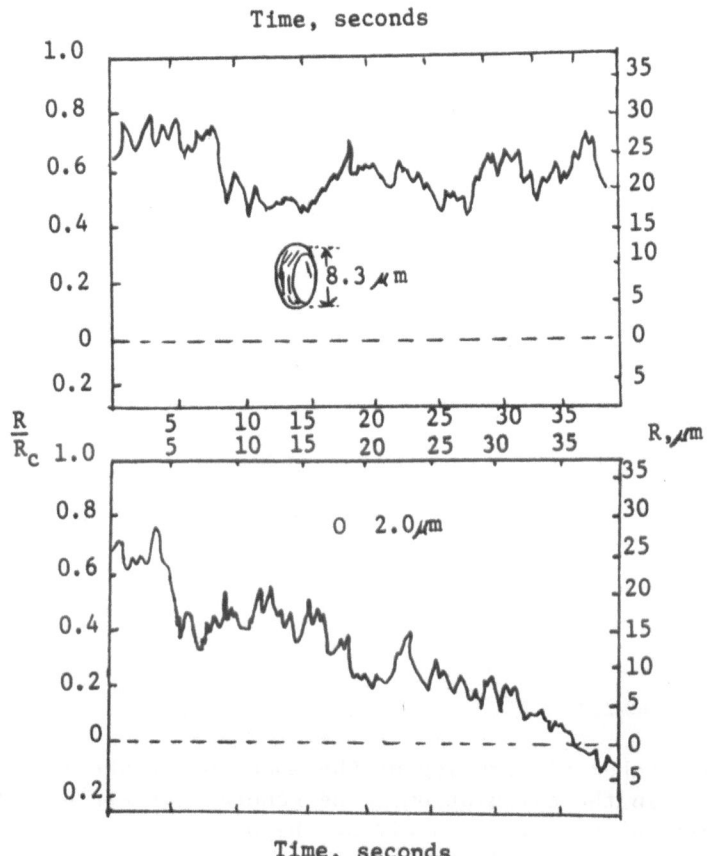

Fig. 7-48: Paths of tracer red cells (top) and of tracer 2 μm latex spheres (bottom) with time in a 40% ghost cell suspension flowing through a 73 um diameter tube (R_0 = 3.65 μm) at a mean velocity of 0.030 cm/sec. The sizes of the particles relative to the tube are shown. After Yu and Goldsmith, in Platelets, Drugs and Thrombosis (J. Hirsch, ed.), pp. 78-93. S. Karger, Basel, 1975.

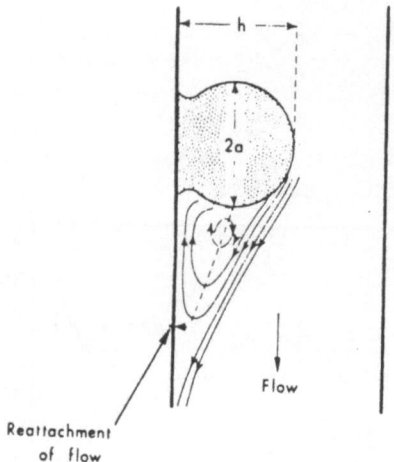

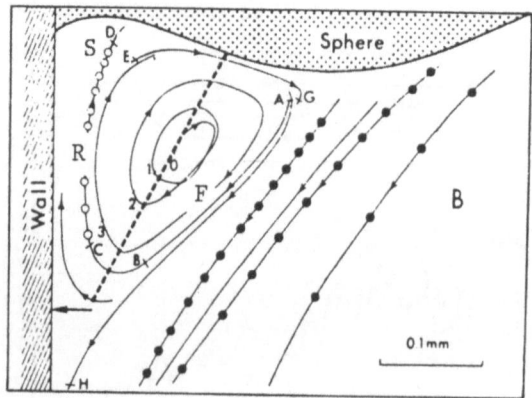

Fig. 7-49: Schematic drawing of the model of a spherical obstruction in the circulation. The general pattern of the streamlines in the vortex is given. The position of reattachment of the flow is indicated.
B: The vortex region is enlarged to show the forward (F), reverse (R), and stagnation (S) regions downstream of the obstruction. The orbits of a red cell as it spiraled out from the center are shown. Large changes in the linear velocity of cells were noted. Open circles show particle positions at 0.12 sec intervals; dots show particle positions at 5.9 msec intervals. From Yu and Goldsmith, Microvascular Research 6:5-31, 1973.

getting into the post-obstruction area, spend a long time recirculating in this area of flow separation. Thus, platelets would have a longer time to undergo various types of chemical interactions. When red cells go into the stagnant, low shear region, they tend to form rouleaux and cause further reductions in flow. Therefore, cells and other solutes spend a long time in such a separated flow region. The reattachment of the flow is marked by arrows in Fig. 7-49.

These considerations indicate the microrheologic behavior of the particles in the blood flowing in our circulatory system may have considerable influence on their interactions with the wall, particularly when there are abnormal situations in the circulatory system. The major determinants of the blood viscosity are plasma viscosity, cell concentration, cell deformability and cell aggregation. There are a number of clinical situations in which the blood viscosity is abnormal due to alterations in one of these factors. Clinically we have classical examples of abnormality for each one of these factors. For example, in multiple myeloma we have plasma viscosity elevation, in polycythemia the cell concentration is high, in sickle cell anemia the cell deformability is abnormal, in macroglobulinemia red cell aggregation is enhanced. I don't know whether there is any statistical information on the correlation between atherosclerosis and these various kinds of disease states. Maybe our colleagues in pathology or epidemiology have some information showing whether there is any correlation between any one of these conditions and atherogenesis. I think it would be interesting to find out if there is any relevance of abnormalities in blood rheology to the problem of atherogenesis.

Relevance of Abnormalities in Blood Rheology to Problem of Atherogenesis

DR. WERTHESSEN: Dr. Chien, on this point of deformability of erythocytes, do you know of Rasmussen and Allen's work? (41). I think it would be a superb tool in these studies to change their deformability by the addition of prostaglandins.

DR. CHIEN: Yes and they used catecholamines too.

DR. SCHWARTZ: I wish to refer back to remarks that Dr. Nerem made about the problems of animal models and Dr. Smith too, and really raise what I think could be an important point in terms of the logic of looking at factors responsible for the development of atherosclerosis. We are tempted to make an assumption which may be quite wrong, that the progression of disease from its initiation to its ultimate development is a continuum. There may be important mechanisms involved in initiation, and different mechanisms involved thereafter.

DR. WOLF: Dr. Mansfield's presentation mentioned the need to have access to early changes and Dr. Smith pointed out the difficulty in distinguishing the difference between early changes and different sites in the structure of the artery for architectural changes, such as cushions and so forth.

Dr. Schwartz just pointed out that one should not assume that one is looking at a long term continuum process and relevant to this I think were the observations that Ted Gillman made at the Lindau Conference, in which he was studying the uterine artery and pointed out that the changes, namely the hyperplasia of smooth muscle cells in the intima occurred in the process of enlargement of the uterine artery with pregnancy and that these reversed after parturition when the uterine artery diminished in size.

With repeated pregnancies there ultimately appeared typical atherosclerotic lesions. Here then an opportunity is offered to look at early lesions, to look at the production and resolution of lesions, and to make distinctions between adaptive changes in the vessel and pathologic changes, if you will. In this connection there is an interesting paper I want to get into the record by Ryan, Clark and Brodie called Neurogenic and Mechanical Control of Canine Uterine Vascular Resistance. It is in the AMERICAN JOURNAL OF PHYSIOLOGY. (42). What they show is that there is cholinergic vasodilator innervation of the uterine artery and adrenergic vasoconstrictor innervation in the uterine artery. During pregnancy the vaso constrictor activity is very severely blunted but reappears following parturition. This is an interesting article and pertinent to all three of these observations cited.

DR. WEINBAUM: We have not mentioned this previously, because the experiments were preliminary, but it is the reason that we initially suspected that we could increase vesicle transport through fluid mechanics or mechanical factors. The experiments are briefly described in a short note that Dr. Caro and I put in PHYSIOLOGICAL PROCEEDINGS. (43). These experiments need to be carefully repeated but their essence is the following. The diffusion velocity of a vesicle, as best we could estimate, is of the order of a hundred angstroms per second. Thus, we tried to design a mechanical disturbance experiment in which we would cause a boundary motion of the endothelial cell which would produce velocities at the plasmalemma which were of that order.

We had known from the stretch experiments of Dr. Fry that if you introduce very small stretches on the order of four or five per cent, that there is almost no change in transport. We attempted to introduce disturbances of the same magnitude as Dr. Fry's but at a frequency such that the boundary motion would be roughly comparable to the diffusion velocity of the vesicle. The results showed that there was a very curious frequency response. When we increased the frequencies to the order of about one Hertz the transport seemed to rise sharply whereas if we decreased the frequency the transport would return to the normal static situation at a frequency of about a tenth of a Hertz. So there was roughly a ten fold range over which there was a very substantial increase in transport of roughly 60 to 100%. Again this data is preliminary. The fascinating feature is that the increase in transport occurs where the boundary velocity of the plasmalemma membrane of the cell is of the same order as is our best estimate of the diffusion velocity of the vesicles. If any experiment has been the motivation for the work that we have done since then, I think this is probably the key one.

DR. DEWEY: How did you make the motion?

DR. CARO: These are very difficult experiments and many more than the 14 we have done need doing, but essentially a dog's common carotid is carefully excised and mounted in a rig at its in vivo length in a bath. A cam is then adjusted which allows it to relax by three or four percent of its length. The motion is simple harmonic and the frequency can be adjusted.

DR. DEWEY: Longitudinal...

DR. CARO: Yes, the extension is longitudinal. Transmural pressure was about one cm. of water.

DR. COLTON: In these experiments what does the backside of the artery look like where you would normally have adventitia?

DR. CARO: I have never done EMs, but to the naked eye it is a tatty piece of adventitia.

DR. COLTON: I suggest that the total uptake depends on the state of the backside of the artery you measure, as well as of the luminal endothelial surface. If there is adventitia and any vasa vasorum, the tissue will be invaginated with lots of vessels that do not communicate well with the bath.

One additional thing that could happen is that the stretching serves to help perfuse the fluid in these vessels, thereby increasing the uptake rate.

DR. CARO: I will accept this absolutely. On the other hand, we do dissect off the adventitia at the end of an experiment and it is not counted as part of the wall. I should also mention that we did some of these experiments with sodium acetate as the tracer and there was no effect of stretching on its uptake.

DR. COLTON: The sodium acetate and albumin are likely to behave quite differently. The sodium acetate may diffuse so readily through the tissue that it is insensitive to the detailed structure of the backside of the artery, whereas the albumin, because it moves much more slowly through plasma and tissue, would be quite sensitive to the anatomical structure and extent of perfusion on the back side.

DR. CARO: But the sodium acetate will presumably come into the vasa vasorum in the same way as the albumin will.

DR. COLTON: The agreement that it is appearing at the endothelium would be more convincing if you had evidence of that.

DR. CARO: I totally agree that it has got to be done by looking, absolutely.

DR. COX: I would like to ask Dr. Caro a question about these studies involving uptake of markers by perfused segments. Do the markers ever appear in the surrounding fluid? I presume there is surrounding fluid.

DR. CARO: Yes they do. We always monitor the bath. The volume of the bath is actually very large (about 50 ml.) compared to the volume contained in the segment, about 0.1 ml. Unfortunately there is no very good solution to the problem of leakage, which we have all encountered. We tried to seal off the vasa vasorum, and test by putting visible tracer and pressurizing the vessel. Then if there is a leak we reject the specimen. In the end I have to carry out most of my studies at zero, or very low, transmural pressure. The conditions are artificial but leakage is avoided.

DR. COX: Could you get around this problem by testing your segment and selecting it from ones where there was no vasa interna originally in your sections so you could eliminate the problem.

Do you have any information that it represents leaking
through the vasa or is it simply continuous diffusion through
the wall?

DR. CARO: This is leakage. No question at all. When
you dissect out the vessel you see the vasa on the surface,
the arteries and the veins and if you are clumsy and cut one
of these and do not tie it securely, when you mount the
segment in the rig a little jet comes out of the vessel.

DR. COLTON: Have you ever thought about coating the
backside with something like beeswax?

DR. WEINBAUM: This is in reference to the questions
that were asked previously about denuding the endothelium.
The adventitia is purposely left on for that reason. The
experiments I described were conducted over a 15 minute
period. This is the shortest time in which one could expect
albumin to diffuse in substantial quantities to the adventitial
surface. If a leak is present it shows up very easily in
the adventitia because we strip it off separately after the
experiment is over. There is never any question as to when
you have a leak because the adventitia will show readings
which are ten fold larger than normal control.

DR. COLTON: Is that data then rejected?

DR. WEINBAUM: Yes.

DR. DEWEY: I have a question for Dr. Smith. I found
it very exciting to look at the data that you presented
earlier regarding the type of
Oxygen Utilization   metabolism within the artery
and how, in fact, it can be
anaerobic and aerobic and how that may in fact be a function
of the diffusion depth to which the oxygen can go in the
artery. One of the rather interesting things I think is that
the diffusion depth of the oxygen and the rate at which the
oxygen is utilized in the metabolic process, will obviously
vary from artery to artery, certainly in terms of the diffusion
coefficient from one artery to another, that should not
change dramatically, I suggest. The utilization rate might,
however, and we do find a dramatic difference in the arterial
wall thickness from, for example, the coronary intermediate
arteries to the aorta and it would suggest to me that
perhaps this balance between aerobic and anaerobic metabolism
may change from one artery to another or, for example,
during vasoconstriction or vasodilation, particularly in the
coronary arteries.

DR. SMITH: This is a very good point and I don't think
there has been any work on this at all. All these measurements
on oxygen uptake and lactate production have been made in
aorta. I would imagine that a very muscular artery like the
coronary, has a much higher metabolic rate so that you might
expect the more adequately perfused coronary artery to have
a higher oxygen utilization and conversely to produce more
lactic acid when deprived of oxygen. I don't think that
there is any data on this and I think this is a very interesting
area indeed. If it was consuming more oxygen then obviously
the critical diffusion distance would become shorter, and if
it was in a state of violent stretch, it would again consume
more oxygen. Certainly, looking at the things that happen
to coronary arteries they seem to have a very rough life
indeed, they might need to consume more oxygen to keep
themselves in shape. I think this is a very interesting
area and does really require further investigation.

DR. CARO: I have a question for Dr. Dewey. You have
said, I think, that you have found on your arteriograms
signs of early changes in the wall in the carotid sinus. Is
the wall there significantly different in thickness than it
is in the parent vessel?

DR. DEWEY: I think the most pertinent data here are
data which Dr. Meyer has on the carotid sinus. I have not
had a chance to analyze them in detail, but I have the
impression from one of the reprints that he furnished to me
that there is a very substantial difference in the wall
properties, between the sinus area and the internal carotid
distal to the sinus itself. In other words, there are very
substantial changes in the elastic properties; and I am sure
there are physiological reasons for this in terms of chemoreceptor
control, but I cannot comment in detail on the actual physiological
differences.

DR. COLTON: Is it known at what PO_2 the smooth muscle
cells of the arterial wall shift over from aerobic to anaerobic
metabolism?

DR. SMITH: I cannot answer that. In the bovine artery
segment data that Arnqvist and Lundholm (44) presented, it
seemded to be a gradual shift. Reducing PO_2 from about 70
mm Hg (normal level for arterial blood) to 35 mm doubled
lactic production, and reducing it from 35 mm to zero,
doubled it again (Fig. 5-2).

DR. BJORKERUD: I think that is different in different situations though. Because we constantly see injury to the plaque tissue when the plaque is completely re-endothelialized. Of course we cannot tell if that is due to a sudden deficiency of oxygen or due to a sudden deficiency of nutriments. We see tissue vary very reproducibly upon re-endothelialization of experimental lesions in the rabbit. Maybe Dr. Mansfield has similar experience from lesions in other species?

DR. COX: I have a question for Dr. Smith in this regard, concerning hypoxia and cold. I have routinely stored blood vessel samples in the icebox overnight. I go back the next day, incubate them at 37 degrees C for a couple of hours. Comparing refrigerated samples, which were between 0 and 4 degrees C, and fresh blood vessels, there was no statistically significant difference in the ability of the smooth muscle to generate force. This is for periods of storage from 24 to 72 hours. So it would seem to me, from a simple point of view, that cold storage is not affecting the contractile ability of cells. These are fairly large vessels which are certainly more than 350 microns in wall thickness. Did you not show data yesterday that indicated, or suggested that storage at 4 degrees had some sort of deleterious effect on arterial smooth muscle?

DR. SMITH: It appears to switch them over from oxidative phosphorylation to the glycolytic pathway. This is the Scott and Morrison data (45,46,47) and this has been pretty amply confirmed (48,49). But this does not mean to say that they can't contract using glycolysis.

DR. COX: I would call everyone's attention to the fact that studies in cardiac muscle mechanics never use capillary muscles more than something like 800 microns in diameter. There have been a number of demonstrations that larger sized capillary muscles studied in vitro have reduced contractile responses.

DR. MEYER: Reminiscent of observations of Gillman on the uterine arteries referred to by Dr. Wolf, (28) I have further evidence of the importance of hemodynamics and associated structural features manifest in the development of some early lesions in the iliac arteries on the side of the obliterated single umbilical artery.

Usually there are two umbilical arteries, but in 0.72 -
1.0 per cent of newborn infants one umbilical artery is
                                missing (49,50). With a
Effect of a Congenital   single umbilical artery a unique
Single Umbilical Artery   hemodynamic situation arises
                                during fetal development: the
entire blood to the placenta is transported from the abdominal
aorta through the common iliac arteries of only one side of
the body (Fig. 7-50). Therefore, the common and internal
iliac arteries on the side of the SUA become exposed to a
higher hemodynamic load during fetal development and,
consequently, assume a larger caliber and thicker wall than
those on the other side of the body which do not participate
in the placental circuit.

The differences in caliber are closely associated with
different structure of the arterial wall (51). On the side
of the single umbilical artery, the common and internal
iliac arteries show the structure of elastic arteries.
Their media consists of tightly packed elastic membranes
(Fig. 7-51a). In contrast, the common and internal arteries
on the opposite side, which do not participate in placental
circuit, display the structural pattern of muscular arteries
(Fig. 7-51b).

Berry et al., (52) measured vessel compliance in vivo
in 18 children born with a single umbilical artery with a
non-invasive method and found significantly different compliance
values in iliac arteries on both sides of the body. These
differences are probably determined by different structural
features of iliac arteries present in children with a single
umbilical artery.

Differences in functional load and structure probably
also account for different patterns of early calcifications
often occurring in iliac arteries of infants and children
with a single umbilical artery. On the side of the closed
or already obliterated single umbilical artery the early
membrane calcifications are usually irregularly distributed
along the luminal surface (Fig. 7-52). In contrast, in the
narrower common iliac artery on the other side of the body,
calcific incrustations often assume a more regular pattern
and appear as transverse streaks. Microscopically, the
streaks represent calcified edges of membrane gaps, a typical
structural feature of muscular arteries. Hence, the calcification
pattern is in accord with the muscular structural pattern of
the narrower common iliac artery.

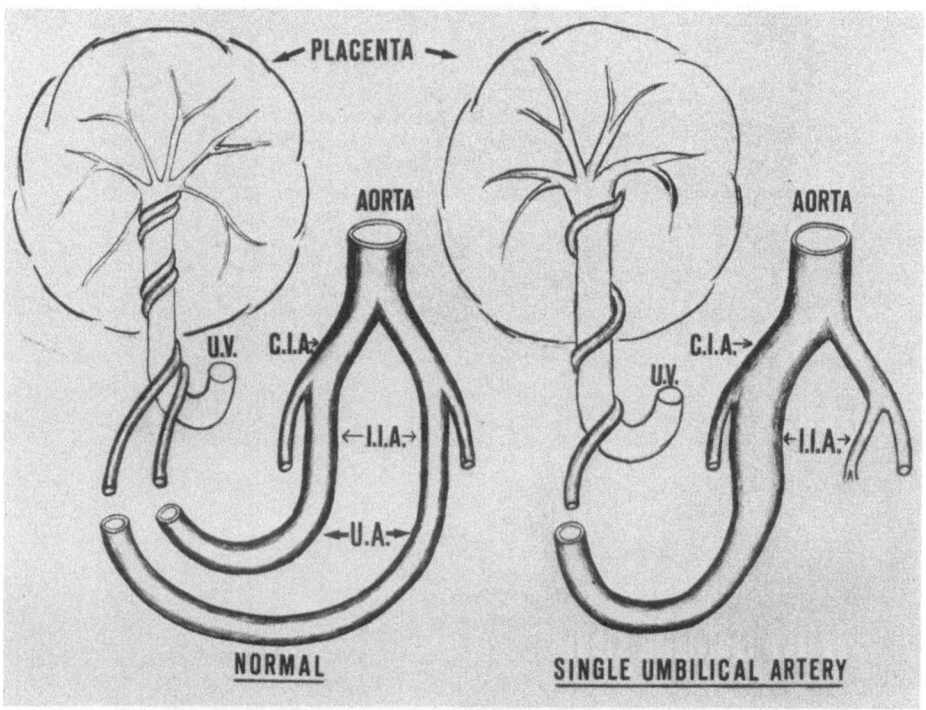

Fig. 7-50: Diagram of a part of the systemic arterial tree in
a fetus with two umbilical arteries (left) and in a fetus with
a single umbilical artery (right) showing different calibers of
the iliac arteries. UA - umbilical artery, IIA - internal
iliac artery, CIA - common iliac artery. UV - umbilical
vein (from Meyer and Lind, 1974).

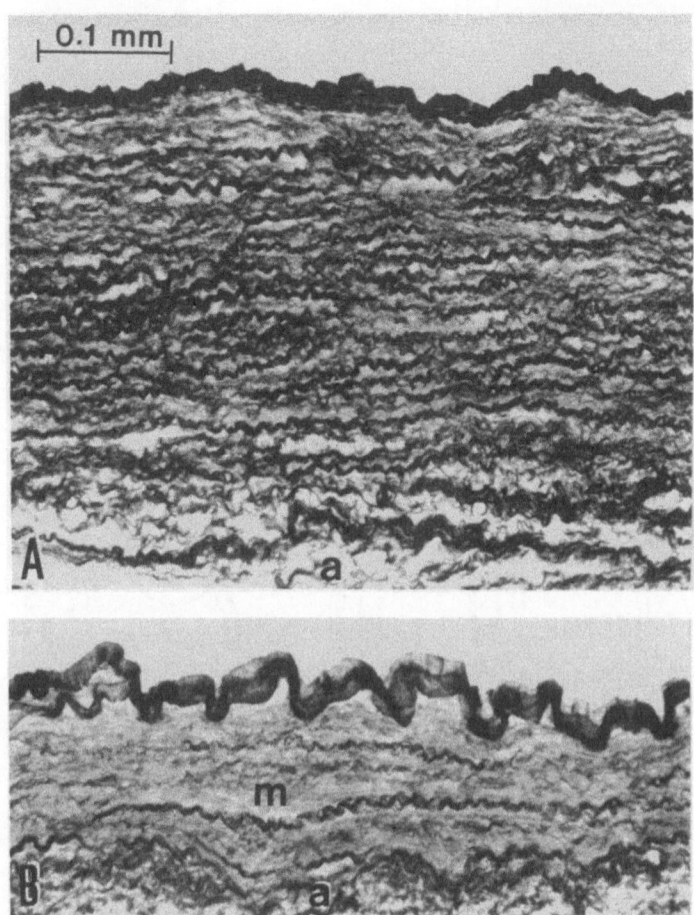

Fig. 7-51: Cross-sections of common iliac arteries of a term
newborn infant. The common iliac artery (A) on the side of the
single umbilical artery is an elastic artery with well-developed
elastic sheets in its media. In contrast, the thin-walled common
iliac artery on the opposite side (B) is a muscular artery with
a media (m) poor in elastic networks. a- adventitia. Cryostat
frozen section. Weigert's resorcin-fuchsin stain. (From Meyer
and Lind, 1974).

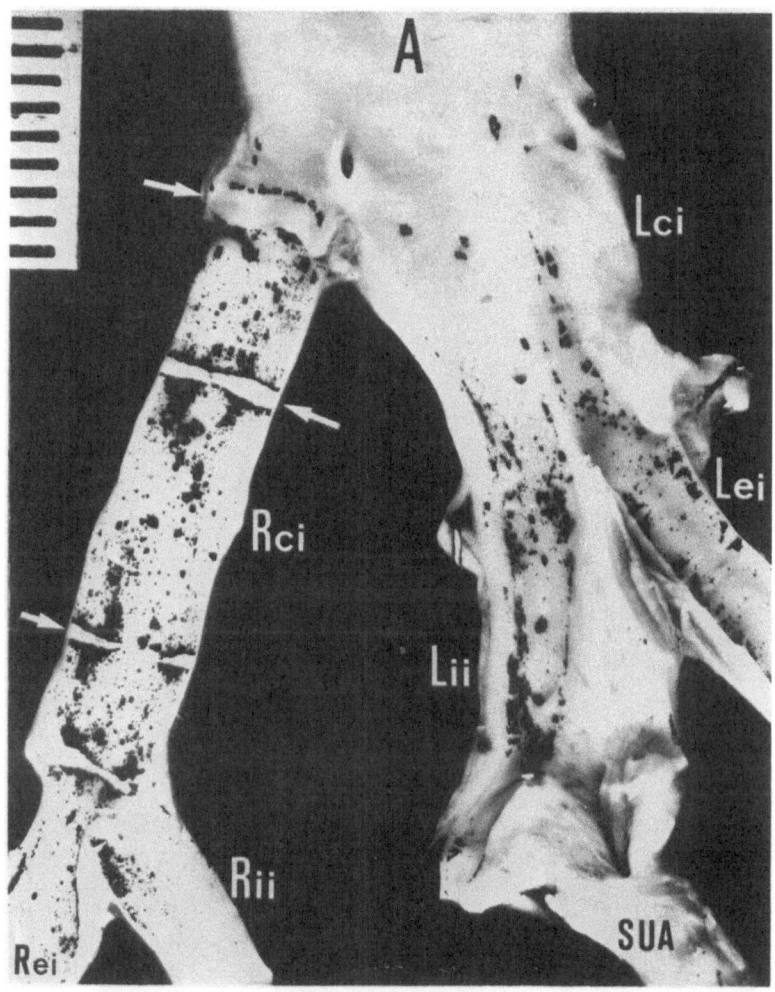

Fig. 7-52: Iliac arteries from a one-month-old infant with a
single left umbilical artery. Note the large caliber of the
common iliac artery (Lci) and that of the internal iliac artery
(Lii) on the side of the obliterated single umbilical artery
(SUA). Conspicuous calcifications (black) are present in both
iliac arteries, but the pattern differs in the iliac arteries on
the side of the single umbilical artery. In the right common
iliac artery (Rci) circular calcium - free bands (arrows) are
seen. Microscopically, they correspond to the gaps in the
internal elastic membrane.
Von Kossa reaction. Millimeter scale at top left. Case 906/73.
(From Meyer and Lind, 1974).

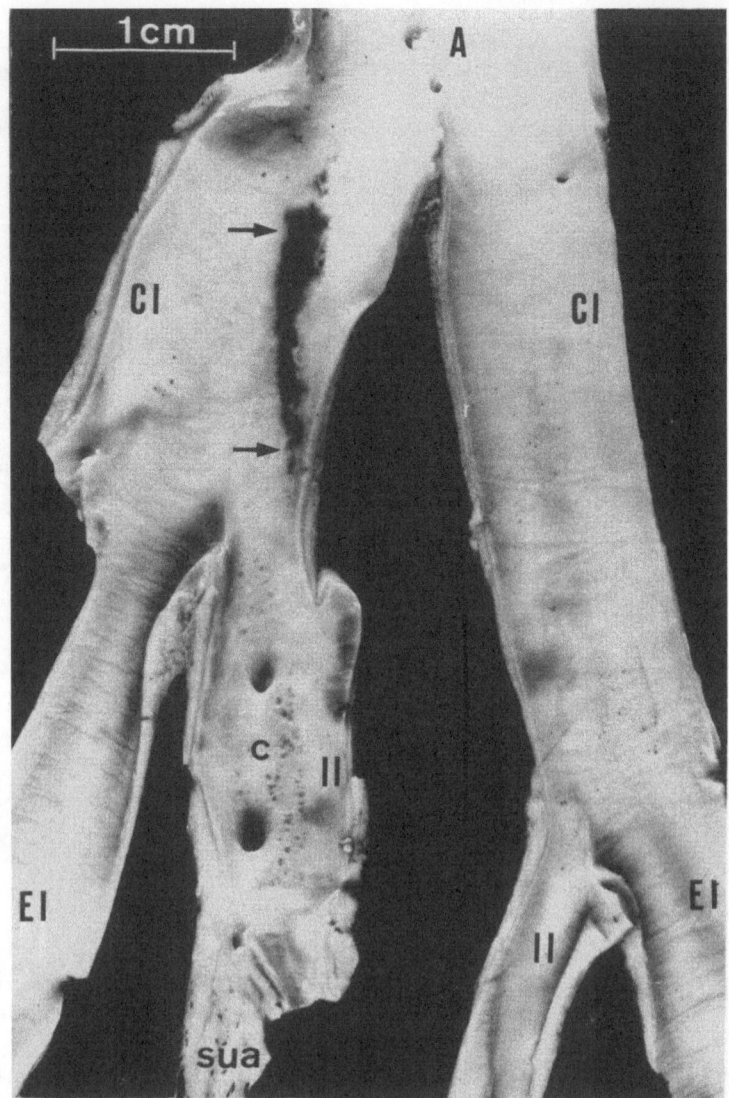

Fig. 7-53: A raised longitudinal atherosclerotic lesion
(between arrows) is seen in the enlarged right common iliac
artery on the side of the obliterated single umbilical artery
(sua) from a four-year-old boy. The red stained lesion
appears black in the photograph. Fine calcific incrustations
(c) are seen in the right internal iliac artery which is
significantly larger than the left internal iliac artery. A -
abdominal aorta, CI - common iliac artery, II - internal iliac
artery, EI - external iliac artery. Case 116/72. Von Kossa
reaction and gross fat staining with Fettrot 7B.

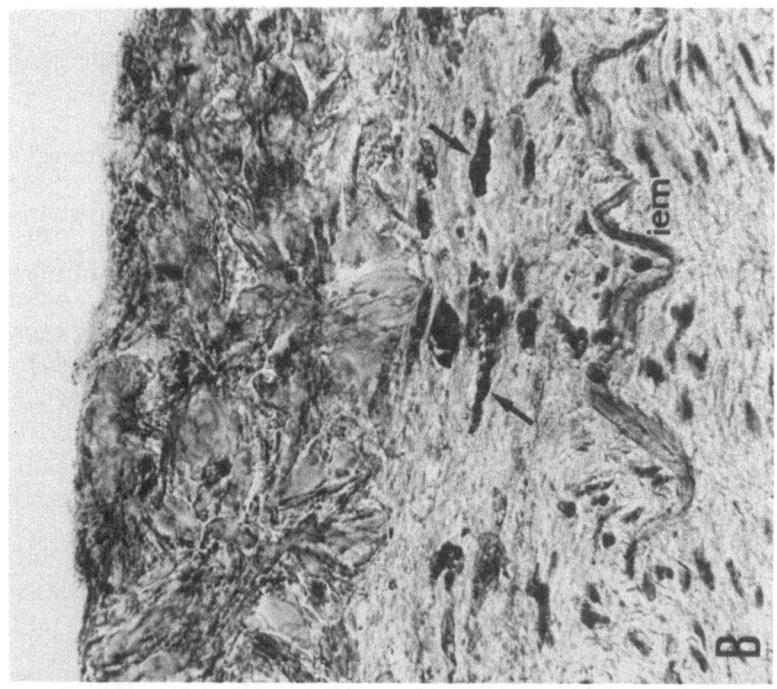

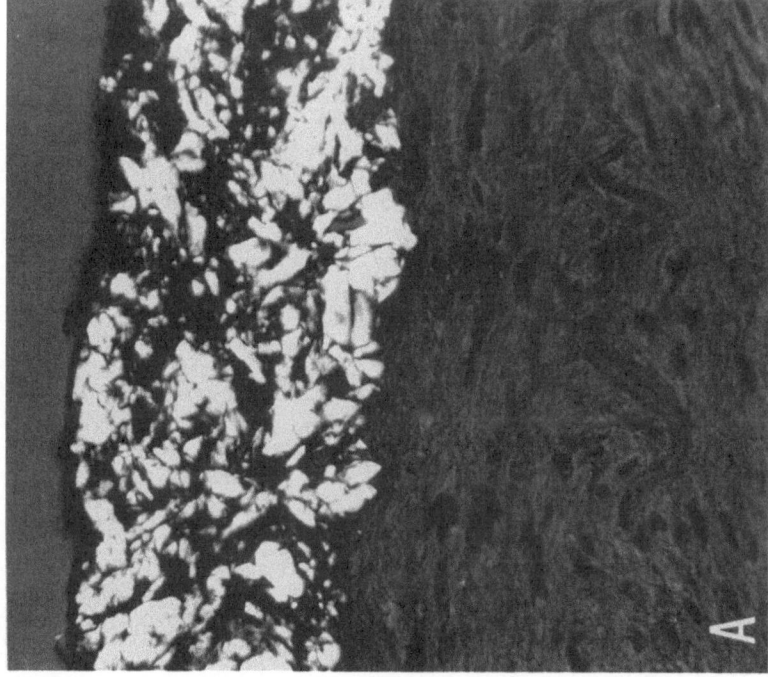

Fig. 7-54: (A) In the luminal layer of the atherosclerotic plaque from the right common iliac artery (on the side of the obliterated single umbilical artery) numerous anisotropic crystals and droplets are seen. B. Same section seen in non-polarized light. The deeper intima includes numerous lipophages (B, arrows). iem - internal elastic membrane. Cryostat frozen section, Fettrot 7B stain. X 500.

   In the enlarged common iliac arteries on the side of a
single umbilical artery established atherosclerotic lesions
have been found in two children aged 18 months and 4 years
(51). (Fig. 7-53 and 7-54). Since fatty streaks were absent
in other arteries, general metabolic factors were probably
not involved. Hence, the development of lesions may essentially
be due to local structural and hemodynamic factors. After
birth and cessation of the umbilical circulation, the enlarged
iliac arteries must accommodate to a considerably diminished
blood flow. This accommodation is associated with a remodeling
of the arterial tube, especially with an intimal thickening
which contributes to the narrowing of the lumen. The prolifera-
ting intima may develop an increased affinity to lipids (53,54)
become the site of lipid infiltration and, in this way, favor
the development of early atherosclerotic lesions.

   DR. WERTHESSEN: I must confess that your Chairman
succumbed to a bit of showmanship in having Dr. Meyer prove
at the end of the conference that nature could do a better
experiment than any of us. I would like to see it repeated
in the laboratory.

   DR. MANSFIELD: I want to emphasize the point that
Dr. Meyer has made so eloquently, that atherosclerotic disease
and arterial changes are surely occurring immediately after
birth, and in fact he finds evidence that they are starting at
parturition. Atherosclerosis is not just a disease of old
age; we only see gross changes at that time, rather it may
be an aspect of vascular adaptation called into play at
any age.

BIBLIOGRAPHY

1. Meyer, W.W. and Lind, J.: Calcifications of the carotid
    siphon--a common finding in infancy and childhood.
    Arch. Dis. Childh. 47:355-363, 1972.

2. Walsh, S.Z., Meyer, W.W. and Lind, J.: The Human Fetal
    and Neonatal Circulation. Function and Structure.
    Charles C. Thomas, Springfield, Ill., 1974.

3. Meyer, W.W.: The mode of calcification in atherosclerotic
    lesions. Internal Workshop Conference on Atherosclerosis,
    London, Ontario, 1975 (In press).

4. Meyer, W.W.: Early forms of calcinosis in human arteries,
    Sandorama, Basel (Switzerland) 11-16, 1975.

5. Meyer, W.W.: The interrelation between the early calci-
    fications and lipid deposits in the carotid siphon
    demonstrated by dual gross staining method. IX.
    International Congress of Angiology, Florence, 1974.

6. Meyer, W.W. and Noll, M.: Gross patterns of early lipid
    deposits in the carotid artery and their relation to
    the preformed arterial structures. Artery 1:31-45,
    1974.

7. Meyer, W.W. and Naujokat, B.: Uber die rhythmische
    Lokalisation der atherosklerotischen Herde im
    cervicalen Abschnitt der Vertebralarterie. Beitr.
    Path. Anat. 130:24-39, 1964.

8. Meyer, W.W. and Lind, J.: Calcifications of iliac arteries
    in newborns and infants. Arch. Dis. Childh. 47:364-
    372, 1972.

9. Meyer, W.W. and Ehlers, U.: Early calcification patterns
    of the iliac arteries and their relation to the
    arterial structure. Z. Zellforsch. 130:378-388, 1972.

10. Keller, S. and Mandl, I.: Non-polar peptides from elastin·
    Protides of the Biological Fluids, 22, 127 (Ed.
    H. Peters) Pergamon Press, 1975.

11. Robert, L.: The macromolecular matrix of the arterial wall:
    collagen, elastin, mucopolysaccharides. In: Athero-
    sclerosis (Ed. R.J. Jones) p. 59 (Springer-Verlag,
    1970.

12. Spain, D.M: Atherosclerosis. Scientific American,

13. Cornhill, J.F. and Roach, M.R.: Quantitative method
     for the evaluation of atherosclerotic lesions.
     Atherosclerosis,

14. Cornhill, J.F. and Roach, M.R.: A Quantitative study of
     the localization of atherosclerotic lesions in the
     rabbit aorta. Atherosclerosis,

15. Pedley, T.J.: Flow in the entrance of the aorta.
     Proceedings from a Specialists Meeting on Fluid
     Dynamic Aspects of Arterial Disease, Ed. by
     R.M. Nerem, held in Columbus, Ohio, Sept. 19-20, 1974.
     (See also: Viscous boundary layers in reversing
     flow. J. Fluid. Mech. Vol 74, Part 1. 59-79, 1976.

16. Nerem, R.M., Seed, W.A. and Wood, N.B.: An experimental
     study of the velocity distribution and transition
     to turbulence in the aorta. J. Fluid. Mech.
     52:137-160, 1972.

17. Lutz, R.J., Cannon, J.N. and Munore, R.E.: Shear stress
     measurements in model arteries during steady and
     pulsatile flow. Proceedings from a Specialists
     Meeting on Fluid Dynamic Aspects of Arterial Disease,
     Ed. by R.M. Nerem, held in Columbus, Ohio,
     Sept. 19-20, 1974.

18. Talkuder, N.: Untersuchung uber die Stromung in arteriellen
     Verzweigungen. Dissertation, Technische Hochschule
     Aachen, 1974.

19. Caro, C.G. and Nerem, R.M: Transport of ^{14}C-4-cholesterol
     between serum and wall in the perfused dog common
     carotid artery. Circ. Res., 32:187-205, 1973.

20. Carew, T.E.: Mechano-Chemical Responses of Canine Aortic
     Endothelium to Elevated Shear Stress In Vitro.
     Thesis. Catholic University of America, Washington,
     D.C., 1971.

21. Reif, T.H., Nerem, R.M. and Kulacki, F.A. An in vitro study
     of transendothelial albumin transport in a steady state
     pipe flow at high shear rates. J. of Fluids Engineering,
     1976.

22. Mack, P.J.: An In Vitro Study of ^{14}C-4-cholesterol
         Transport Between Serum and the Arterial Wall in
         the Presence of a Sinusoidally Oscillating Flow.
         Master's Thesis. The Ohio State University, 1975.

23. Back, L.H.: Analysis of Oxygen Transport in the Vascular
         Region of Arteries. Submitted for publication.

24. Forstrom, R.J., Voss, G.O. and Blackshear, P.L., Jr.:
         Fluid dynamics of particle (platelet) deposition for
         filtering walls: Relationship to atherosclerosis
         ASME Journal of Fluids Engineering, 96-168, 1974.

25. Markle, R.A. and Hollis, T.M.: Regional aortic histamine
         synthesis and transmural albumin uptake following
         focal changes in shearing stress. Presented at the
         60th Annual Meeting of the Federation of American
         Societies for Experimental Biology. Anaheim, Calif.,
         April 11-16, 1976.

26. Haimovici, H., and Maier, N.: Facts of aorta homograph in
         canine atherosclerosis. Arch. of Surg. 89:
         961-969, 1964.

27. Smith, E.B. and Slater, R.S.: Lipids and low-density
         lipoproteins in intima in relation to its morphological
         characteristics. In: Atherogenesis: Initiating
         factors. Ciba Symp. No. 12 (NS) 39-52, 1973.

28. Haimovici, H., Maier, N.: Experiment in canine athero-
         sclerosis in autogenous abdominal aortagraph
         implanted into the jugular vein. Atherosclerosis
         13:375-384, 1971.

29. Bjorkerud, S. and Bondjers, G.: Arterial repair and
         atherosclerosis after mechanical injury. Part I.
         Permeability and light microscopic characteristics
         of endothelium in non-atherosclerotic and athero-
         sclerotic lesions. Atherosclerosis 13:355-363, 1971.

30. Whereat, A.F. and Staple, E.: The preparation of lipo-
         proteins labeled with radioactive cholesterol.
         Arch. of Biochem. 90: 224-228, 1960.

31. Taylor, C.B., Trueheart, R.E. and Cox, G.E.: Athero-
         sclerosis in Rhesus Monkeys. III. The role of
         increased thickness of arterial walls in atherogenesis.
         Arch. Path. 76:14-28, 1963.

32. Ssolowjew, A.: Experimentalle Untersuchungen uber die
        Bedeautung von lokaler Schadigung fur die
        Lipoidablagerung in der Arterienwand. Z. Ges. Exp.
        Med. 69:94-104, 1929.

33. Economou, S.G., Taylor, C.B., Beattie, Jr., E.J. and
        Davis, Jr., C.B.: Persistent experimental aortic
        aneurysms in dogs. Surgery 47:21-28, 1960.

34. Taylor, C.B., Baldwin, D. and Hass, G.M.: Localized
        arteriosclerotic lesions induced in the aorta
        of the juvenile rabbit by freezing. Arch. Path.
        39:623-640, 1950.

35. Stefanovitch, V., and Gore, I.: Cholesterol diet and
        permeability of rabbit aorta. Exp. Molec. Path.
        14:20-29, 1971.

36. Day, A.J. and Proudlock, J.W.: Changes in aortic
        cholesterol-esterifying activity in the rabbits
        fed cholesterol for 3 days. Atherosclerosis
        19:253-258, 1974.

37. Caro, C.G.: Atherogenesis: Initiating factors.
        Associated Scientific Publishers, Amsterdam,
        Ciba Foundation Symposium 12, 1973.

38. Mitchell, J.R.A. and Schwartz, C.J.: Arterial Disease
        Blackwell Scientific Pubications, Oxford, 1965.

39. Schwartz, C.J., Stenhouse, N.S., Taylor, A.E., White, T.A.:
        Coronary disease severity and necropsy. Brit. Heart. J.
        27:731-739, 1965.

40. Goldsmith, H.L.: Blood flow and thrombosis. Thromb.
        Diath. Haemorrh. 32:35-48, 1974.

41. Alan, J.E., Rasmussen, H.: In: Prostaoglandins in cellular
        biology and the inflammatory process. Phariss, B.,
        and Ramwelle, P., (Eds.) Plenum Press, N.Y., 1977

42. Ryan, M.J., Clark, K.E. and Brody, M.J.: Neurogenic and
        mechanical control of canine uterine vascular resistance.
        Am. J. Physiol., 227(3): 547-55, 1974.

43. Caro, C.G., Lewis, C.T., Weinbaum, S.: A mechanism by which
        mechanical disturbances can increase the uptake of macro-
        molecules by the artery wall. Proc. of Phys., C.20,
        p. 77, 1974.

44. Arnqvist, H.J. and Lundholm, L.: Influence of oxygen
     tension on the metabolism of vascular smooth muscle;
     demonstration of a Pasteur effect. Atherosclerosis
     25:245-253, 1976.

45. Scott, R.F., Morrison, E.S., and Kroms, M.: Effect of
     cold shock on respiration and glycolysis in swine
     arterial tissue. Am. J. Physiol. 219:1363-1365,
     1970.

46. Scott, R.F., Morrison, E.S., and Kroms, M.: Aortic
     respiration and glycolysis in the pre-proliferative
     phase of diet-induced atherosclerosis in swine.
     J. Atheroscler. Res. 9:5-16, 1969.

47. Morrison, E.S., Scott, R.F., Kroms, M., and Frick, J.:
     Glucose degradation in normal and atherosclerotic
     aortic intima-media. Atherosclerosis, 16:175-184,
     1972.

48. Morrison, A.D., Berwick, L., Orci, L., and Winegrad, A.I.:
     Morphology and metabolism of an aortic intima-media
     preparation in which an intact endothelium is
     preserved. J. Clin. Invest. 5:650-660, 1976.

49. Benirschke, K. and Bourne, G.L.: The incidence and
     prognostic implication of congenital absence of
     one umbilical artery. Am. J. Obst. Gyn. 79:251-254,
     1960.

50. Bryan, E.M. and Kohler, H.G.: The missing umbilical
     artery. I. Prospective study based on a maternity
     unit. Arch. Dis. Childh., 49:844-852, 1974.

51. Meyer, W.W. and Lind, J.: Iliac arteries in children with
     a single umbilical artery. Structure, calcifications,
     and early atherosclerotic lesions. Arch. Dis. Childh.
     49:671-679, 1974.

52. Berry, C.L., Gosling, R.G., Loagun, A.A. and Bryan, E.:
     Anomalous iliac complicance in children with a
     single umbilical artery. Brit. Heart. J. 38:
     510-515, 1976.

53. Taylor, C.B.: The reaction of arteries to injury by
     physical agents with a discussion of arterial repair
     and its relationship in atheroslcerosis. In Symposium
     on Atherosclerosis, p. 74, National Research Council
     Publ. No. 338, Academy of Sciences, Wash. D.C., 1955.

54. Hass, G.M.: The pathogenesis of human and experimental
     atheroarteriosclerosis. In Cowdry's Arteriosclerosis,
     Survey of the Problem 2nd ed., p. 689. Ed. by
     H.T. Blumenthal. Thomas, Springfield, Ill., 1967

INDEX